PERTURBING THE ORGANISM

The John D. and Catherine T. MacArthur Foundation
Series on Mental Health and Development

PERTURBING THE ORGANISM

The Biology of Stressful Experience

Herbert Weiner

THE UNIVERSITY OF CHICAGO PRESS / CHICAGO AND LONDON

Herbert Weiner is professor of psychiatry and biobehavioral sciences at the
University of California, Los Angeles.

The University of Chicago Press, Chicago 60637
The University of Chicago Press, Ltd., London
© 1992 by The University of Chicago
All rights reserved. Published 1992
Printed in the United States of America

01 00 99 98 97 96 95 94 93 92   5 4 3 2 1

The University of Chicago Press gratefully acknowledges a subvention from the
John D. and Catherine T. MacArthur Foundation in partial support of the costs
of production of this volume.

Library of Congress Cataloging-in-Publication Data

Weiner, Herbert.
    Perturbing the organism : the biology of stressful experience / Herbert
Weiner.
        p.   cm. — (The John D. and Catherine T. MacArthur Foundation
series on mental health and development)
    Includes bibliographical references and index.
    ISBN 0-226-89041-4 (alk. paper)
    1. Stress (Physiology). I. Title. II. Series.
    [DNLM: 1. Stress, Psychological—psychopathology.   WM 172 W423p]
    QP82.2.S8W45   1992
    616.9′8—dc20
    DNLM/DLC
    for Library of Congress   91-838
                                                                        CIP

This book is for those who sustain me:

    Above all, Dora

    And also Tim

           Richard and Jo

           Tony and Priscilla,

    with love and gratitude.

Contents

Illustrations

Acknowledgments

Work on this book began when the Network on Health-Promoting and Health-Damaging Behavior supported by the John D. and Catherine T. MacArthur Foundation asked me to organize a conference on stress, held in West Palm Beach, Florida, in 1986. The proceedings of the conference were not published. But it seemed to many participants at that time that considerable progress had been made in this area of investigation since it was declared in crisis by Rose (1979). On the basis of my report on the conference, I was encouraged by the officers of the foundation and some of the participants in it to write a book on the topic.

I am deeply grateful to the officers of the MacArthur Foundation for a grant-in-aid that has allowed me to devote some of my working hours to the writing and completion of this book.

Further support has come from the officers of the Rockefeller Foundation who invited me to be a Scholar-in-Residence at the Bellagio Study and Conference Center, Lake Como, Italy, in 1990. In an exquisite setting and in the gracious luxury of the Villa Serbelloni, I was able to finish the final draft. I am deeply grateful to Ms. Susan Garfield of the foundation and Mr. and Mrs. Roberto Celli of the center for allowing me to work there and for facilitating the book's completion.

Further impetus for writing yet another book on this topic was given by my friends and colleagues Professors H. C. Hendrie, M. H. Aprison, J. Hingtgen, and D. Hellhammer, who have, over the past several years, conceived and organized an annual series of conferences on the neuronal control of bodily function. In 1987 they asked Professors Hellhammer, I. Florin, and R. C. Murison and me to organize a conference, "Frontiers of Stress Research" (Toronto: Hans Huber, 1989), which was held at the University of Trier, Germany.

In the years between 1987 and 1990, a great deal of further progress has been made. It is encouraging that this area has again attracted basic and clinical scientists from many different disciplines. Some conceptual clarity about stress has been achieved. The neuronal links between the stressful environment and changes in behavior and bodily function are being forged: The "black box"—the brain—is not as impenetrable as it once was!

I am grateful to many colleagues, too numerous to name, for discussions about the topic of stress. They have indirectly contributed to this book. But I am particularly in debt to my many young friends and colleagues—inaccurately called students and research fellows—with whom I have worked in both New York and California. In the past twenty-five years, they have, in seminars and informal interchanges, helped to correct the frequent errors of my ways of thinking.

This book is also the result of the immense labor of my secretary, Mrs. J. Marie Jones. She has checked the bibliography, corrected innumerable errors, and typed and retyped the manuscript of this book in its several versions. She has done so with good cheer, charm, and dispatch.

I thank the following publishers and editors for granting me permission to reprint in amended, modified, and updated form a number of my previous publications which appear in:

Chapters 3 and 4: Weiner, H. 1985. The concept of stress in the light of studies on disasters, unemployment, and loss: A critical analysis. In Stress in health and disease, ed. M. R. Zales, 24–94. New York: Brunner/Mazel.

Chapter 4: Weiner, H. 1985. The psychobiology and pathophysiology of anxiety and fear. In Anxiety and the anxiety disorders, ed. A. H. Tuma and J. D. Maser, 333–54. Hillsdale, NJ: Lawrence Erlbaum.

Chapter 4: Weiner, H. 1987. Human relationships in health, illness, and disease. In Psychopathology: An interactional perspective, ed. D. Magnusson and A. Öhman, 305–23. Orlando, FL: Academic Press.

Chapter 5: Weiner, H. 1988. The functional bowel disorders. In Perspectives in behavioral medicine. Vol. 5, Eating regulation and discontrol, ed. H. Weiner and A. Baum, 137–61. Hillsdale, NJ: Lawrence Erlbaum.

Chapter 6: Weiner, H., and F. Fawzy. 1989. An integrative model of health, disease and illness. In Psychosomatic medicine: Theory, physiology and practice, vol. 1, ed. S. Cheren, 9–44. Madison, CT: International Universities Press.

Chapters 7 and 9: Weiner, H. 1989. Overview of the fourth symposium in Trier, Germany. In Neuronal control of bodily function: Frontiers of stress research, ed. H. Weiner, D. Hellhammer, I. Florin, and R. Murison, 405–18. Toronto: Hans Huber.

Chapter 10: Weiner, H. 1989. The dynamics of the organism. Psychosom. Med. 51:608–35.

Table 1: From Hofer, M. A. 1984. Relationships as regulators: A psychobiologic perspective on bereavement. Psychosom. Med. 46:187.

Figure 5: From Axelrod, J., and T. D. Reisine. 1984. Stress hormones: Their interaction and regulation. Science 224:455. Copyright 1944 by the AAAS.

Figure 9: From Nishizuka, Y. 1986. Studies and perspectives of protein kinase C. Science 233:308. Copyright 1986 by the AAAS.

Figure 11: From Rasmussen, H. 1986. The calcium messenger system. New Engl. J. Med. 314:1098.

The organism is only a living machine constructed in such a fashion that, on the one hand, there is full communication between the external environment and the *milieu intérieur,* and on the other, that there are protective functions of organic elements holding living materials in reserve and maintaining without interruption humidity, heat and other conditions indispensable to vital activity. Sickness and death are only a dislocation or perturbation of that mechanism.

CLAUDE BERNARD (1865)

In looking at Nature, it is most necessary . . . never to forget that every single organic being may be said to be striving to the utmost to increase in numbers; that each lives by a struggle at some period of its life; that heavy destruction inevitably falls either on the young or old, during each generation or at recurrent intervals.

CHARLES R. DARWIN (1859)

1 Introduction

Following a fallow period (Rose 1979), a resurgence of experimental and theoretical interest in stressful experience has occurred in the past decade or so. Major interdisciplinary conferences have recently been dedicated to this topic (Ballieux, Fielding, and L'Abbate 1984; Breznitz and Zinder 1989; Cullen, Siegrist, and Wegman 1984; Taché, Morley, and Brown 1988; Weiner et al. 1989; Zales 1985), and a handbook (Goldberger and Breznitz 1982) and several books have been published about it (Elliott and Eisdorfer 1982; Henry and Stephens 1977; Horowitz 1976; Miller 1989). A reader might well ask: Why should another book be written about this theme? After all, the concept is not rigorously defined; in fact, it is a fuzzy one. Furthermore, no agreed-upon classification of stressful experience exists. The term is applied loosely; at times, it is used so generally that its meaning is lost altogether. Still one might ask why the concept does not simply vanish—like the phlogiston theory, or the concept of the luminiferous ether—if it does not contain some kernel of truth and validity.

This book is written in an attempt to clarify some issues about stress theory and research in order to enhance its validity, supply a definition and a classification, and document the empirical and conceptual advances that have been made. Some of these new findings are contained in the demonstration that acutely stressful situations in young organisms have long-term effects on their behavior, physiology, and health. W. B. Cannon (1929, 1939) and H. Selye (1936) studied acutely stressful "stimuli" and conditions but did not observe the consequences of intermittent or continuously stressful experiences. They were respectively interested in the normal physiology, and in the pathogenetic effects, of stress. Cannon (1939) in particular studied how pain, fear, hunger, or rage disturbed homeostasis. Many students still follow Cannon in defining stress in terms of physiology and of disturbed homeostasis. Selye seemed to remain uninterested in the behavioral effects of his stressors. For reasons that remain unclear neither Cannon nor Selye appears to have been instructed by the writings of C. R. Darwin (1859, 1872).

1

Central to the concept of natural selection (Darwin 1859)—the struggle for existence—is the idea that the dynamic physical and social environments are full of obstacles, dangers, challenges, and threats. They must be met with appropriate, discriminated, integrated (organismic) responses that protect the organism. They must be overcome so that the organism survives to reproduce. But some creatures succumb. Natural selection acts upon behavior, not only upon genes (Mayr 1982). Nature has devised many individual, species-specific and age-related patterns of behaviors appropriate to the tasks of anticipating, protecting against, and mastering the stressful environment and of surviving and reproducing (Crews and Moore 1986).

Significant advances have recently been made in our understanding of how the organism responds in a patterned and integrated, behavioral and physiological manner to new experiences, perturbations, challenges, threats, injury, or complex changes in the environment. One seeks to understand by what means the organism recognizes them, what is the meaningful signal that is perceived, and how that perception is translated and orchestrated into anticipatory and appropriate behavioral and physiological responses designed to ensure survival. But the environment is not only stressful, it is also a source of information and a repository of resources (Levins and Lewontin 1985).

The advances alluded to have occurred on three fronts: conceptual, methodological, and empirical.

Conceptual Advances

Selye (1973) defined stress in the following manner: It "is the non-specific response of the body to any demand made upon it." He stated further that "the stress producing factors . . . are different, and yet they all produce essentially the same biologic stress response."

From 1936 on many of the stressors (stress producing factors) Selye used were designed to damage the integrity of the organism. In his experiments the organism (a rat) was also prevented from making any, or the appropriate, behavioral response. Furthermore, on two scores he was biased toward a medical, not a biological, mode of thought. This bias was brought about by:

a. His demonstration (1936) that a variety of acute and "noxious" stressors produced the same three kinds of anatomical changes. For years thereafter, the connection between stress and disease was, and has continued to be, sought. He assumed that the corticosteroids mediated the anatomical damage he described, despite the fact that it had been demonstrated by the time of his first report that corticosteroids may actually protect animals against injury and infection: Adrenalectomized animals are more susceptible to them (Munck, Guyre, and Holbrook 1984).

b. His clinical observations that diseases in human beings share a commonality of symptoms—malaise, fatigue, lethargy, loss of appetite and weight, sleeplessness, fear, fever, loss of interest in work and people, decreased sexual desire and function—in addition to specific symptoms and signs. They are the general manifestations of the state of being sick. We have only recently learned about their physiological basis. These general symptoms may also occur without actual anatomical changes—i.e., disease—in the body or in the brain.

For a number of years following, the concept of, and interest in, stress fluctuated. A shift in focus on stress can partly be traced to J. W. Mason's (1968, 1971, 1975) and L. E. Hinkle's (1973) insistence on the biological reality that no organism would survive if its integrated behavioral and physiological responses were not exquisitely attuned, and appropriate, to the stressful situation—to danger, challenge, predation, threat, victory, defeat, hunger, heat, cold, or other such experiences confronting it.

Methodological Advances

New and more analytic methods have been developed for studying stressful experiences. Some compare the differential effects of varying the parameters of the stimulus, exemplified by the work of Shavit and his colleagues (1984). They have demonstrated that continuous electric shock produces one form of analgesia in rats, whereas intermittent shock produces another form. The former has no effect on natural killer (NK) cell function; intermittent shock depresses it while enhancing tumor formation. Therefore, subtle changes in applying shock have different effects.

Additionally, potentially life-threatening challenges, such as hypoglycemia and hypoxia, are followed by the secretion of arginine vasopressin (aVP) but not oxytocin (OT) in rats, whereas restraint, hypothermia, or inducing swimming releases only OT. On the other hand, both aVP and OT are released by ether or hemorrhage (Gibbs 1986). The significance of these observations for stress research is that both aVP and OT modulate the release of adrenocorticotropin (ACTH) by corticotropin releasing factor (CRF) (Axelrod and Reisine 1984). These examples, taken from many others, show that physiological responses are exquisitely specific to the stressful experience, contradictory to Selye's contention that they are uniform and nonspecific.

However, one may not generalize across species and genera: In primates, aVP also potentiates the action of CRF to release ACTH. But OT seems to inhibit the role of CRF. In fact, OT and ACTH are released in an inverse, rather than in a positively correlated, manner in stressed primates (Gibbs 1986).

Differences in physiological (and behavioral) responses exist not only between species, but within species. Animal strains susceptible and resistant to stressful experience have been bred. But in utero stressful experiences, not only genetic endowment, occasion individual differences in later behavior.

When pregnant rats are exposed to stressful experience in the last trimester, long-term effects on the mating behavior of their male offspring occur (Ward 1984). In a similar vein, postnatal experience—e.g., the premature weaning of rats—has wide-ranging long-term effects on weight, cardiovascular function, predisposition to hypothermia, gastric erosion formation, and immunopathology on later challenge (Ackerman 1989; Weiner 1987).

Therefore, two sources of variation (individual differences) between individuals of the same species are intrauterine and postnatal experience. Two other sources of individual differences in the response to stressful experience are whether it is unavoidable or inescapable, and whether the animal's avoidant response is punished. If electric shocks are avoidable or escapable, the animal suffers many fewer or less extensive gastric erosions (Weiss 1971, 1972). Selye's original experimental procedures provided no avenue for escape or avoidance. In addition, and with the exception of restraint, they were physically damaging.

In retrospect, Selye's early experiments biased the study of stressful experience in several directions, leading to:

1. The use of overpowering or unavoidable stressful experiences that override the subtler influences of variations in the behavioral and physiological responses of the organism. If the stressed animal's behaviors are not observed, or it is rendered incapable of making behavioral responses—of protecting itself—the observer cannot ascertain whether or not they are appropriate to the experience or are adequate or inadequate, excessive or diminished.

2. Adherence to the concept, still widely held, that only by overwhelming the organism can a stressful experience, or a perturbation, exert its physiological, or tissue-damaging, effects. The fact that in some instances mild, everyday activities or experiences (e.g., public speaking or mental arithmetic) produce myocardial perfusion defects in patients with coronary atherosclerosis (Deanfield et al. 1984) is still dismissed with incredulity. In the minds of many, such an observation raises a question about the definition of a stressful experience (Weiner 1991a, 1991b) because it is banal and not excessive. In fact, such daily perturbations have their effects because they occur in the presence of preexisting disease (or other predisposing risk factors). Stressful experiences does not linearly or by itself produce disease in most instances. Coronary artery disease predisposes to rhythmic disturbances (spasm), which interact with the perturbing influence.

3. The use of controlled experiments in biologically irrelevant, inappropriate, or impoverished social contexts. In their natural habitat, rats do not customarily run across electrified grids. Highly trained monkeys do not exist in the wild, nor do monkeys press levers in their forest homes to get food or avoid pain. Social animals do not usually live in isolated cages; yet they are customarily the subject of experimental procedures after being individually housed. From such unnatural conditions, arranged for the convenience of the experimenter, and in the cause of scientific rigor, conclusions are drawn about how animals (and by extrapolation, human beings) behave in nature in response to naturally occurring experiences, how the brain mediates stressful experiences, and how disease may ensue!

4. An overemphasis on the roles of the corticosteroids (Selye), on the role of the autonomic nervous system (Cannon), and later on the role of the biogenic amines in mediating stressful experiences to produce physiological changes and damage to bodily organs.

Since that time and with the development of new methods (e.g., chromatography, radioimmunoassay), the discovery of peptide hormones, and the description of new phenomena (e.g., "stress analgesia"), the number of mediators of stressful experience has rapidly expanded. Whole families of "stress" hormones have been described. Some are present in both the brain and virtually every other bodily system. Many of them have multiple, not singular, physiological functions. They are colocalized with the classical neurotransmitters in brain and nerve. They integrate and regulate behavior and bodily function, and they promote growth (Sporn and Roberts 1988). They act as communication signals between cells and organs.

Many hormones and neurotransmitters customarily operate in a rhythmic, oscillatory mode. The parameters (frequency, duration, amplitude, and waveform) of their rhythms are individual. One or other of these parameters can be altered by perturbations brought about by stressful experience. Parametric changes in function may occur in one direction or another. New rhythms may appear, or ongoing ones may change and even disappear, when they are perturbed by challenge or changes in the environment. At a cellular (receptor) level, hormones and neurotransmitters interact to modulate each other's activities. A change in one hormonal system alters or modulates the activity of other systems and the rhythms with which they operate. Therefore, changes in levels of a single hormonal variable and at one point in time do not faithfully reflect the complexity of the processes by which they occur. When the organism is perturbed, covarying patterns of hormonal changes are observed (Mason 1971). Many hormones peptides activate or suppress enzyme systems through complex and varied cellular and intracellular mechanisms. Presumably, they do so by altering gene expression and regulation and by other means.

Thus the study of stressful experience moves in new directions as these discoveries are made, and new concepts, to which they give rise, emerge. Until recently stress research was guided by independent (the stressor)/dependent (the physiological change or anatomical lesion) research strategies cast in the traditional mold. As new facts are revealed, the strategy must perforce change to a study of covariances in rhythmically organized systems that are intimately related to each other by communication signals.

Empirical Advances

Until fifteen years ago stress research consisted of correlations between the stressor and the physiological and/or anatomical changes in the body. The discovery of the brain-gut peptides and other advances in neurobiology have changed this unsatisfactory situation. The consequence of this work has been to give a new impetus to stress research by placing it on a firmer basis. To mention just two examples:

1. Two forms of stress analgesia have now been described: One can be reversed by naloxone, the other not. The epoch-making discovery of the presence of endogenous opioid ligands in the brain (Hughes et al. 1975) allows us to begin to understand the first form of stress analgesia.

2. The function of the brain peptides is to produce *patterned* physiological changes, which are exactly what an integrated view of the responses to stressful experiences demands. For example, CRF, in addition to regulating ACTH production and secretion, has diverse behavioral and physiological functions. The CRF is but one example of a peptide involved in regulatory interactions with other hormones and neurotransmitters, and in integrating behavior and physiological patterns. Furthermore, we have learned some of the brain circuitry by which stressful or painful experiences release CRF: The afferent pathways from peripheral receptors to the parvocellular portion of the paraventricular nucleus (PVN) of the hypothalamus have been mapped (Feldman 1985, 1989).

Stress, Ill Health, and Disease

Selye made original observations that different stressful experiences all culminated in anatomical changes in three separate organ systems in rats. Since that time, attempts to link stress to disease have been relentlessly pursued. In this book, disease—the central topic of Western biomedicine—will be defined conventionally as a gross or microscopic alteration in bodily structure(s).

As already mentioned, Selye had also observed that many diseases in human beings are associated with a wide range of shared symptoms that are the hallmark of sickness, ill health, or illness. They reflect disturbances in vital biological functions—e.g., food intake, sexual desire, digestion, elmination, sleep, respiration, and thermoregulation—and are accompanied by aches and pains and by changes in social relationships.

The symptoms of illness or ill health are not necessarily or only the consequences of disease; in fact, most frequently they are not. They are due to changes in (rhythmic) functions such as sleep, body temperature, gastrointestinal motility, menstruation, or respiratory rhythms. These so-called functional disorders have for many years gone by a large variety of constantly changing labels (e.g., neurasthenia, soldier's heart, hyperventilation syndrome, psychogenic rheumatism, fibromyalgia, mucous or spastic colitis). Western biomedicine either dismisses the functional disorders as a figment of the patient's imagination or relentlessly pursues their putative viral, bacterial, immunopathological, or anatomical bases.

Functional symptoms cluster. They are frequently associated with distress, anxiety, sadness and/or depressed feelings or moods (Smith, Monson, and Ray 1986a). They produce disability and markedly raise the annual costs of health care in the United States (Smith, Monson, and Ray 1986b). The symptoms of ill health may last a lifetime. They have been related to acute or chronic stressful experiences. The relationship of ill health to stressful experiences is exemplified by the decline in health that accompanies forced unemployment, which is followed by an increase in illness episodes by 70%, in medical consultations by 150%, and in attendance at medical clinics by 200% (Beale and Nethercott 1986). However, unemployment also raises mortality by exacerbating preexisting but dormant cardiovascular and cardiorespiratory disease and by increasing the incidence of fatal accidents and suicide. The umemployed change their diet and increase their alcohol intake and the use of cigarettes. The families of the unemployed are affected: The school performance declines and the truancy rate increases in their children 12 years of age or younger (Farrow 1984).

The medical implications of stressful experiences go far beyond the pathogenesis of disease. Stressful experiences and the distress they occasion (Levi 1972) seem much more closely associated with the functional disorders, grief reactions, the anxiety syndromes and depressive disorders, or the post-traumatic syndromes, than with anatomical lesions in one or another organ. They are frequently misdiagnosed and neglected by traditional Western biomedicine.

The question of why another book on stress was written and what it is about can now be answered. It will attempt to:

1. Define, specify, and classify stressful experiences. Throughout it the terms *stress*—unless specifically defined—*stress producing factors, stressors, stressful stimuli,* and *state of stress* will be eschewed. The phrase to be used will be *stressful experience* because an active process is being described. It begins with a change in the dynamic environment in the form of an obstacle to be surmounted, a challenge to be met, or a danger or threat to be avoided or overcome. These changes are signaled and interpreted. They may have very different connotations in unlike contexts. The organism is an actor in the environment, not a passive recipient of signals; it experiences them. The word *experience* has three connotations: the perception or apprehension of an external event that has meaning and relevance to the organism; the direct participation in it; and the knowledge, skill, or practice derived from observation or participation.

2. Discuss stressful experiences in broad biological terms as an inevitable part of the struggle for existence.

3. Describe the integrated, discriminated, patterned biological (usually divided into behavioral, psychological, physiological) responses to stressful experiences. They have purpose: ultimately to ensure survival, reproduction, and health. When they fail, injury, ill health, disease, and death ensue.

4. Maintain that each stressful experience must be rigorously described and defined in order to assess whether the patterned responses are appropriate to it or are excessive, inadequate, or absent. The stressful experience may have an acute onset, be expected or not, be chronically present, or occur intermittently. Short- or long-term behavioral and physiological consequences of such experiences may ensue. The outcome may be ill health with or without disease, which in turn may constitute another source of stressful experience.

5. Discuss the role of stressful experience, ill health, and disease. Stressful experiences do *not* by themselves linearly produce or specify the disease; they act as cofactors in predisposed persons. These predispositions are never unitary; they take many forms: (a) genetic defects or genetic variations that increase the risk for disease or limit the appropriate response to the stressor; (b) preexisting but "silent" structural disease; and (c) altered oscillators or feedback systems that generate rhythms.

6. Assert that the experience of, responses to, and outcomes of stressful experience depend on a multitude of factors.

7. Describe the manner in which behavior and bodily function are coordinated. In so doing, this book will present current knowledge about the generation of biobehavioral rhythms and how these are perturbed by stressful situations to alter the pattern of each rhythm. These rhythms are generated by negative, positive, or mixed (negative-positive) feedback that depends on communicaton signals, oscillators ("biological clocks"), or both. New concepts about the perturbation of these subsystems by stressful experience will be presented.

It is not the purpose of this book exhaustively to review the very large literature on this topic; rather, its intent is to highlight and document the assertions listed above by a selective and critical evaluation of data.

2 The History of the Concept of Stress

That the environment is a source of challenge, contains malevolent gods, demons, and spirits, and is the arena of natural disasters and the repository of predators, enemies, pestilence, and poisons that cause death and disease is an ancient idea. The biological significance of some of these categories as the driving forces of evolution was first fully grasped by Darwin. The role of infection in disease and as a threat to organisms was discovered by Pasteur, Koch, and Ehrlich at the end of the nineteenth century. The experimental study of some of the sources and consequences of danger, injury, and challenge was begun by Cannon and Selye in the twentieth century.

Some virtue might be found in going back to Selye's own accounts (1971, 1973) of his original intent: It was to study experimentally a human being's *nonspecific* responses to a wide variety of contingencies—hard work, prolonged exposure to heat or cold, loss of blood, disease, injury, infection, and agonizing fear—that all initially produced the same response: feelings of exhaustion. In the face of such strenuous or potentially damaging situations, most persons go through three stages: They first experience them as a hardship; then they become used to them; finally, they cannot stand them and give up.

Selye relates that while studying medicine he also made the observation that many different acute and chronic diseases were accompanied by the same group of symptoms. Prior to and at that time, physicians sought the diagnosis of disease in specific symptoms and correlated them with a specific pathogen or an anatomical lesion. Selye wanted to understand why patients with many different infections or neoplastic diseases shared the same symptoms, which also accompanied blood loss and burns or followed surgery. What was this general "state of being sick?" he asked.

Based on these clinical observations, Selye (1936) began a series of experiments. He subjected rats to many different stressful experiences—restraining, exercising, or starving them; injecting them with impure glandular and tissue extracts, formalin, bacteria, or croton oil; inducing burns, traumatic wounds, and fractures; exposing them to ionizing radiation; creating anoxia; bleeding them; exposing them to heat and cold—and found that all produced a triad of adrenocortical hypertrophy; atrophy of, and hemorrhage into, the thymus gland and lymph nodes; and gastric erosions. Even local injury produced these three bodily pathologies. They could occur after an animal was merely punctured with a sterile needle.

Somewhat later Selye (1946; Selye and Fortier 1950) formally divided this general reaction to various damaging agents into three stages, which compose the General Adaptation Syndrome (GAS). In (1) the alarm phase, the organism is restless and tense, if the stress is mild; if it is severe, "depression" and shock occur. In both cases the subject loses its desire to eat and to mate. Heat, severe burns, and trauma may produce morphologic changes in the brain. Adrenocortical steroid production and secretion occur in association with the release of aVP and increased autonomic neural discharge (Selye 1950). According to Selye, the effects of the stressful stimuli in producing shock, hyperkalemia, hypothermia, hypotension, hemoconcentration, increased cell-membrane permeability, and gastric erosions are counteracted by neural and hormonal activation, leading to (2) the stage of resistance, during which the subject's appetite is restored to normal but its desire to mate is not, followed by (3) the stage of exhaustion, in which the manifestations of the alarm reaction recur and changes in arterial blood vessels manifest themselves. On reexposure to the stressor, the "defensive" measures of the alarm phase are no longer instituted.

In Selye's earlier writings the line between the beneficial ("defense") and the pathogenic effects of the adrenal corticosteroid hormones was blurred. Initially he postulated that the glucocorticoids damaged the rats. Later he wrote extensively about the pathogenic effects on brain, electrolyte metabolism, muscle function, and blood pressure (BP) of desoxycorticosterone acetate (DOCA) and other mineralocorticosteroids. This muddle continues in the literature: Selye's original thought was that bodily damage was produced by the systemic effects of the stressor, while the defensive ("countershock") reactions attempted to redress the injury. His later work, however, is concerned with the harmful effects of these very defensive reactions.

Selye's Definition of Stress

The main points of Selye's observations have been described in order to highlight the beginnings of a conceptual muddle that was later realized. Note that Selye was interested mainly in the effects of noxious (damaging) agents—infection, radiation, heat or cold, traumatic wounds, fractures, and even danger (to cause fear), etc.:

1. The effect of some of these can be on a local part of the body, but the reaction to all of them is general and identical, regardless of their nature.

2. The stressful agents are nonspecific; they do not determine the generalized response.

3. The physiological response is also nonspecific and stereotyped.

4. The inciting agent—the stressful (damaging) "stimulus"—is external to the organism.

5. The model he proposed is a linear one.

The inference that pain was inflicted on his animals by the procedures was never made; it was abjured in the cause of objectivity!

Yet from Selye's account it is not clear whether stress is defined in terms of the stressor (in his words, "topical" or general stress, which he defined as a "stimulus") or in terms of the response—the GAS—which he called the "biological stress syndrome." This account deemphasized the known fact that in addition to these generalized responses, specific bodily responses also occur to noxious agents or challenges: Cold produces shivering; heat incites sweating, causing loss of electrolytes and body water; blood loss causes hypovolemia and a fall in BP; and infection incites not only an acute phase reaction and inflammation but also a specific immune response. Admittedly, all of them may at times produce the state of shock described in some detail in Stage 1 of the GAS.

After that time, stress, or rather the "state of stress," was defined by Selye in terms of an objective but nonspecific syndrome of bodily changes (the GAS) and not as a "stimulus"—as damage imposed on the organism. It did not just exist as any syndrome, but that combination of changes by which the GAS was circumscribed. In retrospect it has become abundantly clear that stress consisted, in Selye's experiments, of damage to the organism, from which it could not protect itself, or which it could not avoid. It cannot be emphasized too strongly that the stressors employed by Selye were directly damaging, potentially or actually life-threatening. They were unquestionably painful to the animal.

They were (with the exception of exposure to heat, cold, and infection, hemorrhage, and possibly food deprivation) not encountered in nature. Nevertheless, the GAS does seem to occur naturally, even in human beings, but only under the direst life-threatening conditions. In this regard, all of the products of the proopiomelanocortin gene—ACTH (and thus cortisol), β-endorphin, prolactin (PRL), γ-melanocyte-stimulating hormone (γ_3-MSH)—are elevated in patients resuscitated after cardiac arrest, but in ill patients in the same intensive care units only levels of γ_3-MSH (Wortsman et al. 1985) and cortisol are increased (Parker, Levin, and Lifrat 1985).

In 1950, Selye wrote that "even mere [*sic*] emotional stress . . . caused by immobilizing an animal . . . proved to be a suitable routine procedure for the production of a severe alarm reaction." Mason (1971) has written that this statement of Selye's was a point of departure for his own studies of the relationship of psychological factors ("emotional stress") to changes in endocrine function. These psychological influences may be quite subtle. Increases in cortisol levels in humans do not necessarily occur when the body is damaged or when a person has severe pain. But they are especially seen when a person (or animal) loses, or has no, control over a situation (Henry and Stephens 1977). Furthermore, only abrupt elevations in ambient temperature raise urinary 17-hydroxycorticosteroid (17-OHCS) levels in monkeys; a gradual increase actually lowers them (Mason 1971).

For this reason alone (many other exist) it is impossible to define stress only by the physiological changes. Unless the organism is overwhelmed, the (general, nonspecific) physiological pattern may or may not occur. Physiological changes are not indiscriminate, and they cannot be separated either from the nature of the experience, the context in which it occurs, or the behavioral response of the organism. Such considerations make it impossible directly to translate Selye's nonspecificity concept, and the ubiquitous GAS that ensues, to naturally occurring challenges, threats, and changes in social arrangements and relationships that are part and parcel of the everyday lives of people and animals. By virtue of how Selye designed his experiments, he could not study the usual ways in which organisms protect themselves against threat, change, and challenge presented by a dynamic environment.

Many of Selye's contemporaries also defined stress as an internal state. Wolff (1953, 14), for example, wrote that it is a "dynamic state within the organisms . . . not a stimulus, assault, load, symbol, burden, or any aspect of the environment, internal, external, social or otherwise." Others have called it a "trait" (Pearlin et al. 1981), and still others a "physiological state that prepares the organism for action" (Kagan 1971).

This brief account of the history of the stress concept also highlights the fact that there is no agreed-upon definition of stress, in part because one cannot generalize from the effect of damage to other situations of challenge or threat. Nevertheless, Selye (1971) later became aware of the fact that the GAS was not always uniform. Individual responses occur because different agents of equal toxicity do not exactly produce the same syndrome in animals; and individual animals respond to the same agent (the "stressor") with somewhat different lesions. Selye accounted for these individual differences in terms of genetic predisposition, sex, age, diet, and prior exposure to drugs and hormones. The prior social experience of the animal, or the time of day or night when the experience occurs, as additional sources of variation do not appear in his account.

Selye (1971) summarized twenty years of investigation and revised and clarified his pathogenetic hypothesis. He had later shown that aldosterone (but not cortisol and cortisone) secretion raises the resistance of the organism to injury and infection; but it may, in conjunction with other experimental procedures (nephrectomy or salt administration), produce hypertension and myocardial necrosis, whereas corticosterone reduces inflammation.

Several additional aspects of Selye's account are worth recounting:

1. He did not systematically study the behavior of his stressed animals. As noted, he mentioned that the mildly stressed animal in the stage of alarm was

aroused behaviorally. Actually, restrained animals at first fall asleep, and later begin to lose sleep and remain quietly awake (Ackerman, Hofer, and Weiner 1979). They are not restless or aroused, initially or at a later time.

2. He mainly studied physical and pharmacological "stressors," not psychological ones. He believed, however, that fear could produce the GAS, though he never systematically studied its effects.

3. He never explicitly stated that the adrenal gluco- and mineralocorticosteroids and aVP were the only stress hormones, as others have since designated them (Axelrod and Reisine 1984).

4. He also stated that the stage of resistance of the GAS was an attempt of the organism to restore homeostasis. Ever since that time this incorrect concept has pervaded the field: Investigators have attempted to explain some psychobiological responses to stress in this manner. Initially, only Tyhurst (1953) and Rioch (1971) emphasized the fact that stressful experiences, especially if dire, lead to a reorganization of the organism—a concept (to be discussed later) that accords more closely with observation and is at variance with the concept of homeostasis.

The Concept of Stress in the Social and Behavioral Sciences

The concept of stress began to creep into the social and behavioral sciences during and after World War II (Grinker and Spiegel 1945; Hinkle 1973; Arthur 1982). Good reasons exist for this: One-third of the American casualties of that war had sustained no physical injury. They were the victims of the appalling danger, fear, exertion, sleep deprivation, death of colleagues, and exposure to heat, cold, and noise generated by modern warfare. But in addition, the prevalence of duodenal ulcer doubled in the U.S. Army, only to subside to its prewar level after 1945. The civilian victims of the Nazi terror also came under medical scrutiny for a variety of diseases and changes in behavior and cognition (Eitinger 1971). Small wonder then that the concept of stress became fashionable in medicine.

At the same time the concept was used to explain the pathogenesis of a variety of diseases, named by Selye "diseases of adaptation" (Selye 1946; Selye and Fortier 1950; Wolff 1953); their antecedent stressors could be physical or psychological, or both. Currently, there is once again a tendency to revert to this way of thinking. The word *stress* has become synonymous with any event, experience, change, or task likely to be encountered in everyday life, and "stress" is put forward as an explanation of the pathogenesis of disease.

Therefore, the purposes of this chapter are:

1. To argue that *stress* should not only be used in the sense that Selye first meant it—as a damaging agent produced by unavoidable bodily injury, accompanied by wide-ranging physiological effects that are usually, but not necessarily, uniform. The term should also include clearly specified natural and

man-made catastrophes and disasters, which may be threatening but not fatal, and which are known to have different short-term and long-range consequences, implying a total reorganization of the person. But instead of all being called *stress,* they should be designated as *stressful experiences* and clearly specified.

2. To explain the reasons for individual differences in the responses to those events.

3. To suggest that characterizing common events of daily life—separation, bereavement, migration, relocation, working, raising a family, examinations, mental arithmetic, public speaking, indebtedness, leadership, retirement, forced unemployment, jet travel, marriage, widowhood, parenthood, and poverty—as the equivalent of overwhelming infection or trauma has retarded progress in understanding. They are personal experiences with individual meanings, responses, and consequences.

Each of these experiences requires that it be separately analyzed in terms of its impact on different persons and their families—an impact that is age-specific, yet individual. In turn, one may not separate the experience from the meaning it has for the person, or from his/her prior training, intelligence, or manner of dealing with it.

To complete such a program of investigation will require much more data. Despite extensive research on the physiological responses to these various social, psychological, and physical experiences, our ignorance of the manner in which they are perceived, processed, and mediated by the brain is profound, in part because we have largely failed to pay heed to Beach's (1950, 674) injunction "to describe accurately the external events responsible for . . . internal changes." Once such a precise analysis is carried out, we may be able to identify the individual behavioral responses to them, and eventually the neural circuitry that connects the receptor with the brain's output channels regulating action and bodily function. In that way, we shall also be able to understand how the output is modified, and how, in certain circumstances, physiological changes may or may not culminate in ill health or disease. Yet even Beach's prescription is not sufficient. Bereavement or separation does not only lead to grief, depression, or increased visits to physicians; it disrupts the order of a person's life. Social relationships impose a schedule and a structure on people (Moore-Ede, Sulzman, and Fuller 1982).

Selye's Concept of Disease: Diseases of Adaptation

The intimate association between stressful experiences and disease in rats was already apparent in Selye's initial paper. In the next ten years he placed the burden on the glucocorticoids as the main incitors of their anatomical effects, despite evidence to the contrary. At that time, forty years ago, it was quite unclear whether in the normal animal the permissive role of the corticosteroids in endowing the animal with some resistance to stressors was due to the mineralo- or the glucocorticosteroids. Nonetheless, Selye believed that many diseases—hypertension, peptic ulcer, and allergic, rheumatic, and collagen diseases—were the product of excessive or "adaptive" reactions in which the corticosteroids played a pathogenetic role. He called this heterogeneous group of diseases "diseases of adaptation," implying that they were the product of abnormal or excessive responses to stress.

There is, however, no evidence that the most common forms of hypertension are the product of excessive levels of mineralocorticoids (the role of salt in this disease remains enigmatic to this date). But the *coup de grace* to his theory of disease was given by the demonstration that ACTH and the corticosteroids may actually suppress the manifestations of allergic, rheumatic, and collagen diseases (Hench et al. 1949).

In retrospect, it seems unclear why he called these human diseases—while extrapolating from his work on rats—diseases of adaptation, rather than calling them diseases of mal- or failed adaptation. We know today that these varied diseases are not only multifactorial and heterogeneous in their etiology and pathogenesis, but are also characterized by disturbances of the regulation of complex physiological systems (Weiner 1977). Because of their heterogeneity stressful experiences seem to play a variable role in their onset. When stressful experiences do contribute, the person for diverse reasons has failed to cope with them.

Darwin's Concept of Stress as Selective Pressures

Selye did not study the behavior of his animals, yet stressful experiences have behavioral and psychological (in humans), not only bodily, consequences: For example, different animals have a variety of behavioral strategies for survival in dealing with the anticipated or actual threat of predators. These behavioral responses must be appropriate to the threat, danger, change in the environment, or challenge if they are to succeed; were they random or indiscriminate (nonspecific), survival would not be assured. When the threat to survival is an infection, the appropriate response is immunological. If the threat to reproductive success is competition among males for mates, the appropriate response is to fight the rival and win, submit to him if defeated, or flee to find another mating partner.

Despite the fact that the credit for the concept of stress is customarily accorded to Selye and Cannon, the principles briefly enunciated in the previous paragraph were first laid down by Darwin (1859). It is to him that we owe a complete reassessment of the relationship of the organism to its environment, incorporated in the concept of natural selection. According to his view the environment was in constant change (seasonal, climatic, chemical, geological, etc.), or it was continually being altered (e.g., by grazing) by its inhabitants.

In the organism's struggle for existence the environment is potentially threatening or dangerous due to the withdrawal of resources, the disruption of health by infection, starvation, heat, or cold, and the threat of predators and competitors. (People, by virtue of their own activities—the promotion of war, strife, and torture; the pollution of the atmosphere, waters, and ground; and the invention of new and ever more dangerous technologies—add to nature's threats and dangers.)

In Darwin's formulation, the environment was challenging, dangerous, stressful, and full of potential or actual obstacles. Only the fittest survived to reproduce. Thus the question arose: How does the organism deal with these challenges and stressors, prevent and avoid danger, and overcome obstacles in order to survive and reproduce?

Yet the environment also contains resources, cooperative conspecifics, and shelter. It is a source of information for whose reception and processing peripheral receptors and the brain have evolved. This information is analyzed, classified, stored, checked against past stores, and synthesized by the brain, and leads to specific and appropriate actions. These actions include selection of environments by the organism in order to bring it into more favorable conditions than mere random movements would. Animals determine which aspects of the environment are relevant at any one time, and which can be ignored (Griffin 1984); they sense and respond to environmental changes with coordinated physiological and behavioral patterns (Levins and Lewontin 1985).

Biologists study these changing response patterns to some aspect (signal) of the environment or other organisms in it (e.g., the shadow of a predator hawk, or the smell, sight, or sound of a sexually mature mate or a dominant male). Behavioral responses (and their physiological correlates) are usually predictors or indicators of danger, sexual partners, or food; they are often short-term ones, and they are subject to intense selective pressures because they may fail. One reason for their failure is that both individuals and species vary in their capacities to respond to, or prevent, a given environmental challenge—they are differently adapted.

The environmental changes, challenges, and threats to the organism, eliciting specific response patterns, act as signals that may initiate the stressful experiences. Although the physiological responses to stressful experiences are with some exceptions similar (Gibbs 1986) in different species and genera, what differs between similar species is the interpretation of the challenging or threatening signal. As Levins and Lewontin (1985, 43) have pointed out, "the most advantageous response to a signal does not depend on . . . [its] . . . physical form but on its value as a predictor or correlate." Different environments or contexts "require different responses." Conversely, unlike environments may require the same behavioral response as long as it is likely to guarantee survival. Additionally, the very system (the brain) that interprets the environment and upon which the organism depends for survival must (or should) be protected from being disrupted by external forces or internal agents (e.g., the blood-brain barrier).

This digression was intended for the purpose of pointing out that the concept of stress is by no means new. But the physical stressors that Selye (1936) employed in his first study overwhelmed his animals: They were rendered incapable of, or were prevented from, mounting a patterned behavioral response.

Darwin (1859, 1872) entertained the concept that the *whole* organism responds to environmental signals predictive of, or signifying, danger, threat, challenge, or change. Moore-Ede (1986) has pointed out that some hunting or foraging animals anticipate nightfall by returning to the safety of their lairs or nests, in order to be protected from nocturnal predators: The changing illumination, as dusk falls, is the signal for the trip home. Foraging trips during the day are repeated. Other animals anticipate winter by storing food. Thus the anticipation of expectable danger, or of food shortages, is as much of the biology of stressful experience as the response to an actual one.

Darwin's (1872) organismic view went further: Behavior and physiology were one and indivisible. In the response to an enemy (a dog) a cat snarls, assumes a specific bodily posture, shows dilated pupils and erect hair, bares its teeth, or extends its claws. Blood flow through muscle is increased and through the skin is decreased. Blood levels of epinephrine (E), ACTH, and aVP rise (Jänig 1987). A cat about to fight another shows one pattern of cardiovascular responses, which is different than that observed during the fight. Two further response patterns respectively depend on whether it emerges as the victor or the defeated animal (Zanchetti, Baccelli, and Mancia 1976). However, the behavior, pupillary changes, and discriminated cardiovascular responses form an integrated whole: One does not "cause" the other!

If one agrees with Darwin's organismic ideas about the stressful nature of life, then certain consequences follow. Living organisms have special properties that simple matter, or machines, do not have (Mayr 1982). Therefore, they cannot be described by the laws of Boyle, Charles, Hooke, and Newton. Yet the concept of stress originated in mechanics. Mechanical stress—on a piece of metal, or on a gas under pressure—can be measured. But living organisms are not metal bars or gas molecules. They are complex. They are unique and individual by virtue of their genetic endowment and experience. They have a history. They learn. The variability (individual differences) of organisms is the essence. It is the basis of evolution—the very stuff upon which natural selection acts to occasion differential survival and reproductive success or failure. Living organisms are highly organized. Their organization is not merely the product of arithmetically summing their elementary constituents. It is also stable but capable of undergoing change. Stability is not merely a matter of structure: Most of the functions (e.g., circadian rhythms) of the organism manifest it.

Organisms, though complex, can be described by their interacting functional subsystems arranged in feedback loops, or paced by oscillators, and organized in multiple parallel pathways. Though the initial conditions of a subsystem or the whole organism may be determined, the outcome of perturbing it may be quite unpredictable (Glass and Mackey 1988). Some physicists and engineers have recently drawn sharp distinctions between physical systems and organisms and/or social systems. They can be discriminated by counting up the number of variables, parameters, and feedback loops in models of each system; a complexity index is then calculated. Physical systems (e.g., the weather) have low model complexity but high computational complexity. Computer (hardware) networks have moderate model complexity. But models of organisms and their brains, economies, and societies are 10^{12} times more complex than physical systems, and their computational complexity is also very high.

Model complexity is not only a matter of numbers. Physical and hardware systems operate under "invariant rules, are context independent and not self-observing." Human systems (organisms) are, in contrast, context-dependent and self-observing, and they operate according to changes in rules (S. J. Kline, cited in Denning 1990).

Therefore, a comprehensive approach to the biology of stressful experience must (and often does) incorporate some of the known characteristics of organisms, and the changes in their subsystems when perturbed—when the rules change.

Cannon's Concept of Homeostasis and Stress

Since Cannon's and Selye's time many writers have defined stress as "any threat to or disturbance of homeostasis" (Hinkle 1987; Kopin 1989; Munck, Guyre, and Holbrook 1984). This definition is limited to the physiological responses to stressful experiences: It is as problematic as Selye's previously cited definition and for some of the same reasons. Stress research in recent years has taught us that "threats" or "disturbances" are not equivalent (Weiner 1991b). The patterned and coordinated changes in behavior and physiology in response to a stressful experience are exquisitely attuned to it: A patterned disturbance in the circulation produced by orthostasis differs from that produced by exercise or a threatening fight between animals.

The two concepts—homeostasis and stress—were originally brought together by Cannon (1914, 1928, 1935, 1939). In 1914 he wrote about "emotional stress." In a later publication, he mentioned the "stress of excitement" (1928). To make the topic of stress even more mysterious he published a paper on the "stresses and strains of homeostasis" (1935), by which he meant that lack of oxygen, low blood sugar levels, blood loss, and exposure to cold could act as stresses and strains. Once a critical ("homeostatic") level of a variable (e.g., blood glucose or body temperature) was breached, the "stabilizing factors of the organism" (i.e., homeostatic mechanisms) were "strained" to the breaking point.

In the best Newtonian tradition, Cannon's concept of stress was linear and mechanical. The various stresses about which he wrote were some of the emotions and appetites (hunger). But stress, according to his view, could also have social and occupational origins (1939). Furthermore, he believed that stresses were usually acute in nature, entailing fear, hunger, or rage—emergency disturbances in homeostasis mediated by the sympathoadrenal medullary system. These emotions were implicitly causes, not correlates, of the destabilization or "straining" of homeostatic mechanisms.

Cannon's concept of homeostasis (1929, 1935), as Moore-Ede (1986) has recently pointed out, does not imply "fixed and rigid constancy," but rather a range of levels of a physiological variable, maintained by homeostatic constraints. In a figure in his 1929 paper the normal blood sugar levels actually fluctuate within a range of 70 to 130 mg/100 ml—the limits of the "homeostatically defended range" (Moore-Ede 1986).

According to Cannon's vision, rhythmic variation or oscillation of physiological functions was not the primary datum; but the limits within which they fluctuated were. Physiologists have until recently concerned themselves mainly with changes in levels (not in the parameters of the rhythm) of a variable outside the homeostatic range, or with measures of mean or average levels (not the variations about the mean, and the deviations from them).

Of greater relevance for any theory of stress is that behavioral and physiological changes also occur in anticipation of or preparation for challenges, threats, and dangers, and not merely in reaction to them (Moore-Ede 1986). Thus E and free fatty acid (FFA) levels increase in anticipation of driving a racing car (Taggart and Carruthers 1971) or prior to exercise and public speaking (Taggart, Carruthers, and Somerville 1973). Some mammals prepare to hibernate in the autumn. Body temperature rises in anticipation of morning awakening (Moore-Ede, Sulzman, and Fuller 1982).

We know almost nothing about the (possibly stressful) effects on the organism of sudden and/or unexpected or unpredictable events, environments that preclude anticipation or prediction, and ambiguous events or situations in which a sufficiently strong or stable signal is lacking for the appropriate organismic response patterns (including anticipatory ones) to be generated. Equally relevant for any revision of the stress concept is the observation that some regulatory processes (e.g., release of opioid peptides) that seem truly homeostatic come into operation de novo when the organism is perturbed; when it is not they seem not to be secreted into the bloodstream (Bouloux and Grossman 1989). These observations need to be taken into account in any revision of a theory of stress and the concept of homeostasis.

To return to Cannon's ideas: Within a decade or two of the publication of

Cannon's *Wisdom of the Body* (1939), a number of prominent physiologists were taking issue with the universality of the concept of homeostasis. One of the most eminent of these, D. W. Richards, published his thoughts in two papers (1952, 1957) criticizing Cannon. He pointed out that at certain times the body, rather than being "wise," was "stupid." By this he meant that Cannon's concept was mainly limited to normal physiological functioning and failed to account for "abnormal physiology," seen in chronic disease states. Cannon had implied that every bodily reaction was "protective," purposive, and "wise." Richards begged the question: Do "all [physiological] mechanisms have to be called homeostatic mechanisms?" (1952, 50). He commented that the concept of "homeostasis has possessed all our physiological thinking. Other balancing concepts are needed" (1952, 47). Citing instances in which chronic inflammatory and immunological responses lead to cell damage and scarring (as in rheumatoid arthritis, chronic nephritis, and hepatic cirrhosis), or in which the immediate form of hypersensitivity occasions anaphylaxis, shock, and death, he pointed out that physiological processes could be homeostatic in one but not in another direction. Physiological responses, he stated, could be:

a. Excessive (e.g., in anaphylaxis, fibrosis). Richards cited (1957) polycythemia as a homeostatic response to the lack of oxygen at high altitudes. It may, however, at sea level lead to congestive heart failure, with or without pulmonary edema, producing further anoxia and a vicious cycle of further increases in blood volume.

b. Inadequate or deficient (e.g., in infancy, old age, nutritional deficiency, ischemia).

c. Inappropriate, ill-timed, inopportune (e.g., in autoimmune phenomena; in congestive failure when the kidney reabsorbs salt and water excretion to enhance blood volume; or when growth factors are expressed at the inappropriate age to cause the progression of malignant cells).

d. Disordered (i.e., the usual regulatory processes and the functions they control undergo transitions to new modes of functioning, a case in point is the transition from normal cardiac sinus rhythm to ventricular fibrillation).

Richards also pointed out that excessive, inadequate, inappropriate or ill-timed, and disordered responses could characterize behavior, not only physiology. His list of the four categories of failure of homeostasis may today be further lengthened: A physiological function or rhythm may disappear altogether or show a change in its mode of operation by becoming more variable or by manifesting an alteration of one of its parameters. Additionally, new rhythms may appear, or prior ones may reappear.

Richards also contrasted the concept of homeostasis with Claude Bernard's (1865) concept of the constancy of the internal environment, from which the former derives. Bernard had pointed out that the *milieu interieur* was in "full communication" with the "external environment," that "protective functions" existed that maintained the internal environment, and that "sickness and death" result from the "dislocation and perturbation of these functions." He had a clear view that the organism was in free communication with, and was reactive to, the changing environment. It had to "protect" its internal environment from such perturbations by (implicit) regulatory "mechanisms" in order to preserve its "vital activity." When these perturbed (normal) mechanisms go awry, disease may ensue. Richards sided with Bernard and not with Cannon, but he raised the question whether Bernard's version of sickness and death was complete.

Richards was one of the first of Cannon's critics to question the idea that steady states characterize physiological systems and are the basis of homeostasis. A steady state is "a set of values of the variables of a system . . . [that] . . . do not change as time proceeds" (Glass and Mackey 1988, 21). But most physiological and behavioral systems are rhythmic. They oscillate. Each can be described by its characteristic frequency, amplitude, and waveform. Defined in this manner, few functional steady states exist.

The organism's fundamental operating modes are oscillatory. Respiration; body temperature; BP; the heartbeat; sleep stages; chewing; food intake; menstruation; the levels of hormones, neurotransmitters, immunocytes, membrane receptors, and enzyme activity; the cell cycle—all go through regular oscillations on a number of time scales (second by second, hourly, circadian, monthly, seasonal, etc.) (Garfinkel 1983; Rapp, Mees, and Sparrow 1981; Yates 1982).

One reason for the existence of oscillations is that most, if not all, subsystems and systems of the body are arranged in, and regulated by, negative and positive (or mixed) feedback loops: For example, the subsystem controlling ovarian secretion begins with the hypothalamic gonadotropic (GnRH) or luteinizing hormone releasing hormone (LHRH) that stimulates the oscillatory (pulsatile) secretion of luteinizing (LH) and follicle stimulating (FSH) hormone by the anterior pituitary gland, which in turn causes estradiol (E_2) to be produced and secreted by the ovary. Estradiol usually inhibits LHRH secretion (Abraham 1983; Smith 1980). If this inhibition is sufficiently steep the overall system will oscillate. The steepness of the inhibition may increase to critical levels at puberty because the hypothalamic (preoptic and arcuate) neurons become more "sensitive" to E_2. As a result oscillation in the systems begins—a bifurcation has occurred—and menarche is initiated. (Of course, the system is more complexly regulated: Throughout the menstrual cycle E_2 and progesterone levels change, to account in part for intermittence in the menstrual cycle. Additionally, hypothalamic, catecholaminergic, and peptidergic neurons regulate the secretion of LHRH and its [gonadotropin] associated peptide [GAP], while several ovarian peptides (e.g., inhibin] counterregulate FSH.)

The nonlinear concept of bifurcation entails a qualitative change from one

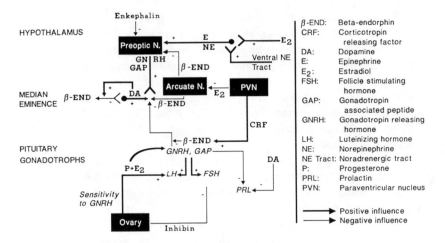

Figure 1.   Regulation of GNRH and GAP Secretion

(stable) oscillatory mode to another. An example of such a transition is the midcycle LH pulse that ends with ovulation—an intermittent process that cannot be accounted for by any single-loop, oscillatory system. (However, the regulation of the pulse of LH differs from its regular pulsatile release). To complicate the matter even further, a single variable may oscillate within two separate time frames: Five to six oscillations (with a mean duration of 28 minutes) in serum cortisol occur in humans during any 24-hour period. These are in turn superimposed on a circadian oscillation (also about 24 hours in length) whose nadir occurs in the first hours of the night. Of equal importance is that ACTH shows a similar circadian oscillation to cortisol's. Yet, and despite its close link to episodic corticosteroid secretion, ACTH levels oscillate ten times in a 24-hour period, each with a duration of about 140 minutes.

Some oscillatory systems may appear to be closely coupled—sleep and the circadian oscillation of cortisol secretion. We know, however, that these two systems may be uncoupled (e.g., by sleep reversal).

Abnormal functioning (illness or disease), in this view, occurs when a system loses the stability of its usual operating mode (engineers call this a "failure mode"). Each form of abnormal functioning can be conceived of as a bifurcation to a mode that "models the dynamical patterns of the pathology" (Garfinkel 1983). The mode may either revert to an earlier one or take the form of an oscillatory instability—tetanic contractions, arrhythmias and dysrhythmias, and various other altered temporal patterns. In other idioms, discontrol or disregulation has occurred.

One may, therefore, reconceptualize the effects of a stressful experience. The perturbations of a system produced by it do not alter the homeostatic steady state; rather they induce bifurcations, forcing a system into oscillatory instability or producing a reversion to an earlier functioning mode.

On the other hand, a subsystem that had previously oscillated by virtue of its participation in a negative feedback loop may be taken out of the loop (e.g., when ectopic tumors produce peptides—pancreatic gastrinomas, lung tumors secreting ACTH, etc.—or when receptors are preempted by an auto-antibody—e.g., in Graves disease—that continually stimulates unregulated thyroid hormone secretion) (Weiner 1989a, 1989b).

Cannon's and Selye's Views on Stress Compared

Selye (1956) wrote that Cannon was his "first critic," questioning the like-lihood that the pituitary and adrenal glands could "help resistance and adaptation in general." Mason (1971) went further: He doubted that the concepts of the GAS and homeostasis were compatible with each other. He questioned that the same corticosteroid response to diametrically opposite stimuli, such as heat and cold, that require different metabolic adjustments could be useful to the organism. How could the same hormone, be asked, "exert both thermogenic . . . and thermolytic effects" in two quite different circumstances? Mason was correct in asking this question. What Selye could not have realized is that brown fat thermogenesis in response to cold is promoted by CRF acting through β-adrenergic sympathetic neurons (LeFeuvre, Roth-well, and Stock 1987); and CRF also stimulates ACTH and thus cortisol secretion. Brown fat thermogenesis and cortisol secretion occur in parallel but are not causally linked.

Cannon's and Selye's concepts about stress are actually incompatible with each other. Cannon, as we have seen, dealt with very specific conditions designed to elicit specific responses to hunger, fear, pain, and rage. He was not interested in the production of disease but in the physiological correlates of hunger and these emotions, and how these in turn were constrained or brought within normal (homeostatic) limits. Selye's experiments terminated in both (thymic) atrophy and (adrenal) hypertrophy in two different organ systems. Presumably, the normal homeostatic range was breached: A *failure* of home-ostasis had occurred, as Richards in his critique of Cannon's concepts concluded. Furthermore, how could such structural alterations be adaptively useful?

Mason's Contributions to Stress Theory and Research

For two decades Mason carried out an extensive program of research using a variety of controlled stressful experiences (conditioned emotional and avoid-ance paradigms, food deprivation, heat, cold, and exercise) while studying a wide range of hormonal variables in the urine and blood serum of monkeys. In

1968 he published a monumental account of his results using a 2- to 72-hour conditioned avoidance procedure. Monkeys were first strapped into a chair in order to get them accustomed to the seat and the laboratory setting. Prior to the actual experiment, they were trained to respond during a 20-second interval to a red light, which was followed by a mild electric shock to the feet unless the animal pressed a lever to avoid it. Once trained, the animal would maintain the action of lever-pressing for as long as 72 hours—a maneuver that required minimal physical effort.

One of the most significant outcomes of this work was the demonstration that endocrine responses are *patterned* and are not confined to any one hormonal system. To exemplify: Urinary E levels increased rapidly and remained high during the entire 72-hour avoidance session, while norepinephrine (NE) levels only rose at the end of the experimental procedure and and remained elevated for three full days after it. Plasma 17-OHCS levels increased throughout the experimental session and fell to below control levels for one day after it. Two of the urinary 17-ketosteroids (etiocholanolone and dehydroepiandrosterone [DHA]) levels showed a negative response, being depressed for the entire avoidance procedure and for three days thereafter. A third 17-ketosteroid, androsterone, however, was usually characterized by a biphasic response, being initially diminished for six days and then elevated. Urinary testosterone levels had a profile similar to aldosterone's. However, changes in aldosterone levels actually showed two patterns—either biphasic or triphasic—characterized by an increase prior to the actual procedure. When the former pattern obtained, urine volume was decreased. Urinary estrogen levels (estrone, E_2, estriol) all fell during the procedure and only recovered to baseline levels over a period of three days or more days after it had ended.

Butanol-extractable-iodine (BEI) (a "state of the art" measure of thyroxins at that time) increased slowly during the 72-hour session and continued elevated for another three weeks. (With repeated exposure to the procedure, no habituation of this response occurred). Plasma insulin levels fell after 2 and 24 hours of the avoidance procedure, while plasma glucose levels rose. But if the monkeys took part in 72-hour sessions, plasma insulin levels showed little change, then fell and increased for the subsequent eight days. The most complex responses were demonstrated by growth hormone, being a function of the initial, baseline level: They fell if initially high, and rose if low (Mason 1968, 774).

Some of these patterns unfolded over time (e.g., NE, insulin) even when the animal was no longer subjected to the experience. They were also quite specific to the stressor; no GAS—Selye's "stress response"—or any part of it occurred in Mason's experiments. If the animal was repeatedly exposed to the same procedure a diminution in the changes in patterns usually occurred (except, for instance, in the case of urinary NE and BEI levels).

Mason (1968, 1971) was sensitively aware that his monkeys were responding behaviorally, not only hormonally, both in anticipation of the experiment and while being acclimated to the experimental chair. During these periods their urinary 17-OHCS levels increased. The pain, discomfort, and fear engendered by the experimental procedures themselves were also potent stimuli, raising 17-OHCS excretion.

His investigations significantly advanced our ideas about stressful experience when he showed that a noxious stimulus had broader parameters to it than a simple stimulus-response (GAS) model implied. Depriving an animal of food in a setting in which its peers were being fed had quite different behavioral and physiological effects than starving it in isolation. Additionally, if the deprived animal was given a tasty but nonnutritious pellet, not totally starved, its hormonal responses were diminished. From these observations, Mason (1971) concluded that "psychological stimuli" were as potent in producing changes in 17-OHCS excretion as the experimental experience was. These "psychological stimuli," including the context in which they were buried, could be quite subtle. They did not necessarily have to entail the animal's experience of severe pain or of discomfort. According to Mason the role of subtle "psychological stimuli" had been grossly underestimasted by Selye, especially when the stressful procedures entailed exercise, fasting, or exposure to cold or heat.

Mason concluded that it was not the GAS per se that was nonspecific. However, ubiquitous emotional responses—fear, pain, discomfort—to many different stressful experiences *were* nonspecific. He stated that "the 'stress concept' should not be regarded primarily as a physiological concept but rather as a behavioral concept" (1971, 331). He thereby called for a reevaluation of the "stress" field, pointing out that it makes a great deal of conceptual difference that "diverse stimuli" elicit a nonspecific endocrine response as contrasted to a nonspecific behavioral response (1971, 328).

Nonetheless, some comments on Mason's clarifying conclusions are warranted. First, pain and fear cannot be directly observed in animals. They can be inferred from behavior or from the development of "stress analgesia" (Lewis, Cannon, and Liebeskind 1980). The analgesia occurs under several conditions—in a male rat intruding into the home cage of another male rat; in rats subjected to unavoidable electric shock or intermittently immersed in cold water, etc.

Second, the idea that it is the emotional experience of the animal that is causal in the hormonal response—a line of thought implicit in Cannon, Selye, and Mason—is fraught with conceptual perils; it raises the problem, still unsolved, that Descartes first posed. A more cautious way of conceptualizing the observation is to say that fear, discomfort, and pain are important signals to the organism of novelty, danger, or injury. They are correlates of, but not necessarily causal to, the hormonal response. The correlation between the emotional and the physiological response can be understood in the following manner: The signal of danger is transduced by, and carried from, various receptors (olfactory, auditory, visual) to the brain by parallel neural pathways that carry the information. The information generates a signal of fear (the emotion) while inducing appropriate physiological responses via parallel, efferent autonomic and endocrine output channels (LeDoux 1989; Weiner 1972).

Third, in Mason's experiments the animal was prevented from making the usual behavioral response that it does in nature: A dog exposed to a hot atmosphere not only pants but seeks out the shade or goes to lie in cool water. In the laboratory the opportunity for such adaptive behaviors is not customarily provided. Therefore, the stressful experience (i.e., heat) cannot be avoided and is more likely to induce discomfort and a hormonal response. The same may be said of the experimental conditions in which only two choices are open to the animal—to receive painful electric shock, or to press a lever to avoid it.

Fourth, Mason believed that the *experience* (the "psychological stimuli" or "emotional response") was nonspecific, but that the physiological response was specific. But he did not make clear that fear is a specific signal of danger, as pain is a signal of bodily injury.

The hormonal response patterns recorded by Mason (1968, 1975) appeared to correlate with specific psychological and behavioral responses to the conditioned avoidance procedure or to chair restraint. But the matter of both specific and nonspecific changes in hormonal patterns occurring simultaneously with two different stressful experiences (other than severe injury or pain) appeared to remain unresolved. Some stressful experiences do seem to elicit the same hormonal patterns in the rat, and several others evoke different ones (Gibbs 1986). The current evidence suggests that nonspecific (general) physiological responses (the GAS) do not occur unless the animal is completely overwhelmed by—incapable of preventing, avoiding, or responding to—the inciting agent (see, however, chapter 6).

One approach to the unanswered question of simultaneous specific and nonspecific responses was suggested by both Mason and Richards: to carry out a precise analysis of the components of the stressful experience. Bleeding an animal produces hypovolemia, hypoxia, hypotension, and hypoproteinemia, each of which is counteracted by a variety of endocrine, autonomic nervous system, renal, circulatory, and respiratory changes. Which of these, Mason (1971) asked, produce increased urinary 17-OCHS levels? What are the afferent pathways by which pain, cold, and exercise activate the hypothalamic-pituitary-adrenal axis? He believed that such afferent inputs acted via the brain (1975), and he suggested a program of research (1971, 1975), some of which has been completed in the past decade (Brown and Fisher, 1985, 1989; Feldman 1985; Reisine 1989; Rivier 1989). Furthermore, he extrapolated from his findings in the laboratory to human stress research (Mason 1975). Both in animals and people, marked individual (both inter- and intraindividual) differences in the responses to stressful experiences occur. Each person appraises potential dangers, threats, and challenges and their contexts differently; each has his/her own manner of dealing with them. Every person's history in responding to these stressors differs; experience, age, knowledge, and training count. Some people react appropriately, some overreact, some react not at all or inappropriately, and some become disorganized in their behavior. These many factors, Mason has pointed out, must be taken into account in any definition of stressful experience. In fact, he clarified many issues in arriving at its definition (1975). And he also implied, but did not explicitly state, that the psychological, behavioral and physiological responses to stressors were inextricable—that is, they were organismic.

3 The Definition and Classification of Stressful Experience

The following definition of stress is based on biological principles, which have frequently been lost sight of by specialists in either biomedicine or the behavioral and social sciences. Specialization tends to isolate scientists, who are traditionally instructed by the concepts and theories guiding their own particular fields and not those of others (Mason 1975, 22).

The physician is predominantly concerned with the relationship of stressful experience to disease onset; if no disease ensues, the experience cannot have been stressful! Physiologists study the impact of stressful experiences in producing changes in measurable bodily functions without necessarily producing disease and illness. Stress is then defined in terms of these (normal) alterations. But stressful experiences also affect behavior without any discernible impact on physiology (and vice versa). Experimental psychologists use observable, readily controlled, quantifiable, independent variables to study single, dependent ones. They rarely study the covariances of physiology and behavior. Individual differences in responses to stressful experiences are a nuisance to be eliminated by rigorous experimental control and statistical means, rather than things to be studied in their own right. But nature is not as simple or pure as the methodology that is used to study its phenomena.

The separate categories of stressful experience, which will be enumerated below, are each made up of many complex components: An earthquake is not only an unexpected, uncontrollable, and frightening event; it may also deprive people of their food and water supplies, property, transportation, place of work, and savings, investments, and income. It may eventuate in injury or death. All facets of such an experience need to be first separately, and later cumulatively, analyzed and assessed. Not only is the actual experience complex, but many other factors in interaction determine what each person experiences and how his/her actions are designed to meet the danger, threat, or challenge and to protect himself or herself against it.

Much of the literature on stressful experiences is concerned with their impact on individuals—that is, physiological and psychological reactions (Lazarus 1971) and their effects on well-being, morale, and health. One of the most popular definitions of stressful experiences is "demands that tax or exceed the resources of the system" (Lazarus 1966; Lazarus and Cohen 1977). The system is defined as an organism or a social system, and the demands (challenges or changes) are such that no automatic adaptive responses are available to it.

This definition implies that stressful experience entails or forecasts a failure of adaptation. The fact remains that even though events may be experienced as stressful, most persons successfully master them by protecting against, removing, negotiating about, or escaping them. "The stress response" is not only "a complex and interactive process" (Elliott and Eisdorfer 1982, 27) but also a mutual one between the organism and its environment. A definition of stressful experience must get away from focusing only on adverse effects. It also should give credence to the fact that the adaptive failure may be due not to the unavailability of responses but to the inappropriate nature of over- or underreactions before, during, and after the experience.

In the past, research on stressful experience has not usually been guided by the biological reality that the natural and social environment is complex and ever-changing. In the laboratory the stressful stimuli or experiences that are used tend to be simple and invariant (e.g., repetitive electric shocks, or signals signifying their onset).

What Stressful Experience Is Not

To recapitulate: The argument was put forward in chapter 2 that stress should be defined in an organismic manner, and not as the stimulus, the contingency, or only one part (either behavioral or physiological) of the response of it. Furthermore, the stressful experience is not everything or anything, nor is the response to it general or indiscriminate.

To speak about physical injury or emotional "stressors" is not correct either, on at least two counts. Injury and pain are experiences with consequences; they are not things in or by themselves. Pain is a signal of injury, or that something is "wrong" in the body; both require corrective measures. Emotions are not per se stressful experiences; they do not usually "do" anything. (Fear and anxiety may on occasion, and when extreme, disrupt rational thinking or disorganize behavior.) They serve as internal signals alerting the organism and requiring a response.

A signal external to the organism is separately processed in parallel by the brain (Hofer 1984; LeDoux 1989; Weiner 1972, 1977). Although the emotional response to the signal may appear to be causally correlated with physiological changes, they are usually only associated in time. To conceptualize emotion and the correlated physiological response in any other manner leads to the insuperable conundrum traditionally designated as one aspect of the mind-brain-body problem.

Both the emotional signal and the physiological changes are biologically purposive, but one does not seem to lead to the other. They may occur independently of each other. Emotions may be pleasant or unpleasant. Pleasant emotions may be experienced in dangerous situations. Therefore, the term *emotional stress* should be eschewed, or discarded as misleading. Another term, *physical stress,* should also be eschewed, for the reason that injury or infection has organismic, not only local, consequences. The totality of experience should be described, not only one of its properties or aspects.

One might also conclude, based on a survey of the literature on stressful experience, that the term should not be expanded without further specification to include any and all threatening, challenging, shifting, "overloading," painful, distressing, or depriving physical or social situations and stimuli. It should not be employed only to signify mental states produced by experiences, the abiding characteristics ("traits") of certain persons, or general or specific physiological responses, hormonal or otherwise. Stimuli (in Selye's sense) or situations such as loud noises, injuries, or a cold climate can hardly be deemed the equivalent of a profound human experience such as the death of a child.

Following stressful experiences people do not of necessity fall ill, nor do they return to their previous state, as the principles laid down by Bernard and Cannon would predict: The experience is stored, and a reorganization of the person occurs. Learning to deal with such experiences also occurs.

In the laboratory Selye exposed his animals to "nonspecific" stimuli, producing physiological responses and counterresponses, which he believed were general; in contrast, human beings usually respond in an integrated, specific, appropriate, and individual manner, even to the most dire and overwhelming experiences. Although commonalities exist, variations in human responses are the rule, not the exception. The statement that human beings vary in their adaptive (or coping) capacities should come as no surprise to anyone conversant with a basic biological truth discovered by Darwin (1859). The nature of the experiences to which Selye subjected his animals made any individual (or other) adaptive responses impossible. Therefore, he concluded that no individual, only general, responses occurred. There are, of course, similarities and commonalities across stressful experiences, especially when they are dire. Panic is a common response to earthquakes or to fires in closed spaces. But not everyone panics. Normative, unfolding responses to bereavement and separation occur (Brown and Stoudemire 1983; Klerman and Izen 1977; Lindemann 1944). Yet individual differences in response to these two profound personal experiences have also been described: No grief may occur after such losses (Wortman and Silver 1989).

Many of the events and experiences that have been called stressful are not physical but are of a personal nature: They result from change in key human relationships. They stem either from humanity's unlimited capacity for inhuman cruelty, or from the disruption of human relationships by death or separation. Conversely, human fellowship buffers the effects of the breaking of the bonds that usually bind human beings together. The study of stressful experience has recently focused upon the vicissitudes of human relationships (Taylor 1987; Weiner 1985a, 1986, 1987). In the course of this endeavor, the general word *stress* has lost its meaning; it cannot conceivably describe the specific subtleties and functions and the individual meanings of personal relationships. The stress theory of the past did not predict that human relationships are crucial to the maintenance, or the restoration, of health, or that social isolation increases morbidity and mortality (House, Landis, and Umberson 1988).

Many of these conclusions and assertions derive from, and continue, the analysis of the concept of stress carried out by Mason (1975). He pointed out that a description of the "stimulus-situation" did not predict the behavioral or physiological response because of individual differences in the eyes of the situation's beholders. Nonetheless, a precise characterization and analysis of the parameters and components of stressful experiences must at all times be made. Many studies done in the past several years show that slight variations of the experimental situation (e.g., exposing rats to different parameters of electric shock, or making them swim in water intermittently, not only continuously) produce subtle differences in the behavior of animals or in the form of analgesia (Ben-Eliyahu et al. 1990; Lewis, Cannon, and Liebeskind 1980; Shavit et al. 1984, 1985).

Experiences are stressful for some and not for others. This observation places the student of stress in the uneasy position of designating as stress a set of stimulus conditions "that may or may not evoke a response" (Mason 1975, 32). But is this really so? In some persons a virus or other pathogen produces no immune response, in others it does. Does that mean that the virus is not usually pathogenic? (It may actually be more so when no immune response is mounted against it.)

Qualitative differences are as important as quantitative ones in studying the mutual interaction of the organism with its environment. Without such an interaction no stimulus, contingency, situation, or event, or its experiences, would be stressful. An interesting question is: Why does a response occur in some persons and not in others?

Mason's (1975) second point flows directly from the first. Stressful experience cannot be defined by the "response parameters" because they are not invariant, universal, or nonspecific. As already mentioned, Selye's investigations suggest that only under the most drastic conditions, during which the animal is unable to make, or is prevented from making, a protective or aversive behavioral response, do general physiological responses occur. But even this inference may not be correct. Furthermore, as Mason (1968) showed, repeating the same severe experimental procedures over and over again leads to diminishing patterns of (some) hormonal responses. (We know today that the receptors of many hormones and neurotransmitters are either "down-regulated" by an excess of their agonists, or desensitized when they are bound by their ligands—but not always.)

Lazarus (1966), Lazarus and Folkman (1984), and Mason (1975) concluded that it was empirically and conceptually unsatisfactory to define stress only in terms of the stimulus or the response parameters; both had to be included in the definition of the process. Mason (1975) suggested that an interactive stimulus-response model was better, but still not wholly adequate. Stressful experience might be defined as specific "evocative conditions" that elicited a "specified set of response[s]." He pointed out that the development of operational and comprehensive criteria would be difficult but not impossible (1975).

This difficulty in part stems from the fact that no response, or inadequate or inappropriate responses, are of equal moment to the organism as those that have been arbitrarily specified to occur. Furthermore, one particular group of expected responses may occur when the "evocative conditions" are first met, and a different set of responses occur later on in time. Mason's stimulus-response model is also too linear; it is not recursive. In most instances the organism's behavioral response—if it is allowed to make one—will be to modify, remove, or flee from the evocative conditions. Thus a recursive, nonlinear model accords more closely with observation (Lazarus and Folkman 1984).

A model of stress must also be time-related, complex, and mutually interactive because of the well-known biological fact that organisms and environments are ever-changing. Therefore, the sources and nature of the subject's variability in response to changing environmental conditions, challenge, and danger must be incorporated in any definition of stress (Appley and Trumbull 1967; Lazarus 1971).

Mutual interactions of all animals with their environments are observable everywhere. Animals select their environments for different activities such as nesting, foraging, feeding, and mating. They alter their environment by grazing, polluting it, or building nests, shelters, dams, and houses to protect themselves and their young. They store food, or fat, in their bodies to ensure supplies. They change their behaviors to accord with ever-changing climatic conditions: When climatic conditions are extreme, such as in the desert, some come out of their shelters only during the coolest part of the day or night. Some animals sleep, hunt, or forage during the day, and others do so only at night. They avoid other predators at certain of these times; conversely, predators prey on their sleeping victims at a particular period of the day or night.

All living creatures have special tasks to perform, which often mutually support and reinforce each other. The balance between success and failure in their execution is delicate and can easily be disrupted by seasonal and environmental changes or unpredictable events. Specific and particular aspects of the change in conditions—the length of the day, the ambient temperature, the amount of sunlight, the size of the prey, or the presence of dominant conspecifics or other predators—act as signals; other signals are ignored. Each signal, whether it is relevant or not, is processed by separate transducing receptors (which change the physical form of the signal) and parallel neural pathways (which activate the appropriate pattern generators of the physiological and behavioral responses). At times the signal is magnified by the organism. At other times it may result in minimal or no physiological or behavioral change (Levins and Lewontin 1985).

Biologists recognize that the environment cannot merely be understood as "surroundings." It is also a way of life; the activity of the organism sets the stage for its own survival and reproduction, that is, "its own evolution" (Levins and Lewontin 1985, 58). The environment is "not a passive 'out there.'" "'Stress' depends on who you are, and on an ensemble of risk factors" (Levins and Lewontin 1985, 245) that differ for each person or creature.

The Definition of Stressful Experience

The concept and definition of stressful experience flow naturally from Darwin's formulation of natural selection. Stressful experiences are inevitable. They consist of selective pressures that derive from the physical and social environment. They are challenging. They threaten the survival, viability, integrity, and reproductive success of individuals and groups. In animals, selective pressures are particularly intense at certain times during the life cycle—for example, during breeding. Breeding requires a chain of favorable or optimal environmental conditions that ensure food supplies, mating, the housing of offspring, the correct temperature conditions, and relative protection from predators (Crews and Moore 1986).

Organisms meet these challenges and dangers by integrated behavioral, physiological patterns of response that are appropriate to the task. Organisms vary in their capacity to respond to, meet, deal with, overcome, or escape from challenges and threats; those who cannot or do not may die, be injured, or fall ill. Therefore, it should not be surprising that individual differences characterize these responses—another principle we owe to Darwin.

Thus the stressful experience is a potential or actual threat or challenge to the integrity, survival, and reproduction of the organism. The threat or challenge may be anticipated. It may be real, imaginary, or an admixture of both. Based on this formulation and in the case of people, it may be possible to suggest an initial and crude taxonomy of stress (Baum, Fleming, and Davidson 1983; Elliott and Eisdorfer 1982; Lazarus and Cohen 1977; Weiner

1985a) as follows: natural occurrences and disasters; man-made disasters; and personal experiences.

Both humans and animals are exposed to one, two, or all of these three categories of stressful experience. By altering or destroying delicately balanced ecologies humans and some animal species place themselves and others at risk for increased competition and for extinction. As overcrowding occurs, or as food supplies shrink, some animals kill their own young.

Social animals establish precise hierarchies. Subordinate or defeated animals are deprived of food and mates and may leave their group. Young animals may lose their parents. Animals prey upon each other; people hunt and butcher them. Animals may be injured or become sick, at which time members of some species display "altruism" to their damaged or ill conspecifics.

Each of the three categories, which are not exclusive, has both general (e.g., injury or death) and individual (e.g., fear or heroism) consequences for human beings, which must be analyzed separately. Each person interprets these experiences in his/her own manner. Each experience has personal meanings and a different impact. Some persons seek out challenges and take undue risks. Some find danger exciting; others shrink or flee from it. Some (e.g., hostages, prisoners) welcome death; others will compromise every principle or go to any length to survive.

Therefore, it is not the event per se that is stressful, but how it is perceived by, and the meaning it has to, the beholder. Whether a response is possible, adequate, and appropriate or not has consequences. A critical variable in the process is a person's sense of control over the experience and over his/her actions in dealing with it. Loss of control over a situation is experienced as helplessness, hopelessness, despair, and "giving-up" (Engel 1968). But most challenges, threats, and dangers are mastered. They may be learning experiences that teach persons to be better prepared to remove, overcome, or flee from them when they recur.

Classification of Stressful Experiences

The Need for Classification

In biology, but not in medicine (Copeland 1977), the taxonomies of plants and animals, begun by Linnaeus and Buffon respectively, have had profound consequences: the theories of Evolution and genetics. Taxonomies in biology are theories that account for common appearances and shared properties but not for common causes; they "create and reflect the deep structure of science." However, species are not essences: Common appearances and shared properties obscure variation—the raw material for natural selection. "Variation is primary; essences are illusory" (Gould 1985, 160–65).

Therefore, variations in the nature, quality, and temporal characteristics of all phenomena affecting human beings are to be expected. The essence of Darwin's revolutionary thought was that differences within and among species were related. But he took as his primary object of study individual differences *within* species, rather than between species (Levins and Lewontin 1985).

Some biologists have had simple ways of telling the difference between species on the basis of the fertility of the offspring of two members of the same species. However, the difference between individuals of the same species is more difficult to classify: The criteria of gender, appearance, and behavior are usually used. But behavior is not a concrete and invariant characteristic, as is gender. It is a set of actions with goals, meanings, intentions, and purposes (Fabrega 1987). Each of these is colored or conditioned by social and cultural conventions, which in turn determine whether it is judged to be normal, appropriate, and adequate in a particular context. Conventions also change, because they are evaluated by shifting religious, historical, social, political, and economic norms or standards. Norms of whatever kind—behavioral, biochemical, immunological, or physiological—are hard to establish. Even these scientific (measurable, observable) "norms" vary—with gender, ethnicity, age, time of day, and season of the year. Actions are subject to an even greater number of variable norms.

Classification must not be too rigid. Consider the time-honored separate categories of physiological function—the autonomic nervous, endocrine, and immune systems. They turn out not to be separate entities. Hormones can act as neurotransmitters or promote growth. Neurotransmitters function as hormones. Lymphokines activate hormonal systems. The products of these systems are communication signals, which act locally and at a distance.

The proposed classification of stressful experiences deals with observable events and contexts that may or may not be experienced as stressful. The categories cited may not be all-inclusive; but they are preferable to a classification based on norms that are hard to establish, change, or may be incorrect. For this reason alone, a classification of stressful experiences based on categories such as "psychic," "emotional," "economic," "occupational," or "physical," should be eschewed, because they are not in fact separate categories.

In what sense do natural and man-made disasters differ, but also resemble each other? Generally speaking, natural disasters, (e.g., earthquakes) often occur suddenly and terminate quickly but may be anticipated. They have a potent impact, causing damage to property and human beings. Their effects are usually acute; they quickly reach a climax, then dissipate. The participants in the disaster are bereft of any sense of control over the event. But its effects are not necessarily limited to those in its immediate vicinity.

Although man-made disasters may be acute, many (e.g., incarceration, or being a hostage) continue for days, weeks, and years. Their effects are also powerful, if largely psychological. They may be quite unpredictable and unanticipated. These events are experienced as the result of a loss of previously held control. Victims lose faith in social or political institutions and agencies (e.g., when the ground is polluted with "dumped" toxins, or when nuclear reactors or dams fail). The long-term effects of such disasters may be unpredictable and chronic. Uncertainty may persist (Baum, Fleming, and Davidson 1983; Baum 1987).

Personal and individual experiences are challenges or changes affecting fewer or only one person(s) (Lazarus and Cohen 1977). They may also have profound personal meanings and implications. Examples include the discovery of an unexpected and potentially fatal disease, the death of relatives, and forced unemployment. They may be self-induced (e.g., HIV-virus infection, alcoholism).

Admittedly, the suggested scheme appears to be based on a separation of environmental events from the organism experiencing it; a separation of this kind has been useful in other areas of biology. But it may also impede progress. Such a classification may be neat or logically satisfying. It may contradict the idea that stress is an interactive, complex process. It may give the impression that one is dealing with mutually exclusive categories, when one is not. In actuality, a classification that consists of mutually exclusive categories is artificial and trivial. As mentioned, many natural and man-made catastrophes lead to injury, loss, disability, death, or bereavement due to the deaths of relatives and friends.

A Classification of Stressful Experiences

1. *Natural occurrences and disasters*

Avalanches	Floods
Droughts	Hurricanes and tornadoes
Earthquakes	Snowstorms
Epidemics	Tidal waves
Fires	Volcanic eruptions

2. *Man-made disasters*
   Acts of terrorism
   Aircraft, ship, train, car, and bus accidents
   Battery
   Child abuse
   Collapse of buildings
   Dangerous sports and occupations
   Discrimination and prejudice
   Economic disaster
   Fires
   Genocide
   Incarceration in POW and concentration camps
   Industrial accidents and explosions
   Mining accidents

Muggings
New technologies
Rape
Torture
Toxic air and water pollution
War

3. *Personal and individual experiences*
Bereavement by death
Birth of children
Change in occupation, school, status
Disability
Disappointments
Disease and illness
Divorce and separation
Economic concerns and hardships
Examinations and other intellectual challenges
Family discord
Forced unemployment or uncertainty about employment
Housing conditions
Incarceration
Injury
Interpersonal discord outside of the family
Losses (including ideals, income, etc.)
Migration or translocation
Monotony
Paced work
Poverty
Pregnancy
Retirement
Social isolation
Shift work

In chapter 4 representative examples of these three main categories will be discussed in some detail, in order to document the assertions about the concept of stressful experience that have already been made.

Sources of Variability in Experienced Stress

Nature and Quality of the Signal Signifying Potential Danger, Challenge, Change, or Threat, and Their Expectation

Many of the categories of actual or potentially stressful experiences are expected or expectable. Human beings can prepare themselves for them realistically and appropriately. They can shore up their homes or move to higher ground as warnings of impending hurricanes, floods, or tidal waves are issued. Chronically ill relatives may be mourned in anticipation of their deaths. Athletes train themselves for demanding and dangerous sports; they have anticipatory physiological responses that carry energy-rich metabolites to muscle in advance of strenuous exercise. Hydrochloric acid and pepsin are secreted by the stomach in anticipation, and by the mere sight, of a meal; their secretion is suppressed during exercise and by fear.

These anticipatory responses, which go by many names (e.g., orienting, alerting, predictive), alert and prepare organisms for the danger or task ahead, focus attention on it, and antecede patterned behaviors (actions) designed to overcome or prevent it. The appropriate behavioral response to danger may either be to become immobile, to flee, or to fight it. In anticipation of certain dangers, protective shelters are reinforced or built.

The coordination between the signal of danger and the behavior can be exquisite: Many wild rodents become immobile when the shadow of the predator hawk falls near or upon them. The hawk's retina is responsive to its prey's movement, not its shape. Thus flight from the predator would be the inappropriate and fatal response. Tonic immobility has been selected out during evolution as the appropriate behavioral response in these species. This signal—the hawk's shadow—is a specific example of the entire potential array of danger signals to other animals emitted by a predator. In other species they may be acoustic, olfactory, or thermal, or consist of threatening gestures and postures displayed by the predator.

Certain categories of stressful experience are unexpected and sudden (e.g., accidental or sudden death of relatives, explosions, fires, accidents, rape, robbery, earthquakes): Unwarned is unarmed and unprotected. The experience of fear and the sense of shock seem more profound in human beings when they are unprepared. But we know little about the nature of the associated physiological changes when the organism is not forewarned: Do they differ in quality and quantity from those produced when preparatory actions and bodily modifications accompany anticipated threats and challenges, etc.?

The signal must be clear and carry specific information in order to be appraised accurately. Ambiguity—inadequate, inaccurate, or unclear information—prevents accurate appraisal of the experience so that no appropriate program of action can be selected or carried out. In fact, ambiguous signals are cited as being a major source of fear (Hamburg and Adams 1967). A person who finds herself/himself on an empty street in an unfamiliar neighborhood at night may conjure up unrealistic dangers that would never appear in familiar surroundings.

The signal is modified by the context in which it occurs. The impact of many stressful experiences is mitigated when they are shared with others. The economic impact of forced unemployment is usually more profound on the divorced, large families, and those with few resources or no savings (Pearlin and Lieberman 1979). Retirement and old age have greater effects on those lower on the economic ladder (Hinkle 1977; Kasl 1977). The danger and horrors of war are mitigated by good leadership and morale, and camaraderie. Even in peacetime, democratic leadership enhances performance and prevents a decline in health (Moos 1979).

Disease and injuries are exacerbated by climate: Mortality in the elderly and the poor from preexisting disease, automobile accidents, and drownings increase during the summer heat (Schumann 1972; Moos 1976). Respiratory distress is increased by seasonal pollens in asthmatic patients, and by irritants in the atmosphere in patients with obstructive pulmonary disease. Inadequate or crowded housing conditions promote distress, depression, and chronic dissatisfaction especially in the poor (Brown and Harris 1978; Kellett 1989).

However, the stability of the social environment and of its institutions seems to protect its inhabitants from stressful experiences and from disease such as hypertensive and ischemic heart disease (Bruhn et al. 1966; Henry and Cassel 1969; Wolf 1969).

The Nature of the Onset, Duration, and Variability of Stressful Experiences

Every category of stressful experience must be assessed in terms of its onset and duration (Cohen et al. 1982; Horowitz 1976; Horowitz et al. 1977). It may be:

1. Acute and time-limited (for example, an examination, a dangerous sporting event, or an acute disease without complications).

2. Acute in onset but with long-term intermittent or continuous antecedents or exacerbations. Many experiences may occur abruptly—a marriage that ends in divorce, the sudden death of a child, or the termination of employment. Although appearing to be sudden, an experience such as a divorce is often the culmination of mounting marital tensions and discord, or long-term suspicions about infidelity, alcoholism in one spouse, etc.; industrial plants shut after a period of rumors about their closing, or in the context of a general economic recession, etc.

Each sudden experience also has individual, social, economic, and familial consequences. A dead child may be mourned for eternity, or particularly on the anniversary of its death. Ex-hostages or veterans may have lifelong nightmares and daytime flashbacks.

3. Chronic and perennially stressful. Examples include chronic, painful disease or disability; poverty and hardship; crowding; caring for a defective, demented, or disabled family member; long-term incarceration or political repression; continuous discord with fellow workers or relatives; or having an alcoholic relative. Many of these may constitute stable, continuous (albeit fluctuating), or repetitive sources of stressful experience.

Some items in this category have been called "hassles" (Lazarus 1971;

Lazarus and Cohen 1977). They are typified by the kinds of routine, daily experiences to which the poor are exposed—lack of money, sanitation, and privacy; poor nutrition; minimal access to health care; and inadequate education (Syme and Berkman 1976). Many poor families are too large; unemployment is rife; several generations live together; work is often menial and meaningless; the streets are "mean" and dangerous (Harburg et al. 1973).

4. Intermittent and repetitive but chronically stressful. Into this category fall repetitive but intermittent discord and fighting among family members, intermittent alcoholism in a family member, intermittent illness, continuously shifting times of work, cycles of unemployment and employment, and repetitive job-related relocations.

Merely to describe the cyclic nature of such events fails to do full justice to their qualities. Work may be unvarying and repetitive and, therefore, monotonous and stressful (Frankenhaeuser and Gandell 1976). Monotonous occupations and work conditions are often imposed by others, or paced by machines. Prescribed, unvarying, time-pressured, and repetitive work of this kind, over which the worker has no control, exists more and more frequently in industrial societies. It is distressing (Siegrist 1984; Siegrist, Matschinger, and Siegrist 1988).

Experiences such as sensory isolation are also deemed stressful by some persons; they produce a decrease, rather than an increase, in stimulation from a relative steady-background state (Zuckerman, Levine, and Biase 1964). Apparently the change in either direction from baseline is experienced as being stressful.

Sources of Individual Variability in Response to,
and Modifiers of the Impact of, Stressful Experiences

One of the main theses of this book is that marked individual differences are seen in response to stressful experiences. This variability makes the outcome unpredictable. It explains the low correlations obtained between stressful experiences and disease onset. People vary in their capacity to appraise, and to respond to, challenge, tasks, danger, and sickness by virtue of many factors—genetic endowment, age, previous life experiences, intelligence, enterprise, courage, capacity for human relationships, economic resources, and the individual meanings that stressful experiences have for them. These individual differences are the topics of much current stress research. They have been studied under the following headings by physicians, behavioral scientists, and epidemiologists:

1. Appraisal of external signals and the correlated internal ones.
2. Genetic factors.
3. Coping—How and why does the manner in which stressful experiences are dealt with enhance or reduce their impact?

4. Social support—Does the help, love, encouragement, and advice that other human beings provide really reduce the impact of stressful experiences?
5. Meaning—What do stressful experiences mean to individuals?
6. Personality—What personal characteristics and resources determine who will overcome and who will succumb?
7. Age—Stressful experiences may have more of an impact at some ages (e.g., in childhood and in old age) than at others.

1. *Appraisal of signals.* It is not the signal of change, challenge, or danger itself but its appraisal as a "predictor and correlate" of the experience that in part determines the outcome. (By *appraisal* is meant an evaluation of the perceived signal and its meaning.) The appraisal of the signal should be accurate. It must be immediate when an acutely dangerous situation is clear and present. Under such conditions it cannot be euphemized or minimized. Many patients delay seeking medical advice and deny that they are sick until their disease is well past treatment. Yet denial of disease may also be valuable in regulating fear in situations that are fraught with the possibility of death. The physiological correlates of excessive fear may enhance cardiac morbidity (Hackett, Cassem, and Wishnie 1968). Conversely, other subjects appraise the signal excessively and inappropriately: Ominous or unrealistic meanings may be attached to it; small dangers are exaggerated or misinterpreted.

These brief remarks are intended to underlie the fact that the manner in which the signal is appraised cannot be divorced from the meaning it has for the appraiser (Lazarus and Cohen 1977). Appraisal of the signal determines whether or not actions are to be taken, and whether the appraiser is able to carry them out. The more realistic it is, the more appropriate the corrective actions are likely to be. Students faced with an examination study for it. If winter is at hand, some animals prepare to hibernate; people insulate their dwellings, store heating supplies, and don warm clothing.

The appraisal of the signal is usually associated with very specific internal communication signals essential to survival. The appropriate signal of danger is fear; pain signals bodily injury, thirst alerts the organism to the need for fluids, and hunger signifies the need for food. Rage accompanies the presence of threatening, dangerous, depriving, or interfering enemies or agents. It prepares the organism to fight a threat. It is also generated when the organism's ongoing activities (such as feeding) are interrupted or interfered with, or when it is deprived of territory, food, or mates. Specific signals are generated in association with having suffered a warmer or colder environment; being defeated; having failed or triumphed; and being separated from, or reunited with, another person.

The organism thus not only responds to external sources of information but also has a specific set of internal signaling systems informing it of its own state. Internal signals are important antecedents of action that is usually carried out if the time and context for doing so are right. They may, however, when excessive, be disruptive.

The literature is replete with the generalization that distressing experiences are more likely than pleasant ones to have unfavorable consequences (Elliott and Eisdorfer 1982). One frequently cited example is that fear eventuating in panic disorganizes and disrupts rational thought and appropriate action. Panics in burning buildings often end in unnecessary death. But there are other examples of inappropriate responses with dire outcomes: In situations of state terrorism and persecution, the victim's desire to survive takes precedence over his/her moral duties—prescribed by the social contract—to others. Many patients do not admit to, or delay seeking help for, a socially unacceptable disease and may continue to spread it. The anger engendered by injustice, prejudice, or jealousy may end in murder.

However, not every distressing experience necessarily has negative consequences. Grief and sadness are the normal response to separation, loss, and bereavement; usually they resolve during the process of mourning.

2. *Genetic factors.* Not enough information exists to confirm or refute the idea that human beings vary genetically in their responses to stressful experiences, such as danger (Shire 1974). However, biological theory would predict that such individual differences would obtain. It has, for example, been observed that fear and anxiety run in families. However, this aggregation in families neither confirms nor refutes genetic heritability of the responses to danger. Some parents who are excessively fearful may teach undue caution. Yet children can and should be taught that fire, knives, and crossing busy streets are dangerous. But they may learn, or disregard the lesson.

Evidence exists that animals can be bred to respond differently to stressful experience (Shire 1979): Strains of rats can be produced that are either stress-resistant or -sensitive. Other rats show increased or decreased behavioral responses (e.g., defecation) to standard tests of their "emotionality." (The validity of these tests is debatable.) Further evidence that animals vary genetically in their physiological responses to stressful experience (Barchas et al. 1974; Ciaranello 1979; Shire 1979) will be reviewed in chapter 7.

3. *Coping.* In response to changing external (environmental) and internal (e.g., thirst, hunger, the need for sleep) conditions, cognitive and behavioral efforts to manage appropriately the specific demand or challenge are carried out, following its appraisal or recognition. Generally speaking, these cognitive and behavioral processes are not automatic (such as swinging arms while walking or running) and are context-dependent (Lazarus and Folkman 1984). Failure to cope has consequences such as apathy, pessimism, and even depression (Lazarus and DeLongis 1983).

The responses and behaviors of the victims of natural disasters are examples of one kind of coping (chapter 4). At first, the realistic fear of danger signals that an emergency is at hand. Most people are initially protected from its full impact and implications by feeling "numb." They are then impelled to save themselves, their kin, and others. Once the emergency is past, they rebuild their destroyed homes and community, with or without the assistance of others. Furthermore, those who perform (or cope) well in acutely dangerous or personally meaningful situations (e.g., examinations) have different physiological responses than those who do not.

In the dire situation of a natural disaster, the tasks at hand to be performed—survival and rebuilding—are clear, and the operations to be performed are specific and defined. In contrast, victims of terrorism and persecution cannot predict that they will survive or escape injury; ambiguity is maximal. All control over their personal destiny is taken away from them. Passivity, capitulation, submission, identification with the persecutor, and massive denial may be the only available ways of coping and surviving: They are the better part of valor. To take steps to attempt to escape or to fight the captor is to court further punishment, pain, or death (chapter 4).

Embedded in these examples are the major components of what is meant by coping. In order fully to understand them, we need to define the nature of the experience, how it is appraised, the individual meanings it has for the person, and the strategies and behavioral programs employed to deal with it. The appraisal of the feasibility, and the meanings, of the task and the manner of tackling it are individual; each person has his/her own style of coping, which also varies with his/her age, experience, knowledge, skill, and sociocultural background.

The process of successful coping entails the appraisal of, and appropriate behavioral programs (actions) for dealing with, and solving, challenges, demands, tasks, and events (Lazarus 1966, 1971; Lazarus and Folkman 1984; Lipowski 1970). The task may realistically be deemed feasible or not. If it is, the person may or may not master it. Success or failure is accompanied by specific emotional signals—hope, pride, fear, shame, disappointment, despair, or helplessness—against which the person may protect himself or herself by "indirect" coping maneuvers, such as self-reassurance, denying that one is afraid, self-deception, resorting to prayer, or seeking the help of others (Lazarus and Folkman 1984).

Alternatively, a task may be appraised unrealistically, and inappropriate, excessive, unproductive, or dangerous actions may be brought into play (such as succumbing to mass panic). There may be no appropriate programs for false information or ambiguous or constantly changing situations. A person or animal confronted with a novel challenge or situation may have no precedent for solving or coping with it. Thus experience and training do count in coping. But some persons are unable to learn from experience, and therefore they never have acquired appropriate coping programs or skills. In many instances, when inappropriate actions are brought into play, damage to the self follows: Some persons cope by resorting to the drinking of alcohol and the abuse of drugs; some cope by displacing their frustrated rage, or their fear and despair, onto innocent bystanders.

The fact that most persons cope with the challenges or demands of their everyday lives, with or without the aid of others, is one reason why there is no relationship between stressful experiences and their outcomes. But the fact remains that we still have no detailed knowledge about how most people cope successfully with migration, unemployment, bereavement, marriage, divorce, illness, and disease. Our information about the stressful nature of these experiences derives mainly from observations made on those who have failed to cope with them, and the consequences that have then followed.

Each category of stressful experiences must also be studied qualitatively. To exemplify: Work means different things to different people; therefore, each person appraises unemployment in a different manner and copes with it in a specific fashion in order to reduce economic hardship, avert a decrease in self-esteem, and forestall depression. If supported by family members or friends, the unemployed person's self-confidence suffers less and he/she has a renewed sense of mastery over the situation (Pearlin and Lieberman 1979; Pearlin et al. 1981); however, coping and support act on separate aspects of the responses to unemployment (chapter 4).

4. *Social support.* A number of social scientists have studied the role of the support provided by other people in buffering the effects of stressful experiences and reducing their deleterious outcomes (Antonovsky 1979; Cassel 1976; Cobb 1976). Conversely, the adverse effect of social isolation—the absence of support—as an independent risk factor for dying has also been documented (House, Landis, and Umberson 1988). By social support is meant the love, reassurance, understanding, help, guidance, advice, and help available, or provided by other persons, to the one who is living through stressful experiences.

Personal relationships may also have additional significance: They act as important mutual regulators of the physiology and behavior of organisms (Hofer 1984). One striking example of this principle was provided by Mc-Clintock (1971). She demonstrated that young women living together in dormitories begin to coordinate the times of their menstrual cycles. Relationships impose other schedules: Spouses, and parents with their children, eat together. Partners go to bed and arise at the same time. Babies have feeding and training schedules. These activities are important *Zeitgebers* of biological "clocks" (Moore-Ede, Sulzman, and Fuller 1982).

The availability of social supports has been shown to lower the correlation between high scores on "life event" questionnaires and the complications of pregnancy (Nuckolls, Cassel, and Kaplan 1972), psychiatric symptoms (Brown and Harris 1978), and the dose of steroid needed to control the symptoms of asthma (de Arauyo et al. 1973). It has also been shown to decrease the number of swollen arthritic joints following the loss of a job (Cobb 1976).

Any resource (including an inanimate one, e.g., money) may be supportive if it is available and sought out (Horowitz and Wilner 1980). Social support has usually been studied quantitatively—by the frequency and number of social interactions, or by the degree of love, trust, advice, comfort, or help the stricken person can obtain from others. But the support does not have to be actual; comfort flows from the belief (or perception) that help or support is potentially available. When that belief cannot be sustained the mortality of elderly persons, for example, increases; it is about one and a half times greater than in those to whom actual or potential interactions or relationships are available (Blazer 1982).

However, social relationships are not necessarily salubrious: Expectations of help may be disappointed; relatives or supposed friends may be unsympathetic or derogatory to the stressed person, or place additional demands upon him or her. A frightened person may scare the very people who might have provided reassurance (Belle 1982, 1987; Wahler 1980).

In our society, men are expected to be more self-reliant and less plaintive than women. Their relationships to other people are also different; they participate more with acquaintances in activities such as sports, whereas women have closer ties with other women, especially within the family, and with women friends. Women seek out, receive, and accept support more graciously. But when men require support they most frequently seek it from their wives. When women require help they go to their friends or seek counsel. But they are also more likely to take care of needy or troubled friends and relatives than are men (Belle 1987; Fischer 1982).

The literature on supportive relationships has assumed their relative uniformity; but this assumption is not correct on the light of the foregoing. Admittedly, good relationships matter. Their absence is a risk factor for the adverse effects of stressful experience. But even when support is at hand, some persons cannot avail themselves of it. The capacity to trust, be intimate with, confide in, have an understanding for, be concerned about, or love another person is not a given. Self-pity, anger, hatred, hostility, cynicism, jealousy, envy, greed, criticism, insincerity, and competitiveness impair relationships both prior to and after stressful experience.

Conclusions drawn from research on social support are liable to a tautology: The death of a spouse is a significant experience for most people, but at the same time, it deprives the survivor of a source of support. In order to avoid confounding bereavement with the loss of support, it is necessary to assess the level of support available to the bereaved prior to or at the time of the death, and not after it has occurred. Only then can it be established that social support truly softens the impact of loss and bereavement (Thoits 1982).

Social support is said to modify the effect of stressful experiences in a variety of ways. Its quality (and not only its quantity), kind, and source need to be evaluated (Thoits 1982). Because this strategy has not been employed so far, the important idea that support buffers the unfortunate against challenge, danger, disease, bereavement, loss, and the winds of change has not yet been firmly established.

Should the buffering hypothesis be upheld, the idea that human relationships are critical for the maintenance of health would further be strengthened. They seem especially important for those who also rely on them for physical well-being—children, the infirm, the aged, the sick, psychiatric patients, and those whose behavior is inappropriate to their age (Mueller 1980).

5. *Meaning.* Physicians do not concern themselves with the healthy; they are predominantly interested in the sick. A large body of literature exists on the stressful nature of being ill. Disease, disability, and illness can have a variety of different meanings for individual patients. By virtue of these meanings being sick may or may not be distressing or disturbing. Sickness may act as a challenge to be met. It may be a source of comfort, like an old "friend": Suffering may be prized or relished. Some persons treat ill health and disease as an enemy to be fought and conquered. Conversely, relief from the everyday cares and problems of life can be obtained by being sick and cared for.

Some diseases (e.g., venereal diseases) are a source of shame or are interpreted by patients as a form of punishment. In young people, chronic disease destroys their hopes, expectations, and plans for the future. The disabled or sick may feel irreparably damaged or disfigured. A pervasive feeling of loss is present in patients in whom a prized function (e.g., memory, vision, or athletic prowess) is impaired or destroyed (Lazarus 1966).

The meaning of illness and disease may have important practical implications. The prognosis in those who need to suffer with a disease is poorer than in those who wish to rid themselves of it. Thus the individual meaning of illness and disease will determine not only its outcome, but also what coping efforts are made to overcome it and how help is obtained and utilized.

6. *Personality.* There is good evidence that some groups of persons are essentially untouched by stressful experiences while others succumb to it. Some people are unusually courageous. (When does courage become foolhardiness?) Some are cowards. Some are prone to fear. People who are purposive, whose lives are meaningful, who are committed to pursuing their goals, and who have a strong sense of controlling their destinies seem least likely to fall ill in the face of adversity and challenge (Kobasa 1979).

Adolescence is a period of life when young people test the limits of their physical and psychological resources to the point of being foolhardy—of courting danger, death, and injury. They drive and ski too fast; engage in strenuous activities; drink and eat too much; stay up at night; use and abuse alcohol, tobacco, and illicit drugs; or deny themselves basic needs—shelter, food, sexual intimacy, clothing, etc. Having tested themselves, they become aware of their personal limitations; a sense of realism in facing challenge or danger is established.

Stressful experiences must be appraised realistically. Personal traits such as optimism and pessimism influence appraisal. Optimists believe that the outcome will be benign and may do little practical to bring it about. Pessimists are certain that every experience will eventuate badly; they may respond by becoming gloomy, by not trying to influence adverse events, or by over-responding to them. Obsessional traits contribute to alternating interpretations of doubts and ruminations about what to do about stressful experiences. The hysterical person may exaggerate or dramatize them or may respond to their emotional impact and not to their actual meanings. The vain take personal umbrage that they would be subjected to them (Horowitz 1976). The suspicious perceive some ominous and hidden agenda behind each experience. Those prone to fear maximize danger.

Personal attributes also influence the prevalence of illness and disease in groups of people. In long-term studies of adults in a similar occupation and over the same period of their lives, Hinkle (1974) found marked differences in the number of illnesses and diseases experienced by the individual members of his cohort. Disease and illness were not independent events randomly distributed in a population. Not every one of his subjects was at equal risk; some were more likely to fall ill than others, from not only one but several illnesses or diseases afflicting several of their organ systems. Furthermore, their disabilities and their several illness and disease episodes occurred frequently in some, and infrequently in other, years. This clustering together of illness and disease coincided with increased demands upon them, disappointment in their work and lot in life, and discontent about their family and other personal relationships. In contrast, the subjects who remained well were people whose social backgrounds, personal aspirations, and interests matched the circumstances in which they found themselves. They fitted into their environments, enjoyed their work, and were fond of their families and associates. They were content. Hinkle's findings accord with those obtained by Brown and Harris (1978, 1986) in their later studies on women with depressed moods in a London community.

Vaillant (1977) carried out a thirty-year, prospective, longitudinal study of Harvard college graduates. He found that age-inappropriate, adaptive-defensive patterns of coping with the environment and of handling personal problems and distress enhanced the likelihood of a significant morbidity and mortality from a variety of diseases. The members of Vaillant's cohort had had the same educational opportunities. But they did not have similar backgrounds, occupations, and personal histories after graduation. His study suggests that variations in psychological maturity play an additional and significant role in determining who remains healthy and who does not over a period of three decades.

Many adult persons who fall ill share certain psychological characteristics. Ruesch (1948) had earlier stressed the age-inappropriate behavioral and psychological features of adult patients that made them particularly unadapted to, and unable to cope with, their (stressful) experiences. He listed their features as impaired or arrested social learning; a propensity for imitating rather than learning from others; a tendency to express thought and feeling in direct physical action; excessive reliance on others; passivity; childlike ways of thinking; lofty and unrealistic aspirations; difficulties in assimilating and integrating life experiences; and a need mainly to secure, and not to give, love and affection. Such people are incapable of mastering changes in their lives, learning new techniques for overcoming challenge, or adapting when they do not get their own way. Additional psychological features characterize them: Many patients do not have the words for, or are unaware of, their own emotions, which serve as signals alerting them to challenge, danger, or change. They do not or cannot recognize their own fears, etc., and therefore cannot take appropriate action. They do not resort to constructive imagination in coping with and solving problems. They are preoccupied with the concrete specifics, rather than the meaning and significance, of (stressful) experiences in their lives (Marty and de M'Uzan 1963; McDougall 1974; Nemiah and Sifneos 1970). They also seem oblivious to the quality and nuances of their interactions with other people.

The kind of person who falls ill is less likely to be mature and has fewer personal coping skills: For different reasons, children, the mentally defective or impaired, widowers, widows, the lonely, and the elderly do not have the education, information, knowledge, social support, or skills that are needed to cope with stressful experiences and to solve personal challenges and change.

The poorer, more immature, or more adaptively inept the person is, the less capable he/she is of coping alone or appropriately, and the stronger the influence of the social environment is on him/her (Bettelheim and Janowitz 1964; Lawton and Nahemow 1973). This is particularly true for the young, who do not usually survive without the protection, care, and feeding of parents or parental surrogates. Studies on the premature separation of animals (e.g., Hofer 1983, 1984) indicate that, at least until the time of weaning, the mother is largely responsible for regulating the behavior and physiology of her offspring. Premature separation has been cited as a risk factor for later illness and disease in both humans and animals (Brown and Harris 1978; Hofer 1981; Weiner 1977, 1982, 1987).

Conversely, reliance on the social environment (and other people who regulate or control one) places a person at risk for the adverse consequences of separation or bereavement. Reliance on one's own personal resources, a sense of being one's own master, and a conviction of being able to control one's own destiny seem to act as protectors against the adverse outcome of stressful experiences (Rotter 1966).

Therefore, stressful experiences are pervaded by the meaning they have. Their outcome depends on the manner of, and capacities for, coping with them, and other personal characteristics. Our understanding of the difference between those who do and do not fall ill is enhanced when the psychological differences between two individuals are specified. These differences also have a history. Psychological maturity and adaptive capacities are maturational and developmental concepts. They are also the product of genetic endowment, adequate nutrition, child-rearing practices, education, and learning, and an "average expectable environment" (Hartmann 1958). They are basic biological concepts that define a person's transactions with his/her ever-changing social, economic, political, human, and physical environment. Conversely, social stability is one factor that protects persons against illness and disease (Bruhn et al. 1966).

7. *Age.* The age of a person is an important variable in determining the impact of stressful experiences. Some are more likely to occur at one period during the life cycle than at another. Children have to learn the dangerous nature of certain situations. They may not have acquired coping skills requisite to mastering demands and challenges. They usually do not know where to obtain needed information; if they do, they may reject advice. Finally, they usually become decreasingly reliant on others as they mature and develop. Normal adolescence is pervaded by academic and social challenges. Upon these are engrafted dramatic and personally meaningful experiences—such as injuries and accidents, falling in and out of love, unemployment, and unwanted pregnancies.

Younger and less-skilled workers in industrial societies are more likely than older and better-trained ones to lose their jobs. Younger people less often fall ill than do the elderly. Younger people marry, and later divorce, more frequently than do older ones; the elderly are, in turn, more likely to lose a spouse to death.

Many elderly persons seem impervious to change but are vulnerable to hardship (Pearlin 1980). As long as they possess a modicum of good health and comfort, interests, some meaningful activity, dignity, and control over their remaining years, they may not become ill; in fact, an inverse relationship may exist between scores on the Schedule of Recent Events (SRE) (Holmes and Rahe 1967) and age (Goldberg and Comstock 1980; Lazarus and DeLongis 1983). However, many older persons experience fatigue, loneliness, unsympathetic relatives and other people, disappointments, and chronic infirmity, none of which is listed in the SRE. Lazarus and DeLongis (1983) have pointed out that either acute or chronic experiences are appraised and experienced differently at different ages. A disease such as cancer may be responded to with rage and hopelessness in the young, and with little fear but with resignation or even relief in older people.

The behavioral programs for coping with tasks and challenges are stored in memory. As memory fades with age, the programs can no longer be retrieved or are lost altogether. Elderly persons tend to restrict their lives and avoid situations with which they cannot cope and that might generate excessive fear (Goldstein 1939). They may pretend that they are more capable than they know themselves to be. They may become irascible when challenged. They may blame others for not being able to perform. In fact, the most frequent coping strategies of the elderly are blaming, avoidance, restriction, denial, minimization, reminiscing about past successes, and complaining about bodily ailments.

Additional factors must also be taken into account. The incidence of fear and anxiety is age- and time-related. It rises precipitously in the fifth decade of life, especially in women. Over a briefer time scale, anxiety and fear vary diurnally; they are more likely to occur in the evening than in the morning hours.

Little or incomplete longitudinal information exists about stressful experiences, their meanings, coping, and social support throughout the entire life cycle (Pearlin 1980); most of the information is based on cross-sectional studies. Furthermore, the same stressful experiences may lead to disease at one age and not another, because the physiological response systems (e.g., the immune system) have or have not developed, are different on first than on subsequent exposure, or become less specifically reactive with age.

The Outcome of Stressful Experiences

The next chapter will take up in some detail selected examples of the immediate and long-term, integrated response patterns and outcomes to the experience of naturally occurring and man-made disasters and personal adversities. These studies are usually biased toward studying their victims. It is as if stressful experience can only be meaningful if it is deleterious!

Those who grow through stressful experience are rarely the object of study. Yet many a person who has recovered from illness or faced adversity becomes more compassionate or understanding. Once experienced, some seek out further danger, adventure, and excitement (Zuckerman 1984). Experience and skill—the development of competence—reduce fear and the associated physiological changes during dangerous occupations. Trained parachute jumpers perform better; they only have anticipatory increases in selected measures of cardiovascular function, which during the actual jump return to resting levels. But novices continue to respond physiologically throughout the duration of the jump (Fenz and Epstein 1967; Fenz and Jones 1972).

Many "native" talents count in the development of competence: Intelligence, special aptitudes, curiosity, a diversity of interests, self-confidence, and trust in others are important personal assets during childhood and later in life (Erikson 1950; Rutter 1979). These traits seem to culminate in the confidence that challenge, change, and danger can be grasped, managed, and overcome (Antonovsky 1979).

Mastering danger, passing examinations, leaving home without feeling lonely and sad, or engaging successfully and without injury in (risky) sports enhances a person's sense of competence and self-assurance. Conversely, parents who overprotect their children from the inevitable vicissitudes of life deprive them of developing the skills needed to master them (Block 1971). Skills can be taught and learned; behavioral programs can become automatized; and personal relationships and friendships can be encouraged. Children can be reassured about their fears, prepared to leave home, encouraged to learn, and buffered against the pain of losing friends and of academic or other failure.

Many highly successful or famous persons have risen from poverty or escaped persecution, or they are the children of unskilled or immigrant parents. Older persons prepare themselves for, or welcome, retirement or face the inevitability of death. Thus many factors combine to determine whether stressful experiences eventuate in personal growth, produce temporary perturbations, or have permanent, deleterious effects (Antonovsky 1979; Hinkle et al. 1959; Benner, Roskies, and Lazarus 1980).

The factors that weigh most heavily in determining these three kinds of outcomes are (1) the nature and duration of the adverse experience; (2) the age of the subject; (3) the subject's intelligence, skills, experience, courage, personal relationships, and ability to plan; (4) the interpretation given to, and meaning of, the experience; (5) the chance to change or escape conditions that are experienced as stressful; (6) the opportunity to make a new life in new settings with the help and guidance of others.

Our ignorance about those who grow with experience and remain healthy with stressful experience is profound. It is further compounded by the lack of an adequate definition of health. Health is not only the absence of illness and disease. Mental and physical health are indivisible: The world of medicine should not artificially be divided into the mental and the physical. To which of these two separate categories are we to assign fatigue; changes in sleep patterns; transient disturbances in sexual desire, menstrual function, or appetite; or fleeting aches and pains? They are frequent manifestations of changes and challenges in people's lives and the distress they occasion. Some functions (sleep and menstruation) seem more readily disrupted by perturbations and stressful experiences: There are probably good biological reasons for this fact. Reproductive success can only occur under optimal environmental conditions (Crews and Moore 1986). Even mothers who breast-feed their infants are usually amenorrheic, presumably because PRL, which is responsible for milk "letdown," is stimulated by suckling and inhibits ovulation. Stressful experiences also release CRF, which, at least in the rat, inhibits the secretion of the gonadotropins (Rivier and Vale 1984; Rivier, Rivier, and Vale 1986).

Most studies emphasize the outcomes of major stressful experiences such as gross physiological or anatomical alterations and marked changes in psychological and behavioral function (chapter 6). The subtle and transient changes in behavior, thought, emotion, or physiology are rarely studied after everyday stressful experiences: Even minor accidents or other frightening experiences may produce sleep disturbance, induce intrusive, repetitive thoughts that cause one to relive the experience, activate dormant fears of injury or dying, or introduce caution, circumspection, and suspicion (Horowitz 1975, 1976; Horowitz, Wilner, and Alvarez 1979).

The linear relationship of stress to illness and disease was emphasized by Selye. Indeed injury, disability, and death are likely under the very dire circumstances of some natural and man-made catastrophes. But many survive, although they may be psychologically "scarred" for life. Thus no linear relationship exists between the most dire circumstances and death, injury, infection, or starvation.

Nonetheless, the probability of morbidity is enhanced when no response to stressful experiences is possible, when the subject is incapable of, prevented from, or punished for making one. This generalization seems to hold true both for humans and animals.

The best manner of conceptualizing the relationship of stressful experiences to illness and disease onset is to consider them as one of a series of risk factors (Orth-Gomer and Ahlbom 1980; Weiner 1977, 1984). Disease is multifactorial (Weiner 1977, 1978, 1982): A combination of risk factors enhances the likelihood of its occurrence (chapter 6). Various specific human lymphocyte antigens (HLAs) and gender enhance the probability for particular autoimmune diseases. Yet the same disease is associated with different HLAs in different ethnic groups (reviewed in Weiner 1990a). An inherited (X-linked) immune deficiency may be expressed in several diseases and at different ages. Each disease, such as duodenal ulcer, is also heterogenous (variability is present) (Rotter and Rimoin 1977); different combinations and proportions of risk factors seem to play a role in the inception of different subforms of a disease (Julius and Esler 1975; Thailer et al. 1985).

The risk factors of ischemic heart disease (IHD) are usually multiple, except, possibly in the genetic forms of hyperlipoproteinemia. Combinations of obesity, essential hypertension, diabetes mellitus or glucose intolerance, increases in low density lipoproteins (LDL), sleep apnea, certain occupations and personal traits, unemployment, and distress predispose or precipitate its various outcomes. No invariant combination of these risk factors will obtain in any one person with IHD. In addition, the natural history and etiology of IHD may differ in women and men. Stressful experience in and by itself does not determine the genesis of outcome of IHD (Weiner 1991a).

Being in possession of one or more risk factors does not necessarily eventuate in disease. Risk factors, including stressful experiences, act as predispositions to illness and disease; when enumerating them a statement is being made about the probability of their outcomes.

Summary

One of the aims of this particular area of stress research should be to describe comprehensively the etiology of disease, with an emphasis on the factors that limit the host's capacity to resist challenges and threats, which may be the product of genetic endowment, or a variety of experiences in the environment during maturation and development, or both. Many factors combine to enhance or impede persons' capacities, promoting health in some, placing others at risk for illness and disease on meeting threats, challenges, infection, or disaster (Weiner and Fawzy 1989). Among the most important of the many key factors influencing the response to stressful experience are the absence or presence, and the quality, of a human relationship to others (Berkman and Syme 1979; House, Landis, and Umberson 1988; Weiner 1987).

Some profound socioeconomic changes may be followed by a change in conduct: The abuse of alcohol and tobacco, for example, increases sharply in men who are forcibly unemployed (Farrow 1984), placing them at risk for a number of serious diseases. Certain sexual practices or intravenous drug abuse frequently antecedes infection with the HIV retrovirus with its inevitable descent into AIDS and death. The smoking and chewing of tobacco products is a hazard contributing to atherosclerosis, pulmonary emphysema and carcinoma, and cancer of the mouth and larynx. Pregnant women who smoke tobacco often deliver babies of low birth weight, as do those who use drugs and alcohol, whose babies may also be addicted to drugs or suffer from the fetal alcohol syndrome, respectively. While alcohol abuse may be one way of dealing with stressful experiences, it can eventuate in disease in virtually every organ of the body. It is also strongly associated with trauma, disability, or death due to automobile accidents and with physical assault on, and sexual abuse of, other persons.

Research on stressful experience must answer the question: Why do persons fall ill at a particular time in their lives, and with one disease and not another? The answers to such questions can only be found by determining the stressful context in which illness and disease begin and by inquiring into the array of predispositions to a particular disease (chapters 5 and 6). When situations of danger, challenge, or change cannot be controlled, illness and disease may ensue. Being able to control a situation means that a person is able to mount the appropriate response to prevent, escape from, or overcome challenge or threat. In part, this ability is a function of knowing how to go about doing so, and in part, it is a function of regulating the cognitive-emotional signals generated by the experience. Many of the stressful experiences that have been correlated with illness and disease onset are dramatic and sudden. Yet a chronic background of distress, irritation, and frustration also conduces to demoralization, a chronically depressed mood, and a variety of diseases (Brown and Harris 1978; Hinkle 1974).

Potentially stressful experiences, although their quantity, quality, and temporal characteristics may vary, are constant. Change is inevitable in the lives of human beings: We grow up, leave home, marry and have children, assume responsibilities, age, become ill, and die. Some experiences are by their very nature uncontrollable by most individuals; we are always at the mercy of climatic, political, social, administrative, and technological changes and upheavals.

Coping with change, challenge, and threat mediates the impact of such stressful experiences. Social cohesion, a close personal relationship, and a slow rate of sociocultural change buffer the effects of risk factors such as a high-fat diet and obesity in the development of IHD, sudden cardiac death, or myocardial infarction (Bruhn et al. 1966; Marmot and Syme 1976).

Missing in the foregoing account is a precise knowledge of how loss of control over, and failure to cope with, a situation are associated with physiological changes that set off events to incite disease in the predisposed person. This subject is very complex. In the past the description of single variables formed the basis of pathogenetic explanations; but they are inadequate. Loss of control in both animals and humans is associated with increases in corticosteroid secretion and levels (Henry and Stephens 1977). But that does not mean that their acute secretion is pathogenic (chapter 8). Failure and defeat lower testosterone (T) levels. The thrill of danger may raise E and NE levels (Ursin, Baade, and Levine 1978). Yet our knowledge about the integrated biology of such a profoundly significant personal experience as bereavement is minimal (Jacobs 1987)—a situation that is especially regrettable in the light of the fact that it may be a codeterminant of the onset of many diseases and altered behaviors (Weiner 1987) when it does not culminate in grief and mourning.

Stress research has added to our understanding about the exacerbations and remissions of disease, which in medicine are usually called "spontaneous." It has also thrown light on prognostic factors in disease. The observations about the correlations of stressful exacerbations to symptom fluctuations not only take the mystery out of such events, but raise the level of the relationship of anatomical lesions to symptoms to a new level of complexity. To illustrate, it is acknowledged that following the initial onset of ulcerative colitis the colonic mucosa remains histologically abnormal forever after in two out of three patients, but the symptoms of the disease may wax and wane (Dick, Holt, and Dalton 1966). Symptom exacerbations in this disease may even occur when the doctor-patient relationship is only briefly disrupted. Remission from symptoms takes place when the patient becomes active and effective rather than remaining hopeless and helpless (Engel 1956). The prognosis after myocardial infarction is determined in part by the marital status of the patient. Single, divorced, or socially isolated persons have an abbreviated life span (House, Landis, and Umberson 1988).

Disease is not sui generis. It cannot be isolated from the person who hosts it: The personal characteristics of patients with rheumatoid arthritis in part determine the prognosis and response to treatment of that disease (McFarlane, Kalucy, and Brooks 1987).

Additionally, patients respond to their diseases both in general ways (e.g., fear) and in idiosyncratic ways that depend on their belief systems and their imaginations. These responses in part determine compliance to treatment; they may shorten or prolong hospital stays, determine reactions to operations, and involve the patients' families (and even lawyers).

These illustrations are the basis of the contention that persons have diseases and that there are not diseases per se (Krehl 1932). Diseases are mere abstractions; they cannot be understood without appreciating the person who is ill.

4 The Outcomes of Natural and Man-made Disasters and of Stressful Personal Experiences

Natural Occurrences and Disasters

The physical environment may suddenly, unexpectedly, and violently erupt to confront its inhabitants with danger and the possibility of destruction, injury, and death. Some of these dangers may occur serially—torrential floods accompany hurricanes, and tidal waves and fires may follow earthquakes.

Fear, panic, terror or horror, and a sense of helplessness are occasioned by these experiences. At times, their potential victims are forewarned of oncoming hurricanes, forest fires, onrushing flood waters and mud slides, or slowly developing droughts. At other times, the dangers are not anticipated. Although the threat may be apprehended, escape from it may or may not be possible. The danger may be sudden and short-lived; or it may mount and be prolonged.

Frederick (1980, 1981, 1987) has described a series of unfolding phases that characterizes the behavior of most but not all individuals and groups who live through such experiences:

1. *The immediate phase of impact.* Persons experience a mixture of "numbing" fear passing over into paralyzing panic and terror. They cannot believe what is happening around and to them. They may be horrified about the disappearance of acquaintances and landmarks and the amount of injury, death, and destruction that surrounds them. A sense of unreality overcomes them. They may be rendered utterly helpless and unable to avert danger, or they may try to flee it. They may attempt to rescue themselves, the lives of others, or their property.

2. *The phase of heroism.* Many make intense efforts to protect or save whom and what they can. Frequently, heroic deeds—feats of great strength or altruism—are performed to ensure survival and, later, to prepare for recovery from the disaster. Many of those engaged in rescue work feel proud of their worthy deeds. They work intensely. They may forego sleep and food. Feelings of exhaustion, irritability, and disappointment eventually begin to overcome them, especially if all their efforts are in vain. During and immediately

after a disaster the social order may break down, and rioting and looting may occur.

3. *The honeymoon phase.* One to several months after the disaster, reminiscences are exchanged among participants in the disaster. The support of rescue missions and charitable, insurance, and governmental agencies is enlisted. Help is promised, and a favorable outcome is anticipated. Hope is engendered for the rebuilding of shattered lives. Future difficulties are minimized or denied.

4. *The phase of disillusionment.* Following the "honeymoon phase," and lasting several months or more, disillusionment sets in as public or private assistance is either inadequate or not forthcoming. The disappointment, bitterness, and anger at broken promises may be intense.

The spirit of sharing danger and working together in a collegial manner is dissipated. Many survivors become depressed. Communal bonds are broken (Erikson 1976; Tyhurst 1957). Those who were more fortunate are the targets of envy and hostility directed at them by those who suffered most.

5. *The phase of reorganization.* As the victims of a disaster begin to realize that recovery is in their own hands, individuals and the community begin to cooperate to rebuild their lives, separately and together. But in those persons in whom animosity, envy, and bitterness continue, and who refuse to participate in cooperative efforts, the incidence and prevalence of chronic posttraumatic stress syndromes increase.

Recent observations and relatively long-term follow-up of victims of natural disasters have further specified and modified these generalizations. Following the volcanic eruption of Mount St. Helens, two groups of survivors were contrasted over a three-year period. The comparison showed that those who lived closest to the volcano, had lost a family member, and had suffered property damage had a higher incidence and prevalence of chronic anxiety, episodes of depression, and a posttraumatic stress disorder than did those who were further removed from the disaster and had lost neither a relative nor property. In the first group, women, but not men, with a history of anxiety or depression prior to the eruption (47%) had a greater (73%) incidence of these complaints than did those (53%) without such a history. This study indicates a crude "dose-response" relationship between the proximity of the victims to the disaster, combined with the presence or absence of loss occasioned by it, and psychological sequelae, especially in those prone to recurrent anxiety and depression (Shore, Tatum, and Vollmer 1986).

Man-made Disasters and Catastrophes

The purpose of listing natural and man-made disasters separately is that their immediate and long-term psychological and behavioral effects on populations and individuals differ somewhat. Each category has its own trajectory over time. But their consequences are also similar: Both carry with them the potential for injury, mutilation, starvation, or death, and lifelong sequelae—especially with man-made disasters—if their victims should survive.

Hostages or the victims of terrorist attacks also become terrified, "numb," and paralyzed. They respond with disbelief and a sense of unreality. Their attention span shortens. Their powers of concentration and their short-term memory are impaired. They are distracted. Their speech drifts off the topic. They cannot sleep. Specific fears of injury, mutilation, torture, and dying mount. Somewhat later they begin to try to interact with their captors. Such attempts may occasion conflicting feelings about being victimized and wanting to propitiate, mollify, or negotiate with them. (Many terrorists blindfold their victims in order to prevent any such exchange.) This second phase is followed by one of acceptance of the situation. Expediency may necessitate that the victim betray his/her friends and jettison his/her own political, moral, religious, or personal opinions and beliefs. He/she may begin to sympathize with the perpetrator's belief and attitudes. The victim may yield to, and imitate, the perpetrator—behavior that is motivated by the desire to survive and to avoid pain and injury. The captor then becomes the victim's protector. A phase of acquiescence finally takes over: Surrender, including sexual submission, may occur in the hope of survival and avoidance of injury. The outcome of such submission may be increasingly ambiguous. Guilt and a sense of personal worthlessness increase, mixed with feelings of impotence, rage, and humiliation, which may far outlast the experience (Frederick 1980, 1981).

Differences between the responses of those subjected to the will of terrorists and prisoners of war (POWs) occur. Identification with and servile submission to the perpetrator do not usually occur in POWs, despite attempts to brainwash them. On the other hand, POWs and concentration camp victims who give up die rapidly.

The immediate consequences of incarceration in concentration camps during the Nazi era consisted of a particularly profound form of the syndrome seen in the other man-made disasters. It is characterized by terror, grading into apathy, mourning, docility, profound denial of the horror, a loss of the capacity to feel ("numbing"), and increasing concern about the self. But some victims acted with heroism (Chodoff 1975), and others were co-opted by the camp guards.

The long-term effects of the Holocaust on its survivors are permanent. The children and grandchildren of its survivors are also affected. The victims continue to manifest an abiding posttraumatic stress syndrome of a special kind. For them, life is meaningless or empty, never again to be enjoyed. Fatigue is permanent. Despair, feelings of inadequacy, hopelessness, guilt of an especially malignant sort, eternal sorrow, bitterness, and feelings of depression recurrently sweep over them. They are mistrustful, cynical, and touchy. They sleep only with interruptions. Their work suffers. They change occupations, often more than once. Their marriages falter. They age and die prematurely.

Symptoms appeared in some survivors with a latency period of several months or years after they were liberated in 1944 or 1945. Cognitive disturbances including concrete thinking and short-term memory disturbances were observed. In 28% of the survivors the electroencephalogram (EEG) was abnormal. Twenty years later they were continually symptomatic; 70% suffered back pain; unpleasant experiences or large meals produced diarrhea in 33%; coronary and cerebral atherosclerosis were diagnosed in 30%; asthma, chronic bronchitis, tuberculosis, and chronic obstructive pulmonary disease were present in another 30% (Eitinger 1971; Thygesen, Hermann, and Willanger 1970; Strom 1968).

One and a half-million children died in concentration camps. Those who survived were irreparably damaged as human beings. Their personal (psychosocial) development was permanently arrested. They were hypersensitive, restless, angry, volatile in their emotional behavior, bitter, cynical, and pessimistic. New experiences caused anxiety. They clung to their peers while mistrusting all adults (Chodoff 1975).

Further differences in the response of the victims of natural and those of man-made disasters and violence are apparent. The victims of natural disasters usually feel no guilt about their failure to prevent the event. Some may feel "survivor" (nonmoral) guilt about having been more fortunate or not helping others enough during the disaster. But they do not feel humiliated or violated and are not necessarily permanently impaired.

Victims of human violence, especially abuse or rape, often blame themselves for not having avoided it. They also feel dehumanized, used, and weak. They are enraged at their violators. If the outcome is more fortunate for them than for other similar victims, their guilt may be intense. The long-term consequences (unless therapeutic intervention helps) are variable: depressive moods; feelings of depersonalization; memory impairment; mistrust of others leading to few or no social contacts; fears of death, assault, or rape; feelings of being in danger; marital discord; fears of, or little or no interest in, sexual intimacy; sleep disturbances; substance abuse. The experience of being held hostage or raped recurs over and over again in dreams and the waking state; it may be a permanent feature of their lives (Notman and Nadelson 1976; Rose 1986).

The Long-Term Behavioral Consequences of Natural and Man-made disasters

The immediate responses (fear, terror, disbelief, etc.) to natural disasters, to being taken hostage, or to being a victim of a terrorist attack are similar. But the subsequent behaviors of people exposed to these two groups of ultimately stressful experiences differ. Additionally, individual variations in responses occur to them—a prediction that would not have been made from earlier stress theory. One would have assumed that every major and severe catastrophe, without regard to its source, would spare none of its victims. The fact is that as much as 10 to 25% of a population seems untouched by disasters (Frederick 1987; Tyhurst 1957), including earthquakes of major proportions (Popovic and Petrovic 1964); they continue to function thereafter without any discernible impairment. Another 25% of adults will immediately succumb to the acute form of the posttraumatic stress disorder (see below), and the rest of the population to fears of objects, panic disorders, major depressions, suspicion of the motives of other people, bodily symptoms, amnesias or fugues, and substance abuse. The posttraumatic stress disorders may become chronic, especially after man-made disasters. Such individual differences are not only a function of the type and severity of the catastrophe, but also of the kind of person experiencing it. The chronic syndrome persists in about 25% of populations for more than one year.

Not all potential or actual disasters are the same: An impending one, such as the Three Mile Island nuclear power plant accident, demonstrates how an ambiguous, intangible, potentially lethal situation may affect a population (Baum 1987; Erikson 1976). For at least one year after the incident, anxiety, worry, and depression overcame the employees of the plant, mothers of young children, and patients attending mental health clinics (Kasl, Chisholm, and Eskenazi 1981; Bromet 1980).

Subjects of different ages at the time of a natural disaster vary considerably. Children manifest a series of disturbances of food intake, sleep, and learned toilet habits. They become disobedient. Their movements, speech, vision, and hearing are altered; for example, they may begin to stutter. They become more childish. They cling to their parents Earlier fears (e.g., of the dark) are reinstituted. They have bodily complaints. They develop tics. They are easily distracted. Their school performance deteriorates. And they avoid their peers.

Somewhat different reactions were discernible in a group of 40 normal schoolchildren who were kidnapped and terrorized for 36 hours but suffered no physical harm. Ten immediately manifested the childhood form of the posttraumatic syndrome. Five months later, 14 still reenacted the kidnapping; 19 were fearful of other people, less spontaneous, and "changed" as persons, and 8 performed less well at school (Terr 1979).

After natural disasters, adolescents manifest retrogressive behaviors in their speech, social relationships, and school performance. They become lethargic. Their sexual desire is dampened. Their powers of concentration decline. Their self-confidence lessens. They develop gastrointestinal symptoms. They demand more attention at home. They avoid both friends and strangers. They express feelings of helplessness. They become obstreperous when made to do what they fear. They may begin to drink or abuse alcohol.

Adults mainly show an increase in the incidence of a variety of diseases, and also disturbances of food intake and sleep. They withdraw, lose interest in their surroundings, become easily angered and more suspicious of others.

Elderly persons, following natural disasters, show many of the same behaviors as adults do, but in addition their mental and physical infirmities and complaints are exacerbated. They appear more easily confused about events around them. Many become more lethargic or depressed.

The Posttraumatic Syndromes

The two forms of posttraumatic disorders differ only in their time course. In the acute form, the onset does not always follow the catastrophe immediately, but it begins within six months and lasts not more than six months. The onset of the chronic form is delayed for at least six months, and it continues for a minimum of six months.

Any of the natural or man-made disasters may precipitate the two forms of the disorder. They occur in rape victims, prisoners of war, survivors of robberies and muggings, victims of torture and concentration camps, after military combat, and in some victims of automobile accidents (Frederick 1987; Kuch, Swinson, and Kirby 1985). The incidence of these two syndromes may be greater if malnutrition or bodily (especially head) injury occurs during the experience.

The central feature of the posttraumatic state is a flashback to the traumatic experience that occurs during waking and/or sleeping hours (Horowitz 1976). Any current experience even faintly reminiscent of the original may invoke its memory and the attendant fear, horror, or terror. The victims of the syndrome are constantly on the alert and on guard. They sleep poorly. They are distracted. They show memory disturbances to the point of developing amnesic and dissociative states. They complain of being estranged from other people. The world and its inhabitants appear hostile, uninteresting, remote, or changed to them. They avoid being reminded of war, natural disasters, rape, and accidents. Their capacities for intimacy, tenderness, and passion are lost. Irritation and anger are poorly controlled.

The intensity of the syndrome varies, being distributed evenly in groups of victims (Frederick 1987). The reexperiencing of traumatic wartime events may be vivid and intense. If the veteran has killed civilians or enemy soldiers, guilt and self-loathing may be extreme. Violence, long after the original episode, may be unpredictable and explosive and is especially likely to occur when the veteran is misunderstood or ostracized by friends and relatives. The feelings of isolation often reenact the loss of, or ostracism by, friends that took place during wartime (Rosenheck 1985).

The manifestations of the posttraumatic syndrome may be combined with guilt over survival, chronic anxiety, depression, suspiciousness, diminished appetite, and bowel disturbances (Tennant, Goulston, and Dent 1986). The victims of these syndromes are at increased risk for later substance abuse (Mellman and David 1985), automobile accidents (by 50%), and suicide (by 65%) (Hearst, Newman, and Hulley 1986).

The probability of posttraumatic stress syndromes becoming chronic was shown to be increased in veterans who had lost a parent before they were 15 years of age, whose fathers drank alcohol, who came from a lower socioeconomic background, who were inducted into service when they were very young, or who, during or after military service, were separated or divorced from their spouses or widowed (Streimer, Cosstick, and Tennant 1985; Tennant, Goulston, and Dent 1986).

Persistent physiological changes accompany the chronic posttraumatic stress disorder. A sample of survivors of the Vietnam War manifested evidence of excessive sympathetic nervous system activity and reactivity (e.g., electrodermal responses) (Blanchard et al. 1982; Brende 1982). The main sources of NE in the body are the neurons of the sympathetic nervous system. Patients suffering from the posttraumatic stress disorder have persistent increases of urinary levels of this catecholamine and also of E, exceeding values obtained from patients suffering from one or other of the major psychoses (Kosten et al. 1987; Mason et al. 1988). However, 24-hour urinary free-cortisol levels (a measure of cortisol production) are lower in patients with the posttraumatic stress disorder than in patients with other categories of major psychiatric disorders (Mason et al. 1986).

With what do these physiological changes correlate? The best hypothesis is that they are associated with persistent vigilance (Frankenhaeuser and Rissler 1970). They differ from those found in the depressive disorders, in which vigilance is not a factor, but in which cortisol production and NE (or its metabolites') levels can be elevated. Until proven otherwise, this explanation of the different features in these two groups seems to be the most attractive one. It is certainly so that patients with chronic posttraumatic stress disorders are constantly alert to any experience that is faintly reminiscent of the original one.

In the literature on the consequences of military combat, the argument is put forward that head trauma, weight loss, and malnutrition are the main causes of the cognitive disturbances seen in veterans. However, some data do not support this conclusion. Askevold (1983) studied the sequelae of World War II by following a series of Norwegian merchant mariners for twenty years. During World War II, they had manned cargo ships that were repeatedly assaulted by German war planes and submarines. Some ships were sunk, and some of the sailors were immersed in the icy waters of the North Atlantic. Some were also injured, but many were not. Within twenty years after the war they became disabled with serious cognitive disturbances reminiscent of presenile dementia, despite the fact that most had not suffered head injuries. Although presenile dementia of the Alzheimer type may occur following head injury, it is also possible that the chronic exposure to danger and uncertainty may produce similar or the same neuropathological changes. In fact, chronic elevations of serum cortisol levels may alone result in damage to hippocampal neurons and also potentiate the effects of head injury (Sapolsky, Krey, and McEwen 1986).

Cognitive disturbances occurred in 87% of 227 Norwegian survivors of Nazi concentration camps, 57% of whom had suffered severe injury (including head injury), to which Eitinger (1965) ascribed these cognitive disturbances; later (1971) he changed his opinion, believing that the appalling personal experiences of the camp survivors were mainly responsible for them or interacted with injury.

Because the victims of the Nazis' unspeakable brutality were also subjected to various combinations of torture, starvation, crowding, cold, frostbite, sleep deprivation, long hours of work, exhaustion, horror, unpredictability, the loss of relatives and friends, and diseases (e.g., typhus, intractable diarrhea, pneumonia, encephalitis, and tuberculosis), it is impossible to decide what were the proximate antecedents of their cognitive disturbances.

Injury, Death, and Disease

Natural and man-made disasters exact a fearful toll on humankind. Automobile accidents and violence are the leading causes of death in American adolescents—especially in black Americans. Fifty million human beings lost their lives in World War II, and at least one million died in the Vietnam War.

Soldiers in wartime throughout history have been exposed, and some have succumbed, to viral, bacterial, parasitic, and fungal diseases. Tuberculosis and typhus devastated the Nazi concentration and prisoner of war camps. Malnutrition predisposes to the threat of infection. Disfigurement, blindness, burns, fractures, and other injuries result from war or are imposed on political and wartime prisoners by torture. The long-term effects of being a POW result in part from a combination of imprisonment, malnutrition, and mistreatment. The morbidity over a fifteen- to twenty-year period of follow-up was higher in American POWs of the Japanese in World War II and of the North Koreans and Chinese in the Korean War than in those captured by the Germans and their allies in World War II. In the latter the sequelae were mainly behavioral (difficulty in readjustment, and the use of alcohol) and psychological (anxiety, depression, and bodily complaints). In the two former, malnutrition, torture, and incarceration combined to produce long-range effects on both physical and mental health, requiring more hospitalization than in those veterans of both wars who were not captured (Beebe 1975).

Eitinger (1965) reported that cardiovascular (and other) diseases were more prevalent in former Norwegian concentration camp survivors than in those not confined. Other dangerous situations or experiences are associated with elevated BP levels. Following the explosion of a munitions ship in Texas City, a predominance of the population examined had elevated BP levels, which were maintained for a period of about two months and then subsided (Ruskin, Beard, and Schaffer 1948). Sustained military combat in the North African desert and at Stalingrad was associated with a disproportionate prevalence of high BP (Gelshteyn 1943; Ehrstrom 1945; Graham 1945). Many factors must have played a role in this phenomenon—danger, malnutrition, dehydration, cold (in Russia), heat (in North Africa), exertion, etc.

But the matter is even more complex. Although piloting a naval combat airplane is extremely dangerous, studies of U.S. naval aviators over a twenty-five year period show that their BP levels do not increase with age—a most unusual circumstance in any population. Henry and Cassel (1969) ascribe this phenomenon to the fact that the subculture in which the pilots live is highly structured and stable with established rules and traditions, despite the danger of their occupation. Conversely, black Americans who are exposed to violence and police brutality, who live in crowded conditions in areas of a city marked by social disorganization and economic deprivation, and whose personal and marital lives are disrupted have higher BP levels than their peers living in the middle-class neighborhoods in which these social conditions do not prevail (Harburg et al. 1973). Thus wartime experiences, civilian disasters, prejudice, and strife may contribute to the development of high BP.

English civilians exposed to German aerial bombing attacks suffered an increase in perforations of peptic ulcer (Stewart and Winser 1942). Fear and anxiety may precipitate asthmatic attacks, the hyperventilation syndrome, and the irritable bowel syndrome (Alpers 1983). Danger and fear may be associated with the onset of Graves disease, especially in its acute form. Many such patients are likely to respond to danger because they have long-standing fears of dying. In the largest series of such patients ever published, 13% of 3,343 patients with Graves disease had been involved in accidents, had been otherwise injured, or had found themselves in a situation of imminent danger. An additional 7% developed the disease following surgery (Bram 1927).

Thyrotoxicosis—a generic name for a hypermetabolic state, of which Graves disease is but one example—often increases in incidence during wartime, as long as nutrition is adequate. Major increases in its incidence and prevalence occurred in Denmark and Norway during the German occupation in World War II (Iversen 1948). In countries not invaded, and in those in which the German invaders starved the population, no such increases were observed.

The Behavioral Biology of Dangerous Occupations and of Challenges in Nature and the Laboratory

Driving a Racing Car

Automobile racing is generally acknowledged to be one of the most dangerous sports ever invented. It entails minimal physical effort, but it may expose drivers to a high ambient temperature and, during prolonged races, deprive them of sleep. Taggart and Carruthers (1971) studied 16 drivers just before, during, and immediately following a 3-hour race. Total catecholamine levels were already raised at the time the contest began, and during the period immediately after it. Most of the increase (86%) was due to elevations of NE levels. Blood levels of FFA rose 125% before the race, peaked at its start, remained high after the race, and returned to resting levels one hour later. Triglyceride levels began to increase when the starter dropped his flag and continued to rise after the race was over. One hour later they were 111% above baseline levels. Cholesterol levels remained unchanged throughout the race. A strong positive correlation ($r = 0.81$) was present between total catecholamine levels below 2 μg/l and FFA levels. When the catecholamine levels were greater than 2 μg/l, the correlation was a mere $r = 0.31$. This study documents that FFAs, which are readily measured in serum, are exquisitely sensitive in anticipation of, and during, a variety of contingencies including dangerous and anxiety-provoking ones (Dimsdale and Herd 1982).

Parachute Jumping

CARDIORESPIRATORY CHANGES. Parachuting from an airplane is a reliable way of inducing fear even in experienced jumpers. Fenz and Epstein (1967) compared 10 novice and 10 experienced jumpers while rating fear and measuring heart rate, (HR) respiratory rate (RR), and skin conductance before, during, and after a descent from 5,000 feet. Most of the novices were frightened to the point of being disorganized in thought and behavior. They found the first jump terrifying, while a minority found it thrilling.

In both experienced and novice jumpers, anticipatory fear manifested itself in the bus on the way to the airfield. But in the experienced jumpers, the fear abated at the point of maximum danger—when jumping out of the aircraft. During the actual fall, they were relatively relaxed. The novices, on the other hand, continued to experience mounting fear until they had landed on the ground. The RR was the first to increase; then the HR rose; and finally skin conductance fell in both groups. In experienced jumpers, the physiological changes peaked and then fell after the men entered the aircraft, but in the inexperienced ones, they continued to increase during the jump and until landing. Precise correlations between fear self-ratings and physiological changes were obtained in the novices. In the experienced jumpers, a dissociation between fear and physiological changes took place while preparing for and engaging in the jump.

Even experienced jumpers do not perform equally well when rated independently by two jumpmasters. Those who performed poorly had the greatest physiological changes. Their RRs rose sharply until the engines of the aircraft were warming up; the RRs then plateaued, but their HRs continued to increase until the jump was completed. By contrast, in the good performers, the RRs first increased, then fell, and the HRs leveled off. The experienced men who performed poorly showed physiological patterns reminiscent of novice jump-ers'. Therefore, the individual manner in which each person responds to a frightening situation depends on both experience and performance (Fenz and Jones 1972).

HORMONAL RESPONSES. Fourteen young soldiers had blood drawn for PRL, thyrotropin (TSH), and human growth hormone (hGH) before and after their first military parachute jump. Baseline values for all three hor-mones were measured at 6 A.M. 13 and 3 days before the jump. On the day of the jump samples were obtained at 6 A.M. and 1 P.M. The jump was made at about noon from an altitude of 366 meters. A final blood sample was obtained on landing. There were significant increases in the mean levels of all three hormones (PRL: 10.4 ng/ml to 19.3 ± 3.1 ng/ml [Range: 6.5 to 40 ng/ml]; TSH: 2.9 ± 0.6 μU/ml to 4.1 ± 0.6 μU/ml [Range: 1.8 to 9 mU/ml]; hGH; 4.2 ± 1.2 ng/ml to 13.6 ± 3.5 ng/ml [Range: 1 to 42 ng/ml]). The effects of cold, exertion, and altitude on the changes in hormone levels were discounted. This study did not attempt to examine the effects of repeated exposure to jumping nor to account for the individual differences in hormonal responses in the 14 recruits (Noel et al. 1976). Ursin, Baade, and Levine (1978) carried out such a study on 44 young, novice soldiers undergoing parachute training. The patterns of fear displayed were similar to those seen in Fenz's and his col-leagues' studies (Fenz and Epstein 1967; Fenz and Jones 1972).

Thirteen of the 44 soldiers quit training after the first jump, during which they had experienced great fear, very high blood levels of E and NE, and ele-vated blood glucose, FFAs, and T levels. The remaining 31 soldiers per-formed variably. The good performers were relatively unafraid. They were impatient to try the jump, which they found thrilling. They had the highest FFAs and moderate E and NE increases during the jump. As they became more adept, the acute increases in these measures became less with each suc-cessive jump. Throughout the series their plasma cortisol levels were low. Those who performed poorly throughout but who did not quit and claimed to be unafraid had the largest increments in plasma cortisol and hGH levels. Only minor increases in E, NE, and PRL levels occurred. Elevations of PRL and a fall in T levels characterized those soldiers who ultimately failed the training course. In conclusion, the novelty of a dangerous exercise, the man-ner in which the person reacts psychologically to it, and his/her performance during it are closely related to the specific nature and the extent of the physio-logical responses.

Until Ursin and his colleagues reported their findings, most studies were devoted to the examination of a single, isolated variable—cortisol, a cate-cholamine, or hGH. The strategy of studying single variables had limited our understanding of the manner in which cardiovascular or hormonal patterns are generated during actual danger, fear, or anxiety. Only recently has it become apparent that different physiological patterns are developed in several different bodily systems depending upon the specific type of frightening situation, the attitude with which it is faced, and the performance and experience of the participants. Each of these modifies an integrated pattern of hormonal response: "Any variable which can be described or measured independently is actually a component of several such patterns" (Hilton 1975).

Training for Military Combat

Underwater demolition training is one of the most dangerous military exercises. It consistently raises serum cortisol levels in men to three times normal levels. In anticipation of the introduction of novel procedures or unfamiliar equipment—for example, scuba tanks and new masks—during such training, further increases of serum cortisol levels occur. As soon as the new equipment is mastered, these additional levels return to steady, high basal levels (Rubin et al. 1969).

Practicing the landing of jet fighter planes on aircraft carriers is associated with a high death or injury rate in pilots and their crews. The successful completion of any landing is always in doubt. Even experienced pilots are fearful; but they rate themselves as less frightened than do the crewmen who operate the plane's radar equipment. Yet the pilots show a threefold increase in serum cortisol levels during flights. The greater increments occur in the pilots during day landings despite the fact that landing at night is even more perilous. Even simulated landings in a laboratory are associated with a rise in cortisol levels in pilots (Miller et al. 1970).

The conclusion that the responsible person is more likely to secrete more corticosteroids than the subordinate one was first described in experienced officers and men of a Green Beret combat unit in Vietnam, who were anticipating and went through a Viet Cong attack (Bourne, Rose, and Mason 1967, 1968). The highest increases in levels of 17-OHCS excretion occurred in the two officers and in the radio operator. In the enlisted men, the levels fell during the attack and then returned to baseline levels.

When soldiers under fire are carrying out their customary duties and rituals with hope, or when they resort to prayer—seemingly oblivious to the threat of injury or death—they have lower urinary 17-OHCS levels than predicted by their body weight (Bourne, Rose, and Mason 1967).

The main metabolite of NE, 3-methoxy, 4-hydroxy phenylglycol (MHPG) —but not urine volume—rises significantly in the pilots and radar officers of U.S. Navy jet fighters making aircraft landings. The highest levels are obtained in pilots during actual night landings. Lesser increases in levels occur during day landings. Simulated landings in a laboratory produce no changes in MHPG levels (Rubin et al. 1970).

The Behavioral Biology of Challenges in daily life

Effects of Examinations

Physiological changes accompany the taking of important tests—such as final, oral, medical-licensure examinations—which habitually cause apprehension, anxiety, and fear in most students. They are associated with significantly raised BP levels to clinically hypertensive levels in young physicians. The BP levels began to rise even before the examination begins. Blood pressure levels in some candidates continue to remain elevated when the interrogation is over, but rise again on requestioning. Individual patterns of BP responses are observed; yet every student shows some degree of BP increases. Von Uexküll and Wick (1962) call this phenomenon "stress-hypertension." They believe that this form of high BP may portend essential hypertension, because the physiological patterns are very similar.

Free fatty acid levels increase significantly only in the most anxious medical students taking examinations (Bogdonoff et al. 1960). Serum cholesterol levels rise in medical students taking a written examination by 10% to 25%, especially in those who perform poorly on it (Bloch and Brackenridge 1972). Oral more than written examination seem to mobilize some hormone levels and not others: In 131 medical students a written test raised hGH levels 33%, and an oral examination raised them 49%. The highest mean levels of hGH occurred in women students. Serum insulin levels increased 45% and 43% in men and women respectively without changing blood glucose levels. Plasma renin activity was enhanced by 44% after a written examination and 27% following an oral examination. Significant increases in HR occurred during the oral examination (Syvalähti, Lammintausta, and Pekkarinen 1976).

In medical students, examination periods produce a number of changes in immune function: a decreased percentage of CD4+ lymphocytes; diminished responses of lymphocytes to mitogenic stimulation; a depression of cytotoxicity activity and the number of NK cells; evidence of reactivation of latent herpes virus infection; and more γ-interferon (γ-IF) production. During examinations cellular immunity may be impaired, leading to reactivation of a latent virus (Glaser et al. 1985a, 1985b, 1986; Kiecolt-Glaser et al. 1984, 1986).

Immunoglobulin levels may also be affected by both examinations and the manner in which students habitually conduct their personal relationships. Salivary secretory immunoglobulin-A levels are higher in students who maintain close and supportive ties with each other and fall less during examinations than in students who are mainly interested in grades and success and not in collegiality. The immunoglobulin levels of the latter group continue to decline even after the examination is over (Jemmott et al. 1983).

On the surface, these observations suggest a direct relationship between immunocompetence and the challenge posed by examinations. However, the matter is again more complex. The altered immune function was greatest in those most challenged (distressed) by the examination, and especially in those who felt most alienated from their fellow students (Kiecolt-Glaser et al. 1984). Based on these reports, one may assume that the relationship to friends and peers modifies the impact on immune function of the challenge of examinations in medical students. However, the changes in immunocompetence do not necessarily have any relevance to changes in the students' health status.

Public Presentations

Every young physician knows that one of the most fearsome experiences he/she must undergo early in his/her career is to present at departmental grand rounds. With the development of reliable techniques for the estimation of E and NE in serum, these catecholamines have been measured in physicians making such presentations (Dimsdale and Moss 1980; Taggart, Carruthers, and Somerville 1973). Epinephrine levels rose sharply before and at the onset of the presentation, and they subsided during its course. Norepinephrine levels gradually increased and remained elevated during the entire period. Marked individual differences in the levels that were attained, and in the patterning of the catecholamine responses, were observed. In fact, in some speakers the levels remained unchanged from the beginning to the end of the talk. The changes in catecholamine levels during the presentation differed from those seen during exercise, when NE levels alone increase.

The Induction of Danger, Fear, and Anxiety in the Laboratory

An abundant literature exists about experimental attempts to study fear, anxiety, and danger in human subjects under rigorous experimental conditions. This area of investigation is confusing because of the difficulty of veridically reproducing naturally occurring dangerous experiences. In addition, Selye's stress theory did not predict the anticipatory and individual nature of changes in HR, BP, and FFA levels.

The relationship of danger to its avoidance is also complex and very difficult to simulate. Avoidance behavior can accompany and follow fear, vary independently of it, or vary inversely with it (Lang 1971). Avoidance behavior may reduce fear, yet it may persist long after fear is no longer felt (Rachman and Hodgson 1974). The persistence of such defensive behavior may also outlast the original fear. Gray (1971) believes that avoidance behavior is accompanied by "safety" signals, which are by themselves secondarily rewarding; they account for the persistence of avoidance maneuvers after fear has diminished.

One would predict that blocking avoidance behavior would produce an upsurge of fear—a phenomenon that is observable only in some people.

Additional reasons for individual differences in physiological responses to danger and fear have partly been identified:

1. The stereotyped yet individual nature of physiological responses in the laboratory. Lacey (1967) has pointed out that different stimuli and contingencies produce similar responses in the same but not in another person. One source of these differences between persons is the relatively characteristic pattern of physiological responses of individuals, without regard to the manner in which they are elicited. Conversely, the same frightening context produces highly individual behavioral and physiological responses across groups of subjects. Individual and species differences also characterize the responses of groups of animals to danger.
2. The novelty or unpredictability of the situation.
3. The previous experiences the individual has had with danger.
4. The role assigned to and carried out by the person in the situation of danger—whether, for instance, he/she is the leader or the follower.
5. The demand characteristics of the situation (Miller and Bernstein 1972). Under conditions of high demand, there may be no intercorrelations among HR, RR, and measures of anxiety. Yet in other situations, high demand characteristics produce positive correlations with hormonal measures, and low demand ones produce negative ones.
6. The quality of the performance: Does the person succeed or fail at the task?
7. The manner in which the person copes with fear and anxiety.

Clinical experience also informs us that fearful and anxious patients differ in their bodily responses; at least four symptom clusters are recognizable. Some patients experience marked increases in muscle tension in various regions of their bodies. A second group has mainly cardiorespiratory symptoms—changes in the rate and frequency of respiration and/or the rate and force of the heartbeat. They may become aware of their heart pounding and beating more rapidly or irregularly. Other anxious persons tremble, wring their hands, have a dry mouth, and complain of upper abdominal sensations ("butterflies"). A fourth group vomits, has diarrhea, or has an increased frequency of urination. A delay in the onset of sleep is observed in many anxious patients belonging to any one of the four groups. Combinations of any or all of these symptoms may occur (see chapter 5). These "response stereotypes" are also seen in the laboratory (Lacey 1967).

The experimental study of fear and anxiety has been fraught with a variety of serious quandaries. Problems of their induction, control, and measurement in a controlled laboratory setting largely remain unsolved, with the result that we know little about the physiology of these emotions. In fact, most of our knowledge about it derives from the study of fear induced in naturalistic settings. Attempts to induce fear and anxiety in normal subjects in the laboratory have been made by exposing them to electrical shocks or sparks of light. Contrived situations have been designed to make subjects fearful; these experiments have usually been unsuccessful because many subjects were not fooled by such maneuvers. Investigators have also attempted to induce anxiety by injecting subjects with sympathomimetic drugs or lactic acid. Phobic subjects have been exposed to the feared object.

When the occurrence and degree of fear or anxiety are assessed in subjects by psychological tests and by recording such physiological measures as pupillary size, cerebral blood flow or metabolism, salivary flow, HR, RR, cardiac output (CO), BP, blood flow through muscle and skin, sweating, gastric motility, or various blood levels of catecholamines, hormones, and FFAs, low correlations are obtained between the two sets of measures (Morrow and Labrum 1978), and marked individual differences are obtained when subjects are compared with each other.

This conclusion is exemplified by studies on the central nervous system (CNS) correlates of fear and anxiety, some of which are contradictory. There is general agreement that the EEG is desynchronized in anxious patients: An increase in low-voltage fast (beta) activity occurs while some theta waves also begin to appear. The slow direct current potential ("contingent negative variation"), which can be recorded over the frontal regions of the skull, is a measure of the subject's expectancy or anticipation of a signal. In anxious patients its amplitude is diminished. The subject's expectancy of the occurrence of a signal is not maintained; that is, the subject is distracted from the signal (Lader 1982), presumably by anxiety.

Various techniques for measuring the cerebral blood flow and oxygen consumption have been developed. Kety (1950) used the nitrous oxide technique and showed that anxious subjects had a cerebral blood flow 21%, and a cerebral oxygen consumption 22%, above those of calm subjects. The newer xenon-inhalation technique is capable of measuring regional (mainly cortical) blood flow. Anxious subjects showed some reduction of cortical blood flow, particularly in the right prefrontal, left precentral, both parietal, and right posterior temporal areas (Mathew, Weinman, and Claghorn 1982). Therefore, these two techniques (nitrous oxide and xenon-inhalation) produce different results that are not easily reconcilable.

Although the correlation between measures of anxiety and many physiological variables is low, and contradictory results have been reported in the literature, certain generalizations are possible: Anxious in contrast to calm subjects tend while resting to show increased RR and HR, enhanced palmar sweating and forearm blood flow, raised systolic BP and pulse pressure, and a decreased ability to habituate their physiological activity—forearm blood flow, BP, skin conductance, muscle tension, and pupillary size. On subsequent challenge these physiological responses are not extinguished (Lader 1970).

Therefore, abundant evidence exists that there is no close correlation in the laboratory between measurable fear or anxiety and its autonomic, hormonal, or behavioral correlates (Lang 1971; Leitenberg et al. 1971)—a fact that has confounded theory. Except under the most intense emotional arousal, the concordance between separate physiological measures is also low (Hodgson and Rachman 1974). Studies of this kind have suggested that fear is multidimensional: Verbal-cognitive, behavioral, and physiological response systems are involved in fear; they may be correlated under certain conditions, but not under others.

More consistent data have been obtained by studying subjects in the field— in dangerous situations such as combat training or actual combat, during examinations or frightening medical procedures. The drawbacks of this approach are that the situational and subject variables are difficult to isolate and control, the methods of measurement are limited, and the data are of a correlational, not an analytic, nature.

Given the constraints on the laboratory study of the emotions, it is not surprising that the question of whether specific physiological patterns accompany an emotion such as fear, sadness, happiness, or anger has not been easy to answer. Some resolution of this problem has recently been obtained (Schwartz, Weinberger, and Singer 1981). The technique of guided imagery was used to induce reminiscences and mental images associated with these four feelings in 32 subjects. The images were recreated during a second period when the subjects were also asked to imagine themselves walking up and down a step, which was followed by rest. A third period ensued when they performed a step-test while again imaging the previous scenes and their associated feelings. A "neutral" control condition followed when they only exercised.

The mean and diastolic BP increments were significantly greater with anger than with fear. But increases in systolic BP were the same for all four emotions. Heart rates rose in equal amounts with anger and fear; this amount was greater than the increase produced by images that elicited feelings of happiness or sadness. When anger was combined with exercise, the greatest increases of all in HR and systolic BP were achieved; these cardiovascular changes returned to baseline levels slower than with any other emotion. Only anger was accompanied by distinctive cardiovascular changes. Fear was not associated with unique cardiovascular effects when compared to periods of induced sadness or happiness.

Electromyography has also been used to discriminate anger and fear. The former produces tonic, regular potential discharges; the latter, phasic ones (Ax 1953). These findings suggest that the electrical potential changes in muscle are biologically meaningful: They prepare angry subjects for a single sustained movement (a blow). When subjects are afraid, their muscles are prepared for intermittent movements (flight).

Another experimental technique in a relatively controlled setting is to show normal subjects films with different themes, intended to provoke fear with suspense films, boredom and fatigue with "neutral" ones, and erotic excitement with pornographic ones. After the showing of each film the subject is asked to fill out a checklist designed to elicit his emotional responses to the film, and blood samples for hormonal measures are obtained. In Brown's and Heninger's study (1975) FFA levels rose 250% in all 8 men 30 minutes after fear was provoked by the suspense film, and 300% 15 minutes after the pornographic one. Cortisol levels increased from baseline levels from 4.0 to 15.1 μg/dl in 4 of 8 subjects after the suspense film, and from 4.2 to 8.1 μg/dl in 3 of 8 subjects after the explicitly erotic one. All three films raised hGH levels in 5 of 8 subjects—increments that were independent of the subjects' aroused feelings.

Another research strategy is to confront fearful (phobic) patients with the feared object or situation in order to induce fear and anxiety while recording their behavior and measuring HR (Leitenberg et al. 1971). A variety of responses was obtained when this was done. In some patients as phobic anxiety decreased the HR increased; in others it decreased or did not change at all. The HR correlates of phobic anxiety do not need to change before anxiety is experienced. But this conclusion must be tentative, as only one cardiovascular measure was taken and gross motor activity was not controlled for. Furthermore, the findings are at variance with those showing that HR responses habituate in some persons but not in others (Grossberg and Wilson 1968).

The same technique has been adapted to study correlated hormonal patterns. Some phobic patients confronted with the feared object or situation responded with extreme manifestations of fear. They wept, screamed, and trembled, and their teeth chattered. When asked to rate their distress before, during, and after the experiment, they all discerned a crescendo of fear during the actual confrontation. The intense fear induced by such "flooding" produced no change in PRL levels (Nesse et al. 1980). Changes in serum cortisol levels were unrelated to "flooding," whether measured at the crest (Curtis et al. 1978) or at the trough of the circadian cortisol cycle (Curtis et al. 1976); they fell progressively during each of five experimental sessions. In one-half of the subjects their elevations occurred in the first and second (baseline) sessions, and only in a minority did the rise occur during the experimental periods. Individual variability characterized the cortisol responses; they seemed mainly to occur in response to the novelty of the situation and in anticipation of the procedure. Human growth hormone changes were also variable in the 11 subjects; the highest levels occurred during the experimental sessions in only 5 subjects. In 4 of these 5 subjects levels remained high even during the recovery period (Curtis et al. 1979).

One source of individual variability in hormonal responses has been identified—i.e., whether or not an anxious or fearful subject interacts with the experimenter during the experiment. During cardiac catheterization, only the most overtly frightened subject had significant increases of serum cortisol. The frightened patients could be divided into two subgroups: Those who talked to the physicians about their concerns during the procedure showed only increments in cortisol levels, while those who did not had significant increases in both hGH levels and cortisol (Greene et al. 1970). Both groups of patients maintained high levels of FFA from the beginning of the procedure. A similar conclusion was arrived at by Brown and Heninger (1976), using the same technique; only one-third of their patients showed hGH responses, those who were "noninvolved" but not frightened.

The results of these many studies are contradictory. They suggest again that in the laboratory physiological responses to the experimental induction of phobic anxiety are unpredictable because many factors influence them. Even when massive phobic anxiety is produced in subjects, no hormonal changes may occur. Under other conditions (e.g., viewing films) the changes that occur do not discriminate fear from erotic arousal. Yet in situations of real danger in a naturalistic setting, more consistent results are obtained, despite the fact that they do not permit control of many other variables: the effects of dietary intake before the experiment, its novelty, muscular movement and exercise during it. Despite these drawbacks, relevant behavioral variables affecting hormone patterns have been isolated in both anticipation and experience of lifelike situations of danger or challenge, especially when the subject has little or no control over them.

Summary

Studies of the physiological responses to acutely dangerous situations in humans do not confirm Selye's concept of a "nonspecific," ubiquitous adaptation syndrome (GAS) without regard to the nature of the stressful experience. Because of a paucity of available biochemical techniques in his day, he emphasized the role of the corticosteroids in response to damaging stressors. Studies in humans suggest that cortisol is produced and secreted in anticipation of a task; in novel and unpredictable situations; with pain, malnutrition, melancholic depression, and anorexia nervosa; and during sustained, uncontrollable danger—but not in everyone. The studies of cortisol responses during real-life situations and occupations that are dangerous begin to reveal the nature of the individual differences in hormone patterns, including cortisol's. What is dangerous to one person is a thrill to another. Novelty, ambiguity, inexperience, and chronic vigilance are more likely to mobilize physiological responses—especially HR, catecholamine, and FFA, rather than cortisol, responses. Good rather than poor performance is more habitually associated with a decline in physiological responses during the task. The demand characteristics of a situation in part determine physiological responses. Leaders are more responsive physiologically than followers in situations of danger. Note, however, that almost all the data on the physiological responses to danger are obtained in acute situations and with men. The long-term physiological effects of danger, fear, and anxiety are largely unknown, and the empirical link of fear and anxiety to bodily disease states is at best tenuous.

An attempt has been made to underline the fact that fear and anxiety are truly biological, not only clinical, phenomena. They play a central role in alerting the organism to danger. Without them, people and animals would not survive predation and bodily harm; they would be selected out. The organism's performance in such situations, including its physiological responses, will determine whether it survives or not.

The Nature of Stressful Personal Experiences: Bereavement, Separation and Loss

The claim that human relationships are crucial to the maintenance of health is based on the observation that bereavement, separation, and loss are associated in (some) predisposed persons with the onset of illness and disease. Presumably they, and the emotional responses they produce, unsettle hidden processes by which health is customarily maintained. Many empirically derived schedules designed to assess important events and experiences in people's lives prior to illness and disease assign the highest weighting to bereavement due to the death of an intimate relative. The study of patients after the onset of a variety of diseases provides abundant evidence that separation, loss, or bereavement is the context in which they begin. Human relationships, it seems, are crucial for many to the maintenance or restoration of physical health and psychological well-being; their disruption is a potent factor in ill health and disease. It also seems likely that human relationships play a central role in the proper development, maintenance, and usual regulation of bodily systems; this assertion also stems from the study of young animals, in which premature separation affects every bodily system and places them at risk for a variety of diseases (Hofer 1984; Taylor 1987; Weiner 1982). The range of disturbances produced is not predicted by previous stress theory.

The Consequences of Bereavement and Separation

The term *bereavement* will be used to denote the death of a person close to the subject. *Separation* signifies the disruption of a bond between two people, but not necessarily by death. Separation or bereavement may be especially poignant for adults if it recapitulates a childhood loss. The usual, or the aberrant, responses to loss may also occur when prized attributes (e.g., beauty, dignity, youth, strength, income, wealth, intelligence, skills, memory, aspirations, ideals, hope, occupations, body functions or parts, health and the sense of well-being) are lost. Bereavement and loss may, however, be anticipated; mourning may be over by the time they actually occur.

Grief

The usual human response to bereavement, separation, and loss is grief (Brown and Stoudemire 1983; Hofer 1984). Grief unfolds in three separate phases.

1. Phase of shock (protest): It begins immediately, lasts from 1 to 14 days, and is usually initiated by a feeling of disbelief and a sense of being "numb," shocked, lost, bereft, or helpless. Grief-stricken persons may grope about. They may not feel like eating or sleeping. They cry. The throat feels tight. They sigh. Nausea and "hollowness" in the chest and abdomen are experienced. The full reality and impact of the experience are hidden by the sense of disbelief, "numbness," and protest that it has taken place.

2. Phase of despair, realization, and grief. After about two weeks, the full impact and actuality of the loss hits the bereaved, as disbelief is dissipated. Crying may increase and come in waves. The bereaved feels drained; the world seems empty; nothing is very enjoyable; none of the basic life functions matter, so eating and sleeping may be neglected or disrupted.

The bereaved repeatedly thinks of, and frequently dreams about, the departed person. The departed person's faults are forgotten; he or she is often idealized. Some survivors reproach themselves for not having done enough for, or regret having held grudges against, the lost one. Anger at, feelings of having been neglected by, and guilt about the deceased may occur in the grieving person, but usually these feelings are fleeting. Brief periods of imagining that the departed person is still alive may occur; strangers may even be misidentified as the departed person.

The second phase usually lasts six to eight months, but there are no rules that state its duration (Parkes 1970); it may last a lifetime. A young couple who loses an only child may grieve for eternity. In other persons, grief recurs on the anniversary of the death or the birthday of the deceased.

3. Phase of resolution. The bereaved person gradually resumes his/her life, interests, work, and relationships. The future no longer seems bleak. He/she returns to the world that seems fuller and more rewarding than before. The emotional bonds that held the survivor to the deceased are loosened, and his/her emotional currency is invested elsewhere. The reality of the loss is accepted; crying spells diminish; and feelings of emptiness are dissipated. The recurrent memories of the departed fade. This phase lasts for weeks or months.

Feelings of grief are attenuated by the support and sympathy of other persons. All cultures makes provisions for sharing bereavement through the agency of mourning rituals. There are, however, individual ways of coping with grief: Gender differences occur; men in our culture find it harder than women do to cry. Angry feelings may supplant grief in some. Physicians notoriously protect themselves against feeling grief, or distract or prevent their patients from expressing it.

The consequences of not being permitted or encouraged to express grief may be dire: Feelings of shame and depression, the resort to drugs such as hypnotics, attempts at suicide, and bodily symptoms designed to elicit attention, sympathy, and help may ensue.

However, grief and mourning do not of necessity have to follow bereavement or separation. Their absence does not inevitably imply "pathology." Some persons have grieved in anticipation of losses; when, for instance, the departed person had been very old, or chronically ill for a very long time. Others are glad to be rid of a hated relative. Such responses may very well be unexpected, and their "inappropriateness" may "shock" others, but they are quite understandable. Grief (or depression) is, therefore, not inevitable, and its absence following bereavement and separation does not necessarily imply "abnormality" then or in the future (Wortman and Silver 1989). Therefore, individual differences to the experience of bereavement or separation are as evident as they are predictable.

"Pathological" Mourning

Bereavement, separation, and loss may incite "pathological" mourning, which may begin immediately after they take place or may be delayed in onset. It consists of a complex mixture of love, longing, and need for lost persons with hatred of, anger at, and the wish to take revenge on them, for leaving. Vengefulness produces a cascade of anguish, guilt, fears of retribution, and the need to make amends to be forgiven. Pathological mourning can be anticipatory. It may occur in childhood and be reinduced in adulthood by seemingly trivial losses (Bowlby 1963; Paulley 1983) or occur in persons customarily incapable of expressing feelings (Lindemann 1944). Its prevalence may be on the order of 10 to 25% in a bereaved population (Zisook 1987).

Pathological mourning occurs when certain kinds of people—those who rely unduly on others and are not capable of mature relationships—are bereaved by unexpected or unusual circumstances such as the murder, suicide, or sudden disappearance of a spouse, lover, or partner (Parkes 1964, 1971; Raphael 1975, 1977). The survivor's guilt stems from the belief that he or she wittingly or unwittingly drove the other person away or to suicide.

Pathological mourning is a risk factor for depression and/or suicide, the silent acquisition of the departed's symptoms and behaviors, or a subsequent life of bitterness and social isolation. Those who mourn in this way may cope by distracting themselves with restless overactivity in order to remain oblivious of the profound sense of loss and the bevy of painful feelings it has engendered. They may deny the death or disappearance of a relative or spouse and live in a make-believe world in which it has never occurred. They may disguise their grief in chronic anger, or they may become touchy or impassive. Some may subsequently become incapable of experiencing or expressing any feelings. Because of their age-inappropriate psychological makeup, those who mourn pathologically are particularly in need of encouragement, help in expressing their complex feelings, and advice (Raphael 1975).

Major depressive syndromes may have their onset in certain patients after a latent period of weeks or months following a bereavement, separation, or loss. Patients of this kind cannot understand the relationship between these events and their illness. They deny their sadness and depression. In other patients delayed grief reactions may be transmuted into a pain syndrome, the chronic hyperventilation syndrome, or the functional bowel disorder; they have been reported in ulcerative colitis.

Following the death of a relative, some survivors, rather than feeling grief and sorrow, remarry quickly after a spouse has died or try to replace a dead child by immediately becoming pregnant or adopting one. Sooner or later they become symptomatic if they have never mourned.

The Physiological Correlates of Bereavement, Separation, and Loss in Adult Humans

The physiological correlates of bereavement, separation, and loss in adult persons have not to date been investigated in much depth or detail. In a pioneer investigation, Wolff and his colleagues (Wolff et al. 1964; Wolff, Hofer, and Mason 1964; and Hofer et al. 1972a, 1972b) studied parents whose children were dying of leukemia. After an initial period of shock, disbelief, and grief on being told the diagnosis and prognosis, they gradually came to accept the illness by seeking information about it. Their sense of responsibility for the illness could be dispelled by the physicians who provided them with the facts about its treatment and advice about coping with, and sympathy for, the impending loss of their child. At each stage of this process, Wolff and his colleagues accurately foretold the 17-OHCS urinary excretion levels in the parents. Their criteria for predicting these levels were twofold: the "integrity" of the parents' inferred psychological "defenses" and ways of coping (such as repression, denial, isolation, and identification), and the intensity of the parents' emotional responses of sadness, grief, depression, or other distressing feelings. Each parent had his/her own individual manner of dealing with the impending loss; the more effective it was, the lower were the mean 17-OHCS urinary excretion levels. In 23 of 31 instances, the 17-OHCS levels (which were all within the normal range) could be correctly predicted by the psychological criteria.

One of the implications of this study was that the baseline level of an individual's 17-OHCS excretion may reflect the effectiveness of psychological "defenses" or other ways of coping with stressful experiences. And indeed the same conclusion using the same criteria was reached in subsequent studies by other investigators (Katz 1982). Alternatively, adrenal cortical excretion levels (or serum cortisol production and secretion) and coping strategies, although temporally correlated, may reflect two separate characteristics of persons; therefore, they may not be causally related. Furthermore, the situation in which the parents found themselves was uncontrollable; they could not alter a fatal outcome.

Other studies in an older age group (Jacobs 1987) do not confirm the idea that "defenses" and coping are critical intervening variables in determining hormonal responses, but show that age and mood status are. Older widowed men and women and those threatened with bereavement were compared: Only the widowed ones who were depressed had higher mean 24-hour mean cortisol excretion levels. Serum E and NE levels were increased in older patients but without regard to their bereavement status or mood scores. Serum PRL levels were higher when all subjects were both anxious and depressed. Their hGH levels were elevated only when the prospect or actuality of bereavement was associated with anxiety. Nevertheless, none of the hormonal changes were reflected in any change in the subjects' health status.

Bereavement is also associated with altered components of the immune system, but probably only if the person becomes depressed. Bartrop and his co-workers (1977) studied the stimulatory effects of phytohemagglutinin (PHA) and concanavalin A (both mitogens) on the incorporation of thymidine into the lymphocytes of widows and an age-matched control population. The lymphocyte responses in the widows were lower six weeks after the bereavement. Similar results were obtained in a longitudinal study on men 33–76 years of age whose wives were dying of breast cancer (Schleifer et al. 1983; Stein, Keller, and Schleifer 1985). Idoxuridine incorporation into lymphocytes after mitogen stimulation was significantly lower in the widowers one month after the wife's demise but not before it. Recovery of lymphocyte function began after that period and was partially completed in one year. Follow-up reports on these widowers to determine if the suppression of this particular T-cell function is clinically, not only biologically, meaningful have not been published to date.

The topic of bereavement, depression, and immune function is subtle and complex. When the bereaved are studied over time, it turns out that only the depressed ones manifest a fall in NK-cell cytotoxic function. But the experience of bereavement by itself is not associated with such a decline. A depressed mood by itself is not associated with changes in other T-cell subpopulations or of ratios of $CD4^+$ (helper/inducer) to $CD8^+$ (suppressor/cytotoxic) cells. However, when the depressed person also shows evidence of anxiety and complains of bodily symptoms, $CD8^+$ cell numbers are reduced and the ratio of $CD4^+$ to $CD8^+$ cells is raised (Irwin et al. 1986, 1987; Irwin and Weiner 1987).

Elderly persons languishing in institutions frequently have little or no contact with relatives, friends, fellow inmates, and staff. The effect of such separation from their family members and such social isolation can be devastating. Systematic attempts at reversing the lack of human interaction have now been made; they show that human contacts can be increased even in the elderly with the result that physical and hormonal changes occurred that were not detected in elderly persons who remained by themselves. The "treated" group did not shrink in physical stature. Estradiol and T levels fell continuously over a period of time in elderly men who remained by themselves and increased in men in the experimental group. Plasma hGH levels increased and DHA levels rose significantly in the first three months of increasing human contact, only to fall back later to baseline levels. The same changes in kind but to a lesser degree in these two hormones were seen in the women who became less isolated (Arnetz et al. 1983). These results are relevant to the topic of separation and bereavement. They show that human relationships can alter hormonal levels in the elderly. But the clinical significance of these changes in unknown.

The evidence, therefore, suggests that the experiences of bereavement and normal grief and sadness (except for crying and a possible sleep disturbance) by themselves are not associated with any significant hormonal or immunological alterations. If the experience of bereavement is, however, followed by a depressed mood, with or without anxiety, such changes do occur. However, the age of the bereft person may play an additional role in determining hormonal responses. Although the experiences of bereavement and normal sadness or grief may not be associated with physiological changes, some other facet of the rupture of important relationships may be. It was mentioned previously that personal relationships structure the day and night; they provide important cues entraining biological rhythms. The investigator who only measures hormone levels at one point in time will remain oblivious to changes in their unfolding patterns over time. In fact, the evidence is that in the depressive disorders many patterned rhythms—in mood, sleep, food intake, and hormones—are altered (for a review see Weiner 1991b).

The Onset of Illness and Disease in the Setting of Bereavement

Abundant observations have been made showing that the health of about 67% of widows declines within one year of bereavement (Maddison and Viola 1968; Parkes and Brown 1972) and psychiatric morbidity increases (Klerman and Izen 1977). Parkes (1964) carried out a study of patients admitted to a psychiatric hospital. He found that the number of patients whose illness followed the loss of a spouse was significantly greater than anticipated for people of that age and social group. Major depressions are particularly frequent in bereaved persons; in one study 45% became severely depressed within one year after their loss (Bornstein et al. 1973; Clayton et al. 1974). Such depressions enhance the risk of suicide, which then becomes another (but not the only) antecedent for the known increases in mortality observed in survivors six months after the bereavement (Bowling and Charlton 1987; Jacobs and Ostfeld 1977; Parkes, Benjamin, and Fitzgerald 1969; Rees and Lutkins 1967). Although suicide is correlated with depressed moods (Paykel 1976; Weissman et al. 1973), it is also associated with disease and with alcohol and illicit drug abuse.

The topic of depressed moods is complex. Generally speaking, those who study bereavement, loss, and separation have focused their attention on grief, pathological mourning, and the onset of disease. Another body of investigators has studied the onset of major depressive disorders following bereavement. Patients are placed at risk for major depressive disorders not only by genetic endowment and family history but also by prior and concurrent stressful experiences. One such factor in these disorders is separation from, or death of, the mother (but not the father) before the child is 17 years of age; another one is belonging to a poor and/or working-class family (Brown and Harris 1986). It is said, albeit incorrectly, that such a history only antedates the "nonendogenous" major depressive disorders (Roy 1987). In only a very few studies has attention been paid to additional factors—e.g., the economic status of the family after bereavement. When poverty continues or is increased it becomes a major risk factor for subsequent psychiatric morbidity, especially depression (Breier et al. 1988).

Additional social background factors place patients at risk for the depressive disorders: An unhappy marriage (defined as the incapacity to confide in a spouse) is a risk factor for both the "endogenous" and "nonendogenous" forms. When the woman is also burdened with caring for three or more children under 14 years of age and is unemployed, the risk is compounded (Brown and Harris 1978, 1986; Roy 1987). These vulnerability factors are based on large-scale samples of patients. Additional risk factors also play a role when individuals are studied in depth: Among the most prominent ones is a chronic medical illness. The prevalence of depression is more than 50% in patients with cancer (especially of the pancreas), rheumatoid arthritis, systemic lupus erythematosus, and ulcerative colitis (for reviews see Weiner 1977, 1989a).

Some patients who develop major depressive disorders are sensitive to the threat or actuality of separation from another person from whom they crave constant love, attention, praise, support, and encouragement. But they give little in return and are oblivious or insensitive to the needs and wishes of others. Criticism and disapproval deeply wound their feelings. Failure makes them feel worthless. When slighted or rejected they become depressed. They demand special treatment; when they do not get it they are enraged, hurt, or depressed. They tend to be moralistic and to be critical of, and at times feel (morally) superior to, others (Cohen et al. 1954; Jacobson 1971).

In recent investigations of the antecedents of the major depressive disorders, the stressful experiences are thought to interact with these special vulnerabilities (Brown and Harris 1986; Paykel 1976). Such experiences are meaningful, profound, and unpleasant. They consist of disappointments in, and losses of, not only actual relationships but roles (as wives and mothers, or workers) and aspirations, hopes, and ideals. Often such experiences are superimposed on long-standing, ongoing, realistic difficulties (e.g., the number of children, economic hardship, poor housing conditions, marital discord). Their impact is attenuated by a supportive, understanding, or dependent relationship to another person (Costello 1982).

Some abrupt events—a sudden bereavement or loss, or an additional disappointment—may immediately precipitate a depression: They are "severe" experiences. The effect of other experiences, judged to be "milder," may take several days to evolve. Of course, both categories (events and difficulties) may be concurrent for prolonged periods of time.

When all these factors are taken into account and combined, it turns out that they antecede major depressive disorder in 89% of all patients. In fact Brown and Harris (1986) have summarized a number of their studies that have also demonstrated that both categories are very similar in kind and number in the milder depressive disorders. In 73% of patients their onset is associated with "severe" events or a major difficulty; when the two categories are combined the number increases.

The depressive disorders are processes occurring over time. A vulnerability factor such as a consistent lack of a close relationship between spouses may increase in magnitude as the marriage deteriorates; one reason for its decline is a spouse's chronically depressed mood that creates a joyless union.

Many studies in Britain have also found that depressed women are more likely to have experienced both events and difficulties than have their male counterparts (Bebbington et al. 1988)—a finding that is not very surprising given the roles assigned to women (especially poor ones) in British society. However, completed suicides increase with age and are more frequent in men (Paykel 1976). Those attempting suicide have experienced significantly more undesirable circumstances in their lives than have patients who only become depressed, or nondepressed, randomly sampled members of the general population. The most frequent experiences prior to suicide are illness in, the death of, or separation from a family member. However, arguments and discord with a spouse, chronic or fatal disease, forced unemployment, incarceration, alcoholism, or business failures also play important roles. Attempted but unsuccessful suicides are also preceded by uncontrollable experiences that persons believe will have a profound and adverse influence on their futures. The attempt is often the culmination of mounting distress in the month before it takes place (Paykel 1976).

Bereaved persons not only show a decline in health and an increase in morbidity and mortality, but they also change their habits. They smoke more cigarettes and drink more alcohol—known risk factors for a variety of diseases— and use more tranquilizers (Parkes and Brown 1972).

Less believable to many physicians are the observations that bereavement and losses are the setting in which many diseases begin. Schmale (1958) studied 42 hospitalized patients, 18–45 years of age, belonging to the same social class. Their assigned diagnoses spanned the range from hysterical conversion symptoms to aseptic meningitis. Shortly after admission, each patient was interviewed with the aim of obtaining a history of the context in which the illness began with a particular focus on events that represented to the patients either an actual, threatened, or symbolic bereavement, separation, or loss, or no loss at all. In 16 of 42 patients significant change in relationships to others had occurred within 24 hours of the appearance of symptoms of the disease. In another 15 patients, a separation or loss occurred within one week prior to the onset of illness. Another 8 patients gave a similar history in the month prior to the onset of illness.

Whether actual or threatened, separation and bereavement have been cited as two contexts that contribute to the onset of a variety of diseases: anorexia and bulimia nervosa (Garfinkel and Garner 1982; Strober 1983), autoimmune diseases (Paulley 1983), bronchial asthma (Rees 1964), malignancies (Bahnson 1969; Kissen 1967), diabetes mellitus (Hinkle and Wolf 1952; Stein and Charles 1971), peptic duodenal (Weiner 1977) and gastric ulcer (Peters and Richardson 1983), leukemia (Greene 1954), Graves disease (Lidz 1949), essential hypertension (Reiser and Ferris 1951), congestive heart failure (Perlman et al. 1971), myocardial infarction (Parkes, Benjamin, and Fitzgerald 1969), abdominal pain (Drossman 1982), ulcerative and granulomatous colitis (Engel 1955, 1968), tuberculosis (Day 1951), complications of pregnancy and postpartum depression (O'Hara, Rehm, and Campbell 1983), and most major psychiatric illnesses (Bornstein et al. 1973; Brown and Harris 1986). In addition the prognosis of a myocardial infarction is considerably worse in widowers than in age-matched married men (Chandra et al. 1983).

Young, Benjamin, and Wallis (1963), studying the mortality among widowers, found that 213 of 4,486 widowers, 55 years old and older, died within the first six months of the loss of their spouse, an increase of about 40% above that expected for married men of the same age. Kraus and Lilienfeld (1959) noted that the mortality rate of persons of both sexes who had lost a spouse was increased and exceeded that expected in those under 35 years of age. In a study reported by Helsing, Szklo, and Comstock (1981), Young and his colleagues', but not Kraus and Lilienfeld's, observation was confirmed: Widowers are considerably more likely to die between the ages of 55 and 74. The death of a spouse in that age group of men enhances the risk of their death, especially from IHD, for reasons and by mechanisms that we do not understand. Bereavement may act as a permissive factor in patients with undetected coronary atherosclerosis. Yet bereavement may also play a more direct pathogenetic role in the onset of other diseases. In none of these studies is it clear whether a fully developed grief, a pathological mourning reaction in its delayed or distorted forms, or depression is associated with the onset of disease.

Developing Schmale's work, Engel (1968) has hypothesized that the "giving-up, given-up" complex (to losses) is the emotional response in which many, if not most disease occurs. He has estimated that this complex precedes the onset of illness and disease in 70 to 80% of patients. Engel notes that as with all other events, it is difficult to predict the meaning of bereavement to a particular person: The determining factors will also be the individual's past experience (of bereavement) and his or her present capacity for coping with it. When bereavement occurs in sensitized persons they may react by experiencing a sense of "psychological impotence"—feelings that they cannot cope with any task and feelings of helplessness and hopelessness. Their self-esteem is low, and they cannot enjoy the company of other people, their work, or their hobbies. Their sense of the continuity of their past, present, and future is disrupted. A reactivation of memories of earlier periods of giving up occurs. Engel believes that in situations in which prompt resolution of this state of mind does not occur, and in which periods of struggling against it alternate with periods of giving up, illness and disease may begin.

Engel's conclusions are based on his studies of patients with ulcerative colitis (1955) and on Greene's (1954) and Schmale's (1958) observations. Paulley (1983), however, finds that pathological mourning specifically antecedes a variety of autoimmune diseases: rheumatoid arthritis, giant cell arteritis, systemic lupus erythematosus, polymyalgia, Sjögren syndrome, and autoimmune thyroid disease.

This area of investigation requires refinement. Specific questions await answers: Are pathological grief reactions, states of depression and helplessness, or states of pathological mourning associated with different physiological patterns that play either indirect, permissive, or more direct roles in the onset of disease? In view of the fact that grief and mourning do not seem to be associated with significant physiological changes or drastic outcomes, it is more likely that the correlates of depression, anxiety, and pathological mourning interact with specific predispositions to precipitate the diseases enumerated.

The "Choice" of Disease Following Bereavement

Linear theories of disease causality would predict that an agent, stimulus, or challenge to humans or animals would produce a specific disease; after all, the *Streptococcus* does incite erysipelas. Yet it only does so, in fact, if the host is also immunosuppressed. Many other factors—the dose of the infectious agent, the age of the patient, the integrity of the immune system, and bereavement with depression (?)—play a role in determining (even infectious) disease onset; a host-agent interaction must occur. A multifactorial theory has better explanatory power than does a unicausal or linear theory of disease.

Those who hold to linear or unicausal hypotheses of the pathogenesis of disease refute the observation that losses and bereavement are associated with the onset of a variety of diseases. Why, they ask, do such events not incite only one disease? The answer is that neither bereavement nor the *Streptococcus* specifies a particular disease. The characteristics of the host's responses determine the specific outcome. Specific predispositions to a particular disease decide its nature following stressful experience. They specify the "choice" of the disease with which the bereaved person will fall ill—if indeed he or she does. They are the source of the variability of outcome. In addition, most diseases are not uniform entities. Various subforms exist whose predispositions differ (see chapter 6).

Stressful Experiences in the Workplace

Two of the stressful experiences that have been most fully studied in an integrated manner are unemployment and specific kinds of working conditions. These observations on workers point up the need to specify with precision the exact nature of these experiences and challenges and the complex responses they engender. They may:

1. Produce job loss, reduction of income, inability to pay the rent and other bills—all undesirable experiences—due to a shrinking economy or during periods of economic instability and in industries that are cyclic in nature.
2. Lead to new job opportunities. If no new job is found, the worker and his/her family may have to relocate.
3. Culminate in wished-for promotions or new jobs, but in enhanced responsibility or a greater work load, which subsequently may end in success or failure. Changes in employment of this kind may occur at times of economic expansion.

Most studies to date examine the consequences of economic contraction and forced unemployment, which increase the incidence of illness, injury, and suicide (Farrow 1984). However, it is still not certain that these associations hold for all countries and all socioeconomic and age groups. Economic contraction is most likely to produce distress, illness, and disease in certain groups of persons—i.e., poorer workers and men over 45 years of age—while economic instability may affect certain individuals only—the unskilled workers and the poor (Brenner 1985).

Unemployment

Forced unemployment uncovers the central role of work in the lives of human beings. Work is valued for reasons other than earning a living. Work ensures mental and physical activity. It may enhance the worker's social status. The goals and purposes of work are shared. Work structures the day. It ensures human contacts and friendships. It promotes shared experiences with persons outside the family.

Unemployment affects people less when they merely depend on their jobs to earn a living than when they also rely on good personal relationships with fellow workers, take pride in their work skills, and work with others towards a common goal. For some, work is an escape from marital discord, a source of pride and dignity, or a way of maintaining authority in the family. The adverse psychosocial consequences of unemployment seem to have a greater impact on some workers than do the economic ones (Jahoda and Rush 1980).

The loss of work is frequently followed by the initial phase of a grief reaction, then a preoccupation with the meaning of work in the several senses just enumerated. Anxiety, insomnia, fatigue, and loss of appetite and weight may occur. Unemployment may be followed in some ex-workers by a depressed mood, accompanied by suicidal thoughts severe enough to require antidepressant treatment. Some unemployed men also drink increasing amounts of alcohol and smoke more tobacco products. The incidence of bodily injury due to various forms of accidents is increased. Unemployed men as a group also perform more acts of violence (Farrow 1984). The incidence of attempted and successful suicide rises in parallel with an increasing unemployment rate (Brenner 1985; Platt and Kreitman 1984). Mental hospital admissions are greater during economic recessions (Brenner 1973).

The unemployed show a marked increase in visits to medical facilities (Beale and Nethercott 1986). In the period between 1965 and 1975 sickness certification increased in England by 77%. (Conversely, unemployment caused by sickness or disability increased 21%.) The nature of the complaints in British men 17–64 years of age ranged all the way from the symptoms of ill health (Farrow 1984)—headaches, backaches, an itching skin—to significant increases in mortality due to cardiovascular disease, suicide, and accidents (Kasl 1979). The prevalence of bronchial asthma, chronic bronchitis, obstructive lung disease, and IHD was raised (Cook et al. 1982; Fox and Goldblatt 1982). Even the threat of unemployment may raise the mortality from IHD in men aged 55–64 years. In another English study, the incidence of peptic duodenal ulcer increased following unemployment (Farrow 1984). Men with prior histories of poor health or recurrent disabilities they had overcome suffered relapses on losing their jobs. Maternal and infant mortality increased in the families of unemployed men.

The metabolic changes that occur with unemployment are some of the very ones that place men at risk for IHD. Kasl and Cobb (1970) found that men who lost their jobs showed increases in their BP. Even the anticipation of the closing of an industrial plant was associated with elevations of serum uric acid (SUA), but not of serum cholesterol levels (SCL). When new employment was found, SUA levels returned to normal. The greater the anguish occasioned by losing the job, the higher the SUA levels. Men who anticipated the closing of the plant by resigning and looking for new employment had high but stable SUA levels. Serum cholesterol levels only rose after the men had lost their jobs; they remained high during the entire period they were without work and only fell on reemployment (Kasl, Cobb, and Brooks 1968). Saxena (1980) reported additional changes: Involuntary unemployment was associated with an increase in serum levels of LDL and a fall in high density lipoproteins (HDL).

The wives of the newly unemployed men, if they themselves were not working, also suffered a decline in their health status. Specifically, an increase in the incidence of peptic duodenal ulcer occurred in these women (Farrow 1984). Yet if the wives worked, their health improved! Children under the age of 12 years are affected in several ways by their fathers' unemployment: increased truancy from school; a fall in the quality of their schoolwork; a greater number of physical injuries; and more visits to the doctor (Farrow 1984).

Not all men who become unemployed become depressed, fall ill, or develop a disease and die. The correlation between job loss and depression is, nonetheless, a significant one (Brenner 1985; Pearlin et al. 1981): 19% of the variance is accounted for by unemployment. In those men who became depressed, a fall in income increased economic problems in their families, causing them to think less of themselves, and reduced their sense of mastery and control over events.

Several ways of coping with unemployment reduce the economic strain and loss of self-confidence, but they do not prevent the loss of the sense of mastery. Successful coping strategies entail seeking information about or looking for a new job, minimizing the importance of money and income, reassuring oneself that one is not so badly off after all. On the other hand, some men make increasing demands upon themselves, feel more pressured, and become more irritable (Siegrist 1984). And other men give up looking for new employment.

The support of family and friends does not reduce the strain of economic worry but prevents the fall in self-confidence and the feeling of loss of control or mastery (Pearlin et al. 1981). These observations underscore the fact that coping and social support act on only two of several aspects of the experience of losing a job. The meaning of work to those who lose their jobs determines their reactions.

Many of the psychological reactions to losing a job share common features with those to other kinds of losses. But the unemployed and their families are at risk for ill health and disease (Lloyd 1983; Weiner 1983, 1985a) and changes in behavior, some of which are inappropriate and damaging.

Working Conditions

Blue-collar workers engaged in heavy manual work, especially if they are exposed to high noise levels (e.g., in foundries), are at increased risk for myocardial infarction (Siegrist 1984). A doubling and tripling of the risk for IHD and myocardial infarction is seen in shift workers, if they rotate their working hours over periods of twenty years (Knutsson et al. 1986). Additional factors play a role: exposure to toxins (such as CO, CS_2), paced work, or excessive workloads (Theorell 1986). However, such working conditions are worsened or mitigated by the absence or presence, respectively, of kindly marital and personal relationships. Social support ameliorates the effects of heavy work schedules and low control over the particular nature of the assigned work (Marmot 1982).

A chronic work overload, especially one over which the worker has no control (e.g., paced work), also conduces to myocardial infarction. Siegrist, Matschinger, and Siegrist (1987) have prospectively studied 416 blue-collar workers exposed to such working conditions. Some of them responded by attempts to enhance their control and increase their commitment to work, which, under the circumstances, led to frustration and irritation but a refusal to quit. These workers were initially free of any discernible signs of IHD. When compared to matched workers not exposed to "forced" work, those who responded with the psychological reactions just described had higher BP levels and lower HDL:LDL ratios than those who did not. In 365 of these blue-collar workers followed prospectively for three years, the incidence of myocardial infarction was 19.2% compared to an incidence of 6.0% in a normal, matched, male control population. Fifty percent of the workers who responded to their work with frustration, irritation, and distress also had sleep disturbances prior to their disease. Twenty percent of the workers not exposed to forced work also had them. Forty percent of the workers with later heart disease whose sleep was disturbed suffered from sleep apnea associated with cardiac arrhythmias. Those at risk who did not have sleep disturbances still maintained high heart rates throughout the night or showed greater heart rate variability during sleep (Siegrist, Klein, and Matschinger 1989).

Summary

A selective review of those categories of personally stressful experiences about which most is known has been carried out. Bereavement, separation, and loss are believed to be the most poignant. They have different outcomes. Grief, along with the (normal) process of mourning by which it resolves, is the most likely to occur and seems to be associated with few physiological perturbations. However, pathological mourning and depression may precede a variety of ominous developments, including the abuse of drugs, an increase in visits to physicians and/or hospitalization, suicide, and disease. The known disease consequences of bereavement may well be mediated through depression, which perturbs or interacts with preexisting, often subclinical, altered function and structure.

However, this sequence of events does not specify the disease that may ensue; other interacting factors do so. But it remains uncertain how many persons in a population of the bereaved grieve, mourn pathologically, or become depressed. Furthermore, much more information is needed in order to specify what a bereaved person is bereft of: What aspect of the past relationship was critically disrupted by the loss?

The information about the acute effects of examinations strongly suggest that patterns of cardiovascular, hormonal, and immune changes occur that vary with gender and are influenced and modified by ongoing collegial relationships. Forced unemployment also has wide-ranging effects on health status—ill health occurs, and dormant disease is expressed. It is accompanied by demoralization, a loss of a sense of control, and an increase in accidents and violence. Several physiological systems are perturbed. The health and well-being of families and the education of children suffer when the breadwinner loses his or her job.

Particular working conditions are conducive to IHD and myocardial infarction. They take control out of the hands of the worker or threaten his or her subsistence. They perturb sleep and the regulation of cardiovascular rhythms.

Despite many gaps in knowledge, a picture emerges of specific experiences that have individual outcomes and are associated with complex behavioral and patterns of physiological changes. They may eventuate in ill health or disease in interaction with specific predispositions.

5 Stressful Experience and Ill Health

One of the purposes in writing this book is to reappraise the relationship of stressful experience to ill health and disease. Ever since Selye's first experiments, students of stress have been inclined to the view that a close link existed between the experience and anatomical damage or lesions, i.e., disease. That conclusion was inevitable because Selye's experiments injured his animals, which were not able to protect themselves against damage.

The crisis and decline of interest in the medical aspects of stress came about because it was realized that stressful experiences did not inevitably, or even frequently, terminate in disease or injury; even in the direst and most catastrophic circumstance, disease was not an inevitable outcome. When everyday stressful experiences, challenges, or tasks occur, such as a bereavement or forced unemployment, only a proportion of persons develop a disease not present beforehand. However, a much larger number show a decline in health: They fall ill, but not with a disease (Morrell 1978). In fact up to 50% of patients seen by physicians are in ill health without having a disease (Juli and Engelbrecht-Greve 1978).

Therefore, the concept of ill health will be the major focus of this chapter. It has been accorded little status in Western biomedicine. And yet its diverse expression is a major source of morbidity, absenteeism from work, and the soaring cost of health care. The ill person also affects his or her family members.

Ill health is not only manifested in the posttraumatic stress disorders, in which sleep disturbances, anxiety attacks, and bodily manifestations occur. The bodily symptoms of the ill person (Mechanic 1980) can be clustered into the hyperventilation, functional bowel, and musculoskeletal syndromes and sleep disturbances. Each of these groups is also strongly associated with anxiety, distress, and depressed moods. These three categories are, however, not mutually exclusive. As the ensuing survey recounts, they are closely linked to stressful experiences.

The importance of these syndromes is considerable. They are often misunderstood and misdiagnosed. Their incorrect diagnosis and inappropriate treatment lead to iatrogenic disease and unnecessary surgery.

The syndromes of ill health may also terminate in disease. Hyperventilating patients with or without coronary artery disease may develop cardiac arrhythmias and other changes in the electrocardiogram. Evidence also exists that anxious and depressed patients have a shortened life span (Coryell, Noyes, and Clarcy 1982; Coryell, Noyes, and House 1986; Haines, Imeson, and Meade 1987; Klerman and Izen 1977).

People who consider themselves to be in poor health have an excess mortality when studied prospectively over a nine-year period. The age-adjusted relative risk for death in those who judge themselves to be in poor health was 5.10 for women and 2.33 for men, when social, educational, familial, economic, and physical health status, depression, and social isolation were controlled for (Kaplan and Camacho 1983). This self-perception acts as a factor per se. The results of the survey do not preclude the roles of other interactive factors in ill health such as smoking, alcohol consumption, job dissatisfaction, and marital discord (Garrity, Somes, and Marx 1978).

This chapter and chapter 6 will attempt to answer the question of why a particular stressful experience may terminate in several different diseases (if it terminates in disease at all) or in ill health. It will put forward the thesis that stressful experiences do not by themselves produce disease; in most instances they constitute one of several interacting risk factors. But such a statement fails to answer the question of how a stressful experience could lead either to physiological ("functional") or anatomical changes in the brain or body: That crucial question remains to be answered.

Stress and Ill Health

Traditional Western medicine is preoccupied with disease. When no alterations in the material structure of organs and cells occur but a patient is in ill health, he/she is either neglected or subjected to unnecessary, repetitive, or inappropriate diagnostic or surgical procedures designed to search out or treat the nonexistent anatomical lesion.

To put it another way: It is customary in medicine to assert that structural changes are the only cause of ill health and the only concern of physicians. Yet a patient may have a disease and either be in good health or be ill. Conversely, a patient may be in ill health without having a disease. But he/she cannot be in both ill and good health at the same time.

Most patients seeking medical care do not have diseases but are in ill health (Morrell 1978). Those in chronically ill health spend seven days a month in bed (in contrast to those in good health, who take off half a day). The annual costs for their care exceeds by a factor of nine the annual expenditure on health care of the average U.S. citizen (Smith, Monson, and Ray 1986b).

They complain of pains in their head, chest, back, gut, and limbs. They vomit or have diarrhea and/or constipation. They over-, under-, or binge-eat. They sigh, swallow air, or breathe excessively or irregularly. They cannot sleep restfully, or they have difficulty falling asleep. Menstruation is sparse, without regularity, or painful. They are fatigued, discontented, depressed, or irritable. They drink too much alcohol. They abuse licit or illicit drugs. Their family life is miserable. They fear disease. They worry about their bodies (Pilowsky 1967; Pilowsky, Smith, and Katsikitis 1987).

As such patients are observed a clear-cut relationship can be found between their ills and their situation in life. They are disappointed and distressed by their lot. They are overwhelmed by the demands placed upon them by unemployment or their work, a low income, poor housing conditions, too many children, and failed dreams. They cannot manage. They appeal to others for advice, help, succor, friendship, and money. If they have nowhere to turn they seek out physicians, who usually do not treat them kindly (Kellner 1986; Lipowski 1986).

Ill health in itself may act as a stressful experience. But very specific experiences also antecede changes in health status (for reviews see Weiner 1983, 1984). They include a mother having to give up her baby for adoption (Condon 1986), losing a spouse (Windholz, Marmar, and Horowitz 1985), forced unemployment (Beale and Nethercott 1986), marital discord, and concerns about children or job security (Chaudhary and Truelove 1962). Uncontrollable and undesirable life experiences are more frequent in patients with functional chest pain (Roll and Theorell 1987). The graver and the more frequent the experience is adjudged to be by the patient, the more days he or she is likely to be symptomatic, to be absent from work, to disrupt daily routine, and to go to physicians (Norman, McFarlane, and Streiner 1985).

As discussed in chapter 4, the threat of, or actual, job loss raises the number of illness episodes, medical consultations, and visits to outpatient clinics (Beale and Nethercott 1986). Previous symptoms of ill health and disability that had abated recur following job loss (Farrow 1984).

Persons in ill health express their distress in bodily symptoms. Attempts to classify and gather these symptoms into mutually exclusive categories are misleading because no one bodily system is their source. The descriptive labels assigned to these clusters have no explanatory power: For example, patients with the functional or irritable bowel disorders have many other symptoms, which cannot possibly have their origin in the gut or any segment thereof (Dotevall 1985). In addition to ubiquitous lower abdominal pain, gas, weight loss, indigestion, and diarrhea and/or constipation, 88% of patients complain of globus, and 87% of nausea, dyspepsia, and heartburn (Dotevall, Svedlund, and Sjödin 1982). They also have headaches, and backaches, and aching muscles. They complain of fatigue and weakness, flushing, worry, anxiety, and depression. They sigh and hyperventilate. Fifty percent fear cancer (Drossman, Powell, and Sessions 1977; Fielding 1984). At least 70% are identifiably anxious (Alpers 1981, 1983; Dotevall 1985); 80% of Hislop's (1971) patients were depressed. At a minimum the whole gut is symptomatic in this disorder. But a change in bowel function cannot possibly account for hyperventilation, headache, or backache. The entire person is afflicted; he or she is in ill health. Yet the relationship of one to another manifestation of ill health—for example, of diarrhea or backache to depression—is largely unsolved.

Some of these manifestations of ill health are also called the somatoform disorders, which have, according to Swartz et al. (1986, 1987), several different subforms: One type is characterized by headache and sexual indifference; a second by headache, oligo- and dysmenorrhea; and a third by headache, depression, and various unpleasant bodily feelings. These three types occur mainly in women (the second, of course, in women exclusively). A fourth group, which occurs predominantly in men, is characterized by musculoskeletal and articular pain, a lump in the throat, hyperventilation, anxiety, and disability. The full gamut of gastrointestinal symptoms, headache, pain, anxiety, depression, unpleasant bodily feelings and disability occurs in a fifth group, also consisting mainly of women. Older men may also have bowel symptoms that they are convinced are the expression of serious disease. A final group is made up of anxious patients who hyperventilate, have fainting spells, have headaches, and eat variably in excess. Headaches, anxiety, pain, and depression may occur in all seven subgroups. Gastrointestinal, menstrual, and hyperventilation symptoms also cluster in women.

Anxiety and fear are known to lead to hyperventilation, which in turn may further heighten fear and anxiety. Episodes of illness may antecede a person's feeling depressed, while high levels of depression result in the increased experience of the symptoms of illness and enhance the risk for subsequent depression (Aneshensel, Frerichs, and Huba 1984).

A more precise analysis of the manifestations of ill health leads to the conclusion that they represent physiological changes in vital biological functions—respiratory and cardiac rhythms, food intake, digestion, elimination, reproduction, sleep rhythms, pain modulation, and mood. Most of these vital functions operate in a rhythmic manner in different time frames. They are disturbed when their usual operating mode undergoes change. They can be perturbed by stressful experiences; in fact such a disruption is the more usual outcome of stressful experiences than is disease. Stressful experiences, as one of the many possible factors involved in the etiology and pathogenesis of disease, has actually a low probability of inciting it: Even in a high-risk population the probability is 0.14 (Mirsky 1958; Weiner et al. 1957). But the accumulated observational evidence is that when stressful experiences are distressing, they manifest themselves as a gamut of bodily symptoms, which are the expression of perturbed biological functions.

These assertions will be supported by a discussion of four of the several syndromes of ill health.

The Hyperventilation Syndrome

This syndrome has been called by many names since it was first described during the American Civil War by DaCosta (1871a). Since 1937 it has been called the hyperventilation syndrome (Kerr, Dalton, and Gliebe 1937) and linked to fear and anxiety. Many controversies still surround it (Paul 1987); nevertheless, some of the main issues about it have been clarified by Magarian (1982).

The acute form of the syndrome is characterized by feelings of weakness, nervousness, fatigue, and headache. Hyperventilating patients sweat, feel weak and giddy, and may faint. Their powers of concentration, and therefore their ability to perform tasks, are impaired. They may panic. They are frightened, tense, and irritable. Their limbs tingle or feel numb. Their perception of the world is altered. Their vision may be blurred or constricted. They feel breathless. They sigh and yawn. They sleep poorly and may awaken out of breath. Their chest muscles ache. They complain that their hearts palpitate and race. They swallow air. They feel bloated, belch, and pass flatus. They complain of heartburn. Their mouth is dry, and their throat feels tight. Their limbs ache and are stiff. They may develop tetanic spasms of their limbs (Magarian 1982).

The acute and chronic, intermittent consequences of fear, anxiety, pain, distress, and depression are expressed in these wide-ranging symptoms. The physiological effects of hyperventilation ensue when the respiratory (ventilatory) effort exceeds the body's need for oxygen. As a result the partial pressure of carbon dioxide ($PaCO_2$) in arterial blood falls, and respiratory alkalosis quickly ensues. The kidney attempts to compensate for the alkalosis by increasing its excretion of bicarbonate, sodium, and potassium ions and by reducing the production of ammonia salts and other acidic metabolites. When hyperventilation continues intermittently, about two-thirds of all patients will show a persistent reduction of $PaCO_2$ (Lum 1976; Magarian 1982, 1989).

If hyperventilation becomes chronic, as it does in many patients, a physiological adaptation occurs: The respiratory center becomes "reset"—it responds to the persistently lower $PaCO_2$ levels in the face of a normalized blood pH (Gennari, Goldstein, and Schwartz 1972). The net effect of this adaptation is to sustain hyperventilation. Further reduction of the $PaCO_2$ sets off a renewed wave of the syndrome. Any sudden change in respiratory rate or in the depth of breathing may start the next bout of symptoms in the chronic hyperventilator: A gasp or sigh may do so. Pain may cause a person to gasp or cry out. Sighing respirations are associated with grief and depression. Fear increases the rate of respiration. Fear and anxiety, in turn, may produce β-adrenergic discharge, conducive to hyperventilation. Beta-adrenergic blocking agents reduce the increased ventilation due to catecholamine release or to breathing CO_2 (Bosisio et al. 1979; Heistad et al. 1972).

One of the metabolic consequences of respiratory alkalosis is hypophosphatemia (Okel and Hurst 1961). A reduction in inorganic phosphorus levels in serum occurs rapidly after the inception of hyperventilation and persists for its duration; it leads to the uptake of phosphorus by cells (Brautbar et al. 1980). Hypophosphatemia can produce a variety of symptoms: disorientation, dizziness, diminished attention, malaise, and paresthesia (Kreisberg 1977)—common manifestations of the hyperventilation syndrome and of the panic-agoraphobic disorder.

Respiratory alkalosis has additional effects on ion fluxes: Extracellular calcium and potassium levels are reduced, leading respectively to heightened neuromuscular excitability and the hyperpolarization of the cell membrane potential. The reduction in $PaCO_2$ tension is also reflected in intracellular alkalosis, leading to increased intracellular calcium concentrations. These in turn stimulate the release of NE from sympathetic neurons, heighten coronary artery tone, and increase peripheral resistance. In myocardial cells, increases in intracellular calcium heighten contractile strength and thus the force of systolic contractions, diminish relaxation, and predispose to arrhythmias by impairing repolarization (Freeman 1987).

Hyperventilating patients may develop sinus tachycardia and arrhythmias at rest. They may show QT interval prolongation, ST-segment elevations or depressions, and T-wave inversion on the electrocardiogram (EKG) (Tzivoni et al. 1980). Supraventricular and ventricular premature beats have been recorded in these patients (Wildenthal, Fuller, and Shapiro 1968).

As a result of hyperventilation vasodilation initially occurs, mean BP falls, and CO and HR increase. A few minutes later vasoconstriction, including of the coronary arteries, occurs (Kontos et al. 1972), and the changes in BP, CO, and HR disappear.

One of the more common symptoms of the hyperventilation syndrome is diffuse chest pain. It can result from the increased respiratory effort and is, therefore, muscular in origin. It can also be due to air swallowing.

In the light of chest pain and changes on the EKG, physicians tend to assume that hyperventilating patients must be suffering from IHD. This assumption may or may not necessarily be correct. The hypocapnic alkalosis of hyperventilation slows coronary blood flow (Neill and Hattenhauer 1975). It produces coronary vasospasm in patients with or without Prinzmetal's variant angina (Mortensen, Vilhelmson, and Sande 1981; Rasmussen et al. 1985; Yasue et al. 1978) or structural coronary artery disease. In fact, hyperventilation in some patients may eventuate in myocardial infarction, probably by producing coronary vasospasm or reducing (coronary) blood flow (Freeman 1987).

It is not known what predisposes to hyperventilation; childhood bronchial asthma may be one factor. Furthermore, the hyperventilation syndrome may start in childhood. Its characteristics and outcome in children have virtually not been studied; the only recent outcome study showed that it continued into adulthood in 40% of children followed for twenty-five years (Herman, Stickler, and Lucas 1981).

Although it is possible to link the onset of episodes of hyperventilation in the individual chronic hyperventilator to certain emotions (Lum 1976)—grief, pain, depression, excitement, fear, and anxiety—no systematic studies have been carried out on the stressful experiences that incite them. Nor do we know what predisposes to hyperventilation in the first place, or why some patients become chronic hyperventilators and others do not.

Additionally, much still needs to be learned about the pathogenetic mechanisms of hyperventilation (rather than its pathophysiology) and the mechanisms that lead to coronary vasospasm.

Stressful Experience and Sudden Death: The Long QT Syndrome

An especially convincing and tragic example of the role of stressful experience is provided by a syndrome that produces sudden death in children and adolescents. This disaster is mediated by the sympathetic nervous system and occurs when an inherited functional disturbance in the electrical activity of the heart is present from birth on. This disorder is called the long QT syndrome. It is characterized by an interval of more than 440 msec between these two EKG waves. These young people also have a low HR. Their EKGs manifest alternating positive and negative T-waves.

As a consequence of the apparent disturbance in electrical conductance, abnormal ventricular repolarization occurs. With sudden perturbations of the patient, the patient faints or may die suddenly. Unless medical intervention takes place, two-thirds of these young people eventually die, having abruptly developed ventricular tachycardia and fibrillation. The triggering events are most often either exercise, fear occasioned by loud, startling noises or frightening games, or excitement; less frequently fainting or death occurs on awakening or during menstrual periods.

These triggering events and exercise are mediated by a specific regulatory disturbance involving the right and left sympathetic cardioaccelerator nerves; the neuronal activity in the former is lower, and in the latter higher, than normal. In dogs, it can be shown that electrical stimulation of the left stellate ganglion produces ventricular tachycardia, whereas stimulating the right ganglion produces sinus tachycardia. (These experiments validate the hypothesis guiding an understanding of the QT syndrome in children and adults.)

Further support for the idea that such inciting events and exercise are mediated by sudden sympathetic discharge through the left stellate ganglion is provided by the demonstration that children who undergo left stellate ganglionectomy are saved from syncope and death. Propanolol also averts this disaster but is a less reliable form of treatment because many of these young patients are noncompliant (Schwartz 1990).

The Irritable Bowel Syndrome: Functional Disturbances of the Gut

There is no agreed-upon definition or subclassification of the irritable bowel syndrome (IBS). In the English and Irish literature "functional gastrointestinal disorders" (Lennard-Jones 1983) and "IBS" (Fielding 1984) are names for symptoms and disturbances that emanate from every part of the alimentary tract—from the mouth to the anus. Other British authors (Chaudhary and Truelove 1962) and most American gastroenterologists prefer to limit these names to the syndrome of pain and diarrhea and/or constipation (Drossman, Powell, and Sessions 1977; Latimer 1983; Schuster 1983) that is ascribed to a disturbance of colonic function.

There is increasing evidence, however, to support the belief that when the predominant symptoms emanate from the colon, disturbances of function (not only symptoms) occur throughout the alimentary tract. This statement is based on several lines of evidence: The lower esophageal sphincter pressure (13.8 vs. 23.8 cm H_2O) is lower in patients with IBS than in control subjects (Whorwell, Clouter, and Smith 1981). Jejunal motility is decreased (Thompson, Laidlaw, and Wingate 1979). Migratory motor complexes (MMCs) are normally as frequent during the day as during the night, but in patients with IBS, jejunal MMCs are reduced. Abdominal pain is then associated with an irregular nocturnal pattern of contraction, which does not, as is the custom, terminate in MMCs. The MMCs are usually abolished by meals and by a procedure such as delayed auditory feedback (Valori, Kumar, and Wingate 1986; Wingate, Valori, and Kumar 1989). In patients with IBS the effect of this stressful experimental procedure on MMCs is much more immediate and long-lasting (McRae et al. 1982). Transit time of a solid meal from mouth to cecum and through the entire gut in patients with IBS whose symptoms were mainly of diarrhea is twice as fast as in normal subjects. The transit time for constipated patients is, however, considerably longer (Read 1980). By a different technique (using radiopaque pellets rather than food) in a mixed group of patients with IBS and other gastrointestinal diseases, no such changes in transit time are observed (Taylor et al. 1978; Taylor, Darby, and Hammond 1978).

The ubiquity of IBS is attested to by the fact that in a nonrandom English population sample 20.6% had the experience of abdominal pain six times in one year. In 13% of this whole population the pain was believed to emanate from the region of the colon. Six percent had painless constipation, whereas 3.7% had diarrhea (Thompson and Heaton 1979). In a U.S. sample of a "healthy" population the figure for the prevalence of abdominal pain and symptoms of IBS in one year was 17% (Drossman 1982). The lifetime prevalence rate of IBS has been estimated to be 50–75% (Texter and Butler 1975); only 10% of sufferers are ever seen by a physician (Wadsworth, Butterfield, and Blaney 1971). Nonetheless, more than half of the clients of gastroenterologists in the United States suffer from one or another form of IBS (Drossman, Powell, and Sessions 1977).

In 1976 the U.S. Digestive Disease Commission reported that 115,000 patients were discharged with the diagnosis of either psychogenic gastrointestinal disorders or IBS as the primary reason for hospitalization. In another 103,000 patients these two diagnostic categories were applied as a secondary diagnosis. Together, the diagnoses accounted for 450,000 hospital days (Mendeloff 1983).

Functional Disturbances of the Esophagus

Patients with disturbances in esophageal motility may also complain of dyspepsia ("heartburn"), while 87% of patients with predominantly colonic symptoms of IBS also complain of dyspeptic symptoms due to acid regurgitation, heartburn, and epigastric pain (Dotevall, Svedlund, and Sjödin 1982). Nonetheless, it is a tradition in medicine to treat each symptom in isolation and to subdivide the IBS into mutually exclusive categories (Truelove and Reynell 1972).

The symptoms of esophageal motility disturbances are, in diminishing order of frequency, difficulty in swallowing (with or without chest pain), nausea and "heartburn," chest pain with "heartburn" alone, or a "lump" in the throat (Clouse and Lustman 1983).

GLOBUS. Globus is a very common symptom, present in about 50% of a population (Thompson and Heaton 1982). The "lump" in the throat may be associated with difficulty in, and pain on, swallowing (emanating from the upper esophagus), an excessive perception of the glossal papillae, and the complaint of "bad breath" (Fielding 1984). It may be present between as well as during meals, and it may not be associated with any swallowing difficulty.

No consensus has been reached as to the psychological correlates of globus. Originally considered to be the prototypical hysterical symptom, it is now believed to occur more frequently in depressed and obsessional patients (Lehtinen and Puhakka 1976). Bereaved persons commonly experience a sensation of tightness in the throat and swallowing difficulty, very often when they are fighting back their tears.

Globus is not a homogeneous or isolated symptom; it may also occur with gastroesophageal reflux (Hunt, Connell, and Smiley 1970); in this instance it is probably associated with the repetitive effort reflexly to clear the esophagus of gastric acid. Gastroenterologists still seek a single cause for globus. Actually, its antecedents are heterogeneous: It has no one "cause." Schuster (1983) considers globus to be due to a heightened awareness of cricopharyngeal contraction. Jacobs and Kirkpatrick (1964) believe that it is merely due to an increase in size of the webs and folds of the hypopharynx in 86% of patients complaining of globus; but they do not tell us what its origin is.

AIR SWALLOWING (aerophagia). Little is known about a tendency to swallow saliva and air during, or independent of, the drinking of liquids or the eating of food. Almy (1983) defines aerophagia as a "habit pattern" associated with anxiety and other emotions. It may produce pain in the neck or behind the lower end of the sternum. The swallowing of air is often accompanied by nausea and belching. (There are many other reasons why gaseousness and eructation may occur; they may accompany diseases of the upper gastrointestinal and biliary tract, sinusitis, the gulping of liquids and bolting of food, the drinking of carbonated liquids and alcohol, the ingestion of bicarbonate, bacterial fermentation, abnormal intestinal bacterial flora or unusual substrates for normal flora [Roth 1973], and the chronic hyperventilation syndrome.)

In most instances air is swallowed through a relaxed upper esophageal sphincter, either at will or unbeknownst to the patient. It then accumulates in the stomach. At times, the lower esophageal sphincter is tonically contracted (Almy 1983), allowing less air to be expelled by mouth than was originally swallowed, leading to a feeling of upper abdominal fullness and dilatation after meals, bloating, substernal or precordial pressure, shortness of breath, and hiccuping or flatulence (Roth 1973).

GASTROESOPHAGEAL REFLUX AND REFLUX ESOPHAGITIS. Gastroesophageal reflux (GER) occurs in virtually everyone but only becomes symptomatic in some persons. It manifests itself as "heartburn," substernal pain, and/or awakening at night with gastric acid in the mouth or coughing spells. It may produce esophagitis and esophageal strictures (Dent et al. 1980). Characteristically the pain is relieved by sitting up or taking neutralizing antacids. But reflux can occur in the upright as well as the recumbent position.

Usually the esophagus is cleared of acids by a reflex, peristaltic wave. In those subject to esophagitis this rhythmic process is less efficient during sleep than it is in normal persons (Johnson and DeMeester 1974; Orr, Robinson, and Johnson 1981). A diminished resting tone of the lower esophageal sphincter is present in patients (Orr 1983). But the matter may be even more complex (Dent et al. 1980). In sleep there is little relationship between the refluxing of acid and the resting pressure of the lower sphincter. Rather, patients with GER awaken too briefly during the night to clear their esophagus of acid, nor do they constrict the sphincter protectively. Thus, in addition to local disturbance in function, GER appears to be a form of sleep disturbance.

DIFFUSE ESOPHAGEAL SPASM. Intermittent, sharp substernal pain and dysphagia are associated with this form of spasm. In one-half of all patients spasm is precipitated by swallowing a meal (Castell 1976; Cohen 1979; Vantrappen and Hellemans 1983); in other patients it is not. Diffuse esophageal spasm is brought on by nonperistaltic, repetitive waves, which occur especially in the lower portions of the esophagus. They may become long in duration and high in amplitude. Other abnormalities of esophageal motility have also been recorded: "tetanic" responses to a single swallow (Gillies, Nicks, and Skyring 1967; Roth and Fleshler 1964); spontaneous contractions independent of the act of swallowing; and interrupted peristalsis.

These motility disturbances can be conceptualized in new ways: The nonperistaltic tetanus is a form of oscillatory instability. The parameters of the usual waves have also undergone a transition into a new frequency, amplitude, and form. They may suddenly and unpredictably be abolished (interrupted). In about one-third of all patients the lower esophageal sphincter does not relax during the spasm (DiMarino and Cohen 1974); in the remainder it does. The lower sphincter may be under higher pressure, or it may go into rhythmic contractions at normal pressures (Gillies, Nicks, and Skyring 1967; Graham 1978).

Thus various of transitions in rhythmic motility patterns are associated with esophageal spasm. Spasm can also be produced by gastric acid reflux. It may be stress-related (Cohen 1973) or occur for unknown reasons in elderly patients (Ingelfinger 1958; Schuster 1983) and during pregnancy (Nagler and Spiro 1961).

SYMPTOMATIC PERISTALSIS. Another variant of an esophageal motility disorder is associated with normal, progressive, peristaltic waves, which are, however, increased in amplitude and/or longer in duration. Substernal (angina-like) pain and dysphagia are also complained of. In these patients, the drug ergonovine induces the larger, longer-lasting waves (Benjamin, Gerhardt, and Castell 1977; London et al. 1981). Patients with noncardiac chest pain in whom the parameters of esophageal motion go through various transitions also have a lower pain threshold to artificial distention of the organ (Richter, Barish, and Castell 1986). Thus both the sensory and motor functions of the esophagus are altered.

MOTILITY DISTURBANCES AND CHEST PAIN. The clinical importance of esophageal motility disturbances, particularly in esophagitis, diffuse spasm, and symptomatic peristalsis, cannot be overemphasized, because they may mimic IHD (Bennett and Atkinson 1966; Brand, Martin, and Pope 1977; Vantrappen and Hellemans 1983). In 100 consecutive emergency-room patients with anterior chest pain, 77 complained of the symptoms of angina pectoris. In 61 of these the pain was due to IHD, and in 16 it was due to an esophageal motility disturbance. In 4 of the 16 the disturbance consisted of diffuse esophageal spasm, and 8 had esophagitis on endoscopy. Acid perfusion of the esophagus reproduced the pain in 5 patients (Davies, Jones, and Rhodes 1982). A predominant number of them were also anxious and depressed (Clouse and Lustman 1983).

But the matter becomes even more complex because chest pain can occur with normal esophageal manometrics. And other patients do not complain of such pain despite having diffuse-spasm, high-amplitude, or long-lasting esophageal peristaltic waves. Presumably, patients vary in their thresholds to pain.

Dysphagia may also occur with normal manometric tracings; when they are abnormal they take the form of diffuse spasm in one-quarter of patients and of high-amplitude long-lasting waves in the remainder (Brand, Martin, and Pope 1977).

PHYSIOLOGY, PHARMACOLOGY, AND PSYCHOPHYSIOLOGY OF ESOPHAGEAL FUNCTION. The usual stepwise primary and secondary peristaltic movements of the esophagus and its sphincters are regulated and coordinated by brain stem reticular mechanisms, which are under volitional control. Esophageal sphincters and motility are under the control of multiple neurotransmitters and hormones. Lower esophageal resting pressure is raised by metoclopromide, a dopamine antagonist, and cholinergic agonists (Mellow 1977). Esophageal spasm may be induced by α-adrenergic agonists in some predisposed persons. The resting pressure of the lower esophageal sphincter is reduced by secretin, nicotine, alcohol, anticholinergics, and the female sex hormones.

It has been known for years that nonpropulsive esophageal waves may occur with stressful experience (Jacobson 1927; Rubin et al. 1962). They are reduced by relaxation and during sleep. On the other hand, heightened anxiety enhances dysphagia when esophageal motility is already disturbed (Rubin et al. 1962). Sounds above 1,000 Hz produce nonpropulsive contractions of the esophagus, which are part of the "defense" reaction and habituate in time

(Stacher 1983). Additionally, it has been shown that aerophagia can be eliminated (Johnson, DeMeester, and Haggitt 1978), and the resting pressure of the lower esophageal sphincter can be reduced, by biofeedback (Schuster, Nikoomanesh, and Wells 1973).

ESOPHAGEAL CONTRACTION ABNORMALITIES AND PSYCHOPATHOLOGY. Clouse and Lustman (1983) carried out esophageal manometry on 50 patients, of whom 25 were found to have contraction abnormalities: 13 of them complained of chest pain only, 31 had dysphagia with chest pain or heartburn, and 2 experienced only heartburn. Not one but four kinds of manometric abnormalities were discovered in the 25 patients: 5 had diffuse spasm; 18 had an increase in the duration and amplitude of the contractions, abnormal motor responses, and triphasic waves; 1 had esophageal refluxing; and 1 had a distal esophageal ring.

All of the 25 patients were depressed, suffered from an anxiety, phobic, or somatization disorder, and/or were alcohol- or drug-dependent. Seventeen of 25 other patients (with normal manometric patterns, or minor and "nonspecific" motility disturbances, reflux esophagitis, or achalasia) were free of any discernible psychopathology.

NONULCER DYSPEPSIA. The symptoms of another supposedly distinct form of IBS—dyspepsia—are nausea and/or vomiting, eructation, and heartburn, retrosternal pain, epigastric bloating and/or pain, acid regurgitation, rapid satiety, and occasionally weight loss. They may either be aggravated or relieved by eating food. The diagnosis rests upon the exclusion of one of the many forms of gastritis, of liver, heart, kidney, and gall bladder disease, and of alcoholism, and peptic ulceration; it is also made when a patient fails to respond to a drug such as cimetidine. (An increasingly frequent cause of dyspepsia is the use of nonsteroidal antiinflammatory drugs.)

The usual symptoms of nonulcer dyspepsia enumerated above are frequently accompanied by loose or frequent stools, lower abdominal pain relieved by defecation, and abdominal distention (Hill and Blendis 1967; Manning et al. 1978; Möllman et al. 1976). These additional symptoms are only reported by some patients; when they are present they clearly suggest that (some?) forms of nonulcer dyspepsia are part of a more general IBS.

According to some authorities the only true discriminant between nonulcer dyspepsia and peptic ulcer is that patients with the former are younger, tend to complain of nausea and vomiting, and do not have epigastric pain at night or a family history of peptic ulcer disease (Crean et al. 1982; Dotevall 1985; Horrocks and DeDomball 1978).

Sixty percent of 775 patients with dyspepsia do not demonstrate a peptic ulcer or other structural gastric or duodenal disease. In 45% of 200 patients with nonulcer dyspepsia the gastric mucosa is normal; 36% show slight mucosal surface erosions; in 14.5% a chronic atrophic gastritis is present; and a chronic superficial gastritis occurs in 4.5% (Williams et al. 1957). Dyspeptic patients who do, and those who do not, show gastritis cannot be differentiated on the basis of their symptoms. Furthermore, only 65 to 70% of patients with demonstrable gastritis complain of any symptoms (Edwards and Coghill 1968; Kreuning et al. 1978; Volpicelli, Yardley, and Hendrix 1977).

Until recently, these anatomical data were in all likelihood the product of sampling errors: A single mucosal biopsy may miss patches of gastritis; multiple biopsy samples need to be taken. In those patients with nonulcer dyspepsia the gastritis when present consists of polymorphonuclear infiltration of the gastric epithelium and lamina propria. It is often associated with esophagitis and duodenitis, for which there are no agreed-upon anatomical criteria. Duodenitis may antecede, or occur with or without, peptic duodenal ulceration. Twelve of 18 patients with nonulcer dyspepsia had a greater number of gastrin-containing cells (G-cells) in the gastric antrum than normal subjects. Only 4 of the 12 had a superficial gastritis. Nine showed only a duodenitis with normal serum gastrin levels. Six patients had an atrophic gastritis of various degrees, and in 4 of these a duodenitis was also present. The number of antral G-cells was the same in the 6 as in the control subjects, but they had elevated serum gastrin levels (Piris and Whitehead 1975). In this small group of patients with nonulcer dyspepsia, heterogeneity exists, both anatomically and physiologically.

Regrettably, the clinical histories of these patients are not available. Therefore, it is not possible to assess whether their symptoms were incited by alcohol or other liquids, solids, a particular component of food, or stressful experiences. The question of whether liquids or solids produce symptoms is no trivial matter. The tonic activity of the gastric fundus is mainly responsible for the emptying of liquids, whereas the grinding and emptying of solids is carried out by the antrum (Kelly 1983).

Various forms of changes in gastric motility have been described in one-half of 70 patients with nonulcer dyspepsia. They were especially prone to nausea on awakening, often associated with retching, dry "heaves" and the vomiting of bile (Chey et al. 1983). They tolerated liquids better than solids. (Eleven of the 31 patients also had lower abdominal cramps or pain and diarrhea and/or constipation—symptoms of IBS.) Instead of the usual rhythmic 3–4 cycles per minutes (cpm) pacesetter potential recorded from the antrum of the stomach, two different kinds of transitions in motility were recorded: an irregular 5 cpm rhythm (tachyarrhythmia); or a regular 7 cpm rhythm followed by silent periods (tachygastria). Backward propagation of slow waves also occurred. A third change in rhythm was seen in 2 patients—an intermittent 1–2 cpm pacesetter potential (You et al. 1980, 1981). Thus in patients with this form of dyspepsia, several kinds of parametric changes in gastric motility are seen—in its regular form and its frequency.

Patients with nonulcer dyspepsia share another feature in common with patients with esophageal motility disturbances and IBS: They become aware of gastric discomfort and pain at much lower volumes of fluid infused to distend the stomach (Dotevall 1985).

Irritable Colon Syndrome

Patients with IBS of the so-called colonic variety mainly suffer from clusters of symptoms: colicky abdominal pain (in 85–90%), which is often much enhanced by eating (in 75%) and relieved by a bowel movement; constipation and/or diarrhea (in 80%); gas; mucous in the stool (in 25%), and weight loss (in 20%) (Drossman, Powell, and Sessions 1977; Fielding 1984). Characteristically the physician focuses on these symptoms while failing to take note of the fact that a considerable proportion of these patients also complain of globus, nausea and vomiting, bloating sensations after meals, headache, backache, flushing, fatigue, anxiety and depression, sighing respirations, and hyperventilation (Dotevall 1985; Drossman, Powell, and Sessions 1977). They frequently have cool and sweaty palms and brisk reflexes. They smile (often in embarrassment) and describe their symptoms vaguely. They fear that they have cancer (50%). They have had unnecessary and repeated abdominal operations, which result from incorrect diagnosis (Chaudhary and Truelove 1962; Fielding 1984).

These facts should alert physicians that IBS is an illness of distressed persons, not of the colon (Weiner 1988). Nonetheless, the diarrhea may be the result of lactase deficiency (McMichael, Webb, and Dawson 1965; Weser et al. 1965) or the malabsorption of bile salts (Thayson and Pedersen 1976). Yet lactase deficiency may occur without symptoms (Peña and Truelove 1972).

It is often forgotten that DaCosta (1871b) reported what is now called IBS. (He also described soldier's heart—the hyperventilation syndrome.) Both syndromes were found in soldiers exposed to the danger of battle. But later physicians drew no conclusions from the self-evident connection of danger, fear, and bowel symptoms. It remained for Chaudhary and Truelove (1962) in their series of 130 patients to explicate the fact that fear and worry were associated with the onset or exacerbations of this chronic, yet intermittent, disorder. These emotions were identifiable in 77% of patients with IBS and in 87.5% of patients with painless diarrhea. They appeared more commonly in women patients who were concerned about their children or worried about their (unhappy) marriages; these women had always been worriers or fearful people. The men were more likely to be concerned about their occupations and job security. Many reported a prior history of bacterial dysentery, in addition to their current worries and fears; when both were present the prognosis of the disorder was considerably worse.

Many patients with IBS have identifiable psychiatric illness and also describe antecedent stressful experiences at its onset. The diagnosis of psychopathology does not, however, tell us what role it plays in IBS: Does it precede, or is it the consequence of, being overly concerned about the bowel symptoms, which may be frightening, painful, embarrassing, and inconvenient? Nonetheless, a frequent association exists between IBS and the incidence of anxiety (Esler and Goulston 1973) and depression (Hislop 1971). In Hislop's series (1971) 80% were depressed. A similar incidence (72%) of depression occurred in patients with IBS when they were compared to patients with other forms of chronic bowel disease, in whom it occurred in 18% (Alpers 1981, 1983; Young et al. 1976).

Fourteen percent of patients with anxiety neurosis and the hyperventilation syndrome complained of diarrhea as a solitary symptom (Wheeler et al. 1950). In view of the much greater aggregation (72–80%) of anxiety disorders and IBS some additional factors must be present, but it is not clear what they are. Patients whose IBS was characterized mainly by diarrhea can be classified independently as suffering from an anxiety or a somatization disorder. When constipation and pain predominated patients were either depressed or suffering from a somatization disorder. In two-thirds of both groups of patients the psychiatric symptoms anteceded IBS (Alpers 1981, 1983).

PSYCHOGENIC ABDOMINAL PAIN. Another group of patients suffers only from abdominal pain (Drossman 1982), headaches, joint and back pains, and fatigue. Not every specialist recognizes this syndrome, which occurs mainly in young women. The abdominal pain is recurrent. The illness is of 6 months' duration or more. The women tend to be either histrionic, pain-prone, hypochondriacal, or depressed. In some of these patients the abdominal pain began in a setting of bereavement or separation (Drossman 1982; Gomez and Dally 1977). (A history in childhood of bereavement or illness is also more frequent in IBS patients than in those with inflammatory bowel disease or in a healthy control population [Mendeloff et al. 1970].)

The Physiology and Psychophysiology
of the Irritable Colon Syndrome

The topic of the physiology of the colonic variety of the IBS falls into a number of different categories—attempts to understand the basis of symptoms, to identify some especial physiological feature of the IBS that might help as a diagnostic criterion, or to explain its etiology, pathogenesis, or pathophysiology.

PAIN. The cramping abdominal pain that is a feature of IBS is believed to be a correlate of an increase in the frequency of small-bowel or colonic contractions (Connell, Jones, and Rowlands 1965; Holdstock, Misiewicz, and Waller 1969; Horowitz and Farrar 1962). But the matter may be more complex than merely a matter of motility. Patients with IBS may have lower tolerance to pain or, alternatively, a heightened sensitivity to it. Although they frequently complain of gaseous bloating accompanied by pain, the quantity and quality of intestinal gas is the same as in normal subjects (Lasser, Bond, and Levitt 1975, Levitt and Bond 1983). When the colon is experimentally distended in a stepwise manner with 60 to 160 cc of air, pain is likely to be produced at lower volumes in more IBS patients (55%) than in normal subjects (6%) (Ritchie 1973; Whitehead, Engel, and Schuster 1980)—a finding that could not be confirmed by Latimer et al. (1979, 1981). The perception of pain appears to be the same in IBS patients as in normal persons, but the tolerance to it differs (Whitehead, Engel, and Schuster 1980). This conclusion is supported by the fact that some patients with functional abdominal pain may otherwise also be pain-prone.

ALTERED COLONIC MOTILITY. Almy and his colleagues (1947, 1949a, 1949b, 1950) first demonstrated that constipated patients with IBS were prone to altered parameters (increased frequency, amplitude, and duration) of sigmoid-colonic contractions, whereas in those with diarrhea the parameters were decreased—observations that have repeatedly been confirmed by other investigators (Bloom, LoPresti, and Farrar 1968; Chaudhary and Truelove 1961; Misiewicz, Connell, and Pontes 1966; Waller, Misiewicz, and Kiley 1972; Wangel and Deller 1965). These changed patterns can also be induced by meals, which in some IBS patients are particularly likely to lead to diarrhea. These observations are not surprising, because many different drugs and toxins producing diarrhea in animals and man are associated with hypomotility, but with obstipating agents and in patients with simple constipation, hypermotile colonic patterns occur (Powell 1977; Truelove 1966).

Other transitions in motility have been observed: The response of the colon to fecal matter or air may be different in IBS patients than in the normal person. The response of distending the rectosigmoid colon with 20 cc of air in a stepwise manner produces an immediate, solitary contraction in normal persons. In both symptomatic and nonsymptomatic patients with IBS, the response is delayed and multiple contractions take place; in other words, dilating the colon produces oscillatory instability, for reasons poorly understood (Whitehead, Engel, and Schuster 1980). But these findings have not been replicated in all patients. Connell, Jones, and Rowlands (1965) found no differences in colonic motility between patients with the "spastic" form of IBS and patients with duodenal ulcer. But they did find that patients with both diagnoses who suffered abdominal pain after meals showed a doubling of the frequency of colonic motility after eating.

Latimer (1983) has pointed out that no consistent differences have been found between normal persons and those with IBS, even when patients with painless diarrhea or diarrhea-prone patients (who do not have IBS) are excluded from studies. Based on his own recent work and that with his colleagues (1979), comparing IBS patients and psychoneurotic, normal subjects, during baseline monitoring, a neutral stimulus, and then a stressful interview, a meal, or an intramuscular injection of neostigmine (0.5 mg), he has concluded that no contractile differences exist between these various groups. Marked individual variation in motor activity characterizes each group of patients (Latimer et al. 1981). It is also quite likely that IBS is heterogeneous in nature. Therefore, intergroup and intragroup differences exist. In fact, the foregoing review already suggests that IBS consists of a minimum of two groups—a predominantly sensory one and a predominantly motor one (Weiner 1988).

MYOELECTRICAL ACTIVITY OF THE COLON. The colon has pacemaker, electrical activities that differ from those of the rest of the gut. Whereas only two types of electrical activity are known in the stomach, the colon has four kinds (Sarna 1983). But only two of these four activities have been extensively studied in IBS: a slower (2.5–4 cpm) and a faster (6–9 cpm) basic electrical rhythm (Christensen 1971; Daniel 1975; Misiewicz 1975). Normally 10 to 15% of a unit of time is occupied by the slower rhythm, and the remainder of the time by the faster one. In patients with IBS, the proportion of slow electrical activity is increased threefold, leading to increased segmental motor activity (Snape, Carlson, and Cohen 1976; Snape et al. 1977; Snape and Cohen 1979; Taylor et al. 1974). Injections of pentagastrin and cholecystokinin (CCK) enhance, and glucagon diminishes, the incidence of low-frequency waves in normal persons and in IBS patients (Snape et al. 1977; Taylor et al. 1974, 1975). However, the increased incidence of the slow waves is unrelated to the symptoms of IBS, because it also occurs in patients who either suffer from diarrhea or constipation or are asymptomatic (Taylor, Darby, and Hammond 1978; Taylor et al. 1978).

Latimer (1983) has pointed out that Snape, Carlson, and Cohen (1976) had claimed that the peak distributions of the two frequencies were discontinuous. But Taylor and colleagues (1978) found a continuous spectrum of frequencies, and that peak frequencies were simultaneously present. In fact, no differences were detected in IBS patients and controls with respect to the incidence of low-frequency myoelectric activity (Latimer et al. 1979; Sarna et al. 1980). The heterogeneity among IBS patients in regard to the various parameters of the duration of spike bursting electrical activity rather than in their frequency is likely (Bueno et al. 1980). One must conclude that the matter of a specific myoelectric abnormality in IBS is by no means settled, because the syndrome may not constitute a uniform entity.

EFFECTS OF MEALS IN IBS. A subgroup of IBS patients exists in which meals bring on abdominal pain and/or diarrhea. But the role of meals in producing such symptoms remains unsettled (Waller, Misiewicz, and Kiley 1972; Wangel and Deller 1965). Sullivan, Cohen, and Snape (1978) and Snape and Cohen (1979) found that patients show a delay in the onset of colonic motility with a 1,000-calorie meal. The contractions also last much longer (80 vs. 50 minutes) than in normal persons and are associated with myoelectric activity at a predominant frequency of 6–7 cpm (rather than 10–11 cpm).

MEDIATORS OF STRESSFUL EXPERIENCE IN IBS. We are only at the beginning of our understanding of how stressful experiences could possibly alter the parameters of gastrointestinal contractions, abolish MMCs, and produce oscillatory instability in the esophagus, stomach, and colon. Some experts maintain that these phenomena are merely the expression of the enteric nervous system or gut peptides—i.e., of local processes. Other students of the problem hold to the view that they are the direct expression of vagally mediated phenomena affecting contractions (Dotevall 1985). A third group emphasizes that the enteric nervous system is perturbed by superordinate neural and hormonal influences: For example, CRF increases colonic transport in rats (Taché, Stephens, and Ishikawa 1989).

At first, these "descending" influences were mainly laid at the door of the biogenic amines. Yet Latimer (1983) found no effect of neostigmine on colonic motility in patients with IBS. But others have demonstrated that parasympathomimetic agents do increase sigmoid activity in patients with a "spastic" colon and painless diarrhea (Chaudhary and Truelove 1961) and in normal control patients (Wangel and Deller 1965). In fact, the effect of neostigmine is by no means settled (Champion 1973; Connell et al. 1964; Misiewicz, Connell, and Pontes 1966). When it acts, it also does so in patients with diverticulosis (Chowdhury, Dinoso, and Lorber 1976; Painter and Truelove 1964).

Segmental rectosigmoid contractions are observed in two-thirds of patients with constipation regardless of whether it is associated with diverticulosis or IBS (Powell 1977; Truelove 1966). They are abolished by atropine and glucagon (Chowdhury, Dinoso, and Lorber 1976). Conversely, bradykinin and serotonin (5-HT) produce diarrhea and colonic hypomotility in subjects with both constipation and diarrhea (Murrell and Deller 1967).

The prostaglandins (PGS, both of the E and F series), injected intravenously, also decrease motility and cause diarrhea (Hunt, Delawari, and Misiewicz 1975; Konturek 1978). Prostaglandin E_2 (PGE$_2$), levels in the jejunal fluid in patients with IBS have been measured: In 2 of 15 with alternating diarrhea and constipation, and in 10 of 17 with chronic "nervous" diarrhea, they were elevated. In 6 of the latter group of patients, indomethacin (a PG antagonist) decreased stool volume and frequency, and in 2 it lowered PGE$_2$ levels (Bukhave and Rask-Madsen 1980). Elevated levels of PGs have also been found in the blood of children with diarrhea (Dodge et al. 1981) and in the stools of food-intolerant patients with IBS (Jones et al. 1982).

A potential role for gut peptides is suspected in IBS; some alter gut motility and are also released by food. The gastric inhibitory polypeptide (GIP) is released by protein and carbohydrate. Cholecystokinin secretion by the pancreas is stimulated by fat and protein. Both of these, and calcitonin, glucagon, secretin, neurotensin (NT), substance P, and vasoactive intestinal peptide (VIP) induce intestinal fluid and electrolyte secretion. (They can also produce diarrhea.) At the same time these peptides have opposite effects on motility: Gastrin, bombesin (Porreca, Sheldon, and Burks 1989), CCK, and motilin increase it; and secretin, glucagon, GIP, VIP, and pancreatic polypeptide (PP) diminish it (Harvey 1979).

Nonetheless, there is no established evidence that levels of any of these gut hormones are altered in IBS. Neither in the fasting, nor in the postprandial, state are blood levels of gastrin, insulin, GIP, PP, motilin, enteroglucagon, or NT significantly different than in control subjects (Besterman et al. 1981). Yet in another study, motilin and PP were raised in response to drinking water in patients with the constipation and diarrhea of IBS (Preston et al. 1983).

It is of course possible that blood levels of peptides remain normal, but that some of these peptides have local effects on the gut, that the intestinal musculature or mucosal cells have a heightened sensitivity to normal levels of one or other of them, or that their interactions or regulatory and counterregulatory effects on motility and secretion are altered.

Cholecystokinin increases small-intestinal and colonic motor activity in animals and humans (Dinoso et al. 1973; Glossi et al. 1966; Gutierrez, Chey, and Dinoso 1974). In 4 of 8 patients with IBS who showed marked increases in the duration and amplitude of colonic contractions and complained of abdominal pain on eating, the injection of CCK reproduced the pain and change in contractions (Harvey and Read 1973). However, Chowdhury, Dinoso, and Lorber (1976) found that a hyperactive colonic segment in constipated IBS patients was unaffected by CCK and secretin. Thus CCK may play a role in inducing the abdominal pain induced by eating, but not in any other symptom of IBS.

PSYCHOPHYSIOLOGY. That some emotions may change gastrointestinal motility, mucosal blood flow, or mucous secretion has been known since the time of Pavlov (1910) and Cannon (1929). These observations were significantly extended in normal human beings by Almy and various colleagues (1947, 1949a, 1949b, 1950), and many others, since that time. Specific correlations between increases in colonic contractions and mucosal engorgement and pain, fear, anger, excitement, tenseness, withholding, and coping have been made. Giving up and hopelessness produce a diminution of contractions (Chowdhury, Dinoso, and Lorber 1976; Connell 1962; Wangel and Deller 1965). Indeed, deeply depressed patients are constipated, yet giving up, depression, and hopelessness are associated with diminished colonic contractions, which should theoretically produce diarrhea!

In all likelihood, the changes associated with the emotions have no specificity; they occur in normal persons and those with IBS or ulcerative colitis (Almy, Abbott, and Hinkle 1950; Chaudhary and Truelove 1962). Furthermore, marked individual differences are seen in the colonic response to generating strong, short-term emotions in IBS patients and in normal subjects (Almy, Abbott, and Hinkle 1950; Latimer et al. 1981). In fact, the laboratory may not be the place in which these relationships can, or should be sought. To add to the puzzle further, both the arousal of an emotional response and food produce the same colonic responses in patients with IBS of various categories (Wangel and Deller 1965).

Studies on the psychophysiology of the colon have not identified any specific characteristic of IBS patients. But no other kinds of studies to date have done so either. Thus one must conclude that pain or emotion may change colonic motility over the short term. The common occurrence of anxiety and depression in patients does not, however, explain the etiology or the pathogenesis of IBS.

Fibromyositis (Fibrositis, Fibromyalgia)

Two groups of symptoms—(1) pain, discomfort, and stiffness in the muscles supporting the head, in the neck and shoulders, and in the lower back radiating rather diffusely into the legs, and (2) sleep disturbances associated with fatigue during the day, and feeling unrefreshed on awakening—are among the commonest complaints made by patients with fibromyositis. They constitute one of the main manifestations of ill health.

In one Canadian study of 500 families picked at random, 36% had such pains, which in 11% were chronic (Crook, Rideout, and Browne 1984). Other kinds of surveys have revealed that 32% of a population had some kind of sleep disturbance (Bixler et al. 1979), including the one already described.

On the surface, the relationship of pain and discomfort to disturbed sleep seems self-evident. But it is not. A reciprocal relationship exists between the two (Moldofsky 1989). On the other hand, it could be argued that their relationship is a chance one: Both occur frequently; therefore, they are bound to overlap. However, this argument is not correct either.

The current name given to the first group of symptoms is fibrositis, fibromyositis, or fibromyalgia. Fibromyositis is extremely common. It has been estimated that up to 6 million persons (usually young and middle-aged women) in the United States are afflicted with it (Wallace 1984). Given the fact that in the Canadian survey about one-third of the population complained of such pains, it is likely that the figure of 6 million is a gross underestimate of the actual prevalence of this syndrome.

The most characteristic feature of fibromyositis is that the pain and stiffness are at their worst on arising in the morning. As the day wears on, after a warm bath, massage, or the taking of a mild analgesic, partial relief is obtained. At first, exercise seems to intensify the pain and stiffness; later it relieves it. Because examining physicians often find small, tender nodules localized in the neck, shoulders, chest, lower back, and buttocks and around the elbows and knees of their patients, they traditionally believe that some regional, possibly inflammatory, "rheumatic"-like process is affecting muscle and tendons, or their sheaths (Campbell et al. 1983). However, this local hypothesis is un-proven, especially in the light of the fact that these patients additionally com-plain of sleeping poorly and awakening unrefreshed. Furthermore, many of them suffer from the IBS and/or are hyperventilators. No local process could possibly explain such a wide variety of symptoms: The entire person is in ill health.

In a brilliant inductive leap, Moldofsky and his colleagues (1975) related the morning symptoms of fibromyositis to an antecedent sleep disturbance. They demonstrated that in fibromyositis an EEG-defined alteration occurs. It consists of the intrusion of α-rhythm (7.5 to 11 Hz) during any phase of non-REM. Their original observation has been confirmed on several occasions (Shackell and Horne 1987; Ware, Russell, and Campos 1986).

Of particular moment is the fact that the validity of these observations has been experimentally established. When normal, sleeping subjects are sub-jected to white noise for three consecutive nights while in a non-REM, slow-wave sleep stage, α-rhythm intrudes into it. On awakening, these subjects complain of poor sleep, aches and pains in muscles, and fatigue. If the sleep of the same subject is not disturbed in this manner, the triad of complaints either remits or is not further manifested. When the same noise is presented during REM sleep in normal subjects, the subjects do not develop any symp-toms (Moldofsky and Scarisbrick 1976).

Potential treatment for fibromyositis and its related symptoms is implied in this study by the observation that athletes subjected to noise during non-REM sleep develop no symptoms. And indeed, fitness training, when tolerated by patients with fibromyositis, appears to improve or abolish the triad of their symptoms (McCain 1986) and abolish the EEG anomaly (as do tricyclic anti-depressants) (Carette et al. 1986; Russell et al. 1987).

Stressful Experience and Fibromyositis

Stressful experiences are more often followed by sleep disturbances, anxiety, fibromyositis, the IBS, and hyperventilation, singly or in combination, than by disease. This assertion requires empirical support. Even if it is proven to be correct it does not answer the question why one or another or all of these clus-ters of symptoms appear in one patient and not the next one.

In one study, patients with fibromyositis, sleep disturbances, and α-rhythm intrusion into non-REM sleep developed their symptoms after automobile and industrial accidents, in which, however, they had not sustained a bodily injury (Moldofsky et al. 1975). They remained symptomatic for two and a half years after these experiences (Saskin, Moldofsky, and Lue 1986). The triad of symptoms has also been described in one-third of a small group of Israeli veterans of the 1973 war, who had neither been injured nor captured (Lavie et al. 1979). It should not be assumed, however, that fibromyositis is merely a product of any form of sleep disturbance, associated for example with fear and anxiety or the major depressive disorders (Saskin et al. 1987). In fact, it can be differentiated from the many other sleep disorders by virtue of the appearance of α-rhythm intrusion into non-REM sleep. Furthermore, fibromyositis with its related sleep disorder is not merely a matter of a depressed mood or certain specific personal characteristics (Gupta and Moldofsky 1986).

The fibromyositis syndrome is not a homogenous entity. It may occur with or without another form of sleep disturbance, during which periodic and repetitive, involuntary jerking limb movements (myoclonus) occur. These myoclonic movements arouse patients; the arousal is also evidenced by EEG criteria (Moldofsky et al. 1984). Patients with this second, myoclonic, form of sleep disorder are older than those first described. But they are just as symptomatic as younger patients are; they also complain of musculoskeletal pain and daytime fatigue and sleepiness (Moldofsky, Lue, and Smythe 1983; Moldofsky et al. 1984).

The case should not be made that (1) the α-EEG intrusion in non-REM is specific to fibromyositis or that (2) stressful experiences alone antecede it. The fact is that relationship of pain to the sleep disturbance is bidirectional, and probably recursive. The anomalous appearance of α-rhythm during non-REM sleep occurs under other conditions than stressful experiences: in persons with no apparent complaints (Scheuler, Stinshoff, and Kubicki 1983); during the withdrawal of addicting opiate drugs (Kay et al. 1979); and in patients with complex partial seizures due to temporal lobe disease (Greenberg and Pearlman 1968). But in these three groups of patients no attempt was made to determine whether pain, fatigue, or nonrestorative sleep accompanied the changed EEG patterns.

Fibromyositic symptoms, poor sleep, irritability, fatigue, and depression have been associated with living near a major airport (Tarnapolsky, Watkin, and Hand 1980). Some residents only are partially or fully awakened by the noise. Apparently some additional feature must characterize all those who are sensitive to noise and become symptomatic. Actually, some of the asymptomatic persons also demonstrate α-rhythm during non-REM sleep. But those who develop the fibromyositic symptoms appear to have a lower threshold for noise (Gerster and Hadj-Djilani 1984) and pain (Scudds et al. 1987).

Other experiences besides airport noise play a role in inciting the EEG changes with which fibromyositis is associated. The most important of these is pain itself, which may interfere with sleep. The articular pain of both rheumatoid and osteoarthritis is worse in the morning, especially during acute exacerbations or after exercise. The pain of both diseases is often associated with early morning stiffness, fatigue, weakness, and the appearance of α-rhythm during non-REM sleep (Mahowald et al. 1987; Moldofsky, Lue, and Saskin

1987; Wolfe et al. 1984). But only a minority (14%) of patients with chronic rheumatoid arthritis also have fibromyositic symptoms. Those that do are single, lonely women who are more fearful and depressed than others are. Their arthritis is chronically more active. Their disability is greater (Wolfe, Cathey, and Kleinheksel 1984; Wolfe et al. 1984).

Fibromyositic-like symptoms have been ascribed to various infectious agents, especially viral ones. In medicine's continuous search for the physical explanation of all ill health and disease, recent attention has been focused on the Epstein-Barr (EB) virus as the pathogenetic agent for a syndrome that has every feature of fibromyositis (Buchwald, Sullivan, and Komaroff 1987; Salit 1985). In fact, the triad of symptoms that characterizes the (misnamed) chronic EB syndrome is associated with the same EEG anomaly as is fibromyositis (Moldofsky et al. 1987). Nonetheless, there may be some as yet dimly understood connection between viral infection and the sleep disturbance, which is possibly mediated by immunoregulatory lymphokines (Moldofsky 1989).

Sleep apnea is a common disorder, particularly in middle-aged, overweight men, many of whom imbibe too much alcohol. It is characterized by periodic breathing and snoring during which the soft palate partly or completely obstructs the passage of inspired air. As a result the patient stops breathing. During apnea, repeated cycles of desaturation of oxygen in the blood occur. The BP increases, and cardiac acceleration and arrhythmias occur. The patient partly awakens during apneic cycles and is restless during sleep. Some sleep apneic patients, but not all, develop the triad of symptoms, including the EEG anomaly, characteristic of fibromyositis (Molony et al. 1986).

Mechanisms of Fibromyositis and the EEG Anomaly

The regulation of sleep and wakefulness, and of the various sleep stages, is complex. At least three pacemakers in the brain stem and the hypothalamus have been implicated. A variety of peptides (interleukin-1β [IL-1β], α-2 interferon, the tumor necrosis factor [TNF], the muramyl peptides, etc.) promote slow-wave sleep. The interactions of several biogenic amines (e.g., 5-HT and acetylcholine) also do.

Nonopioid and opioid pain systems are present in animals and probably in humans. They may be implicated in fibromyositis. The effects of these systems may be mediated by 5-HT (Dewey et al. 1970; Major and Pleuvry 1971). But the relevance of all these potential mediators for our understanding of fibromyositis is unclear (Moldofsky and Lue 1980; Moldofsky and Warsh 1978).

Summary

The evidence that stressful experiences are related to the various functional and overlapping disorders just reviewed is more than tentative and tantalizing.

The predominant emphasis in this area has to date been on studying the correlation of their symptoms with anxiety and depression, but not on studying what elicits them. Much more information on the stressful antecedents of ill health is needed (Dotevall 1989). Only a few reports have clearly linked stressful experiences with the hyperventilation syndrome and the IBS.

In the case of fibromyositis, the evidence is more convincing. Yet Moldofsky (1989) has pointed out clearly that not only stressful experiences are associated with its onset and recurrences. Its etiology is multifactorial. The experimental studies of Wingate, Valori, and Kumar (1989) have underlined the subtlety by which experimentally produced stressful experiences alter one particular form of gut motility; meals also do.

New concepts are needed that will allow us to understand how respiratory, gastrointestinal, and sleep rhythms are altered by stressful experience: New rhythms may appear; old ones may vanish, and their parameters may change (chapter 10).

Stressful experiences perturb some vital biological functions more than others. Sleep and menstrual cycle (Weiner 1989c) appear to be the most sensitive to perturbations. The possible evolutionary significance of this observation—should it be borne out—is not easily understood.

6 Stressful Experience and Disease

Selye's investigations, as previously discussed, assigned a predominant and direct role to stressful experience in the genesis of disease—a line of endeavor that is still being vigorously pursued. The procedures he used were injurious to his animals. The subjects could neither prevent, nor protect themselves from, harm. And, as noted, he concluded from his experiments that stressful experiences were not specific, that they were mediated by a general process (the general adaptation syndrome) to terminate in an invariant triad of anatomical changes. The particular stressful experience did not specify the anatomical changes. But the argument has been put forward that this result was due to the overwhelming and injurious nature of his procedures. Under other and less stringent conditions it does not occur.

We know, however, that in most instances the integrated response of the organism to stressful experience is exquisitely attuned, and is appropriate, to the specific experience, and no disease ensues. But the question of the occurrence of both a general and a specific response to a particular stressful experience is still unsettled.

The fact that a certain stressful experience does not specify a particular disease has also been a major source of criticism of its role in disease onset; it would seem, on the surface, to support the idea of the nonspecificity of stressful experience. For example, many different diseases begin in a setting of bereavement, separation, or loss (chapter 4). Forced unemployment also has several different possible disease outcomes. But why should such facts lead to a refutation of the role of these experiences in contributing to the genesis of disease? Many examples show that a particular virus or bacterium does not specify a particular disease (see also chapter 4). The hepatitis B virus may incite acute hepatitis in one person. Other people become the well carriers of the virus; in fact, millions of them exist around the world. Some of these carriers develop mild symptoms of a "subclinical" disease, manifested by slight biochemical deviations of their liver functions. Still other persons succumb to a progressive, chronic hepatitis, or a malignant tumor (hepatoma) of the liver, many years after the initial infection. Both the carrier state and the ability of carriers to transmit the virus are, in part, genetically determined (Blumberg 1977).

The EB virus also has different outcomes. In temperate climates it may produce infectious mononucleosis. Yet almost every living adult carries antibodies against it, suggesting prior infection but not disease. In tropical Africa, the EB virus may incite two different forms of malignant tumors—nasopharyngeal carcinomas or Burkitt's lymphoma.

The outcomes of many specific bacterial infections—with the hemolytic *Streptococcus,* the *Mycobacterium* of tuberculosis, or the *Treponema* of syphilis—are different and variable. Why should this be so? The answer is that a particular infectious agent does not directly specify a particular disease. That specification depends on complex interactions between the agent and the host (Copeland 1977). Multiple host factors coexist that either place him/her at risk for disease, or are protective and, therefore, endow resistance to it.

One of the main functions of the immune system is to protect the organism from infectious agents. Hereditary forms of immunodeficiency exist: In one of these, which is X-chromosome linked, antibody formation is profoundly impaired because gammaglobulins (Ig) are not synthesized. Children with this disease develop frequent infections, from which they may not recover. If they do, they are especially liable to rheumatoid arthritis or malignant tumors. Therefore, this specific, genetically determined deficiency does not have one outcome either. Furthermore, immunodeficiency can be acquired—e.g., after infection with a specific immunodeficiency virus (HIV-1).

Neither a particular stressful experience, a specific virus or bacterium, nor a particular immunodeficiency specifies the disease outcome. Only in the case of certain natural or man-made disasters does the experience terminate directly, but not inevitably, in injury, disability, or death. Thus linear theories cannot account for disease outcome: Only multifactorial models do justice to the problem (Ader 1980; Engel 1977; McKeown 1976; von Uexküll 1979; Weiner 1977, 1978, 1979a). These multiple factors include genetic, developmental, maturational, nutritional, psychological and sociocultural ones. Stressful experience is only one (risk) factor in disease outcome.

The Question of Specific versus General Responses to Stressful Experience

The argument so far has been put forward that Selye's nonspecific definition of injurious or noxious experience was overstated. Very specific, integrated, appropriate responses to each stressful experience occur. At times, however, they may be inappropriate, excessive, or inadequate, in which case disease or injury may ensue. But in many cases, they may be entirely appropriate in response to a task or challenge. Life-threatening disturbances of function may still occur, as is the case when mental activity or exercise is followed by myocardial ischemia and cardiac arrhythmias, which are in turn most often, but not always, associated with preexisting coronary artery disease (Deanfield et al. 1983, 1984; Maseri et al. 1978).

In this instance, preexisting disease and a challenge or task interact to perturb regular cardiac rhythms and/or incite spasm in the coronary arteries. However, if the heart stops, massive secretion of multiple hormones occurs—a general response to a potentially fatal event has occurred.

There are those who believe that some common denominator also connects the many different socioenvironmental factors that either reduce or increase the incidence and prevalence of many different diseases. Although some conditions and diseases (e.g., smoking, obesity, diabetes mellitus, and IHD; or obesity and BP) are clearly related to each other, many are not. The nature, etiology, and pathogenesis of many diseases and conditions are very different, yet they covary with specific, stressful socioeconomic or environmental situations and experiences, which do not, however, define the specific diseases, illnesses, or conditions (Najman 1980; Syme 1979; Syme and Berkman 1976).

Low or high socioeconomic status, urban or rural living, industrialization, unemployment, immigration, social mobility, divorce, widowhood, bereavement, and other life changes, obesity, and smoking, are according to this view responsible for diminishing the resistance of the host to various diseases. While all of these increase the vulnerability to disease, other factors intervene to determine its specific nature. It is also important to understand why only certain persons become ill when exposed to these ubiquitous socioenvironmental or personal experiences. These seemingly separate questions are actually closely linked. The partial answer to them is that persons differ in their genetic makeup and past experiences, which allow them to resist, or make them succumb to, the impact of challenge, change, migration, poverty, job loss, dissatisfaction, or bereavement.

But we do not know what this general susceptibility to disease might entail. In the case of infectious disease both specific and general responses do occur. The former consists of the production of specific antibodies to viral, bacterial, and other antigens by specialized (B−) lymphocytes and plasma cells. But a general response—the acute phase reaction—also takes place, incited by a variety of different infectious agents. (The reactions to viral and bacterial infection differ somewhat.) It begins within hours or days and may continue as long as the infectious disease is active. As the infectious agents are ingested and digested by macrophages and monocytes (and possibly other cells in the brain, kidney, and skin), IL-1 is released. This lymphokine has a broad range of activities. It produces fever by causing PGE_2 secretion that acts on the thermoregulatory centers of the hypothalamus. It induces slow-wave sleep. It promotes the secretion of CRF and ACTF, and thus cortisol. Insulin, glucagon, GH, TSH, and aVP are released into the bloodstream. It directly stimulates bone marrow cells to increase the production of neutrophilic leukocytes, and it then enhances their metabolic activity. It is chemotactic, attracting leukocytes to the site of infection. But it depresses serum iron levels and iron metabolism, resulting in anemia. It triggers the transcription and synthesis of a variety of liver proteins, including C-reactive and serum amyloid A protein, haptoglobulins, fibrinogen, ceruloplasmin, complement proteins, and protease inhibitors, while depressing albumin synthesis.

It activates B-lymphocytes to produce antibodies, and also T-cells, which in turn secrete IL-2. Interleuken-2 causes CD4$^+$ (helper), CD8$^+$ (suppressor), and cytotoxic T-lymphocytes to increase in number; it also augments NK-cell cytotoxic activity.

Interleukin-1 causes fibroblasts to proliferate and collagen to be produced, both of which are crucial in tissue repair. However, it also incites muscle wasting and weight loss by enhancing protein catabolism, and the release of amino acids and glucose from stores of muscle glycogen (Dinarello 1984).

In summary, IL-1 is a humoral and paracrine communication signal with wide-ranging, general properties designed in part to alert and mobilize the body to fight infection and to promote the repair of damaged tissue. In so doing, it has both beneficial and deleterious effects.

Another general response to many acute and chronic diseases, malnutrition, starvation, and weight loss is known as the low-triiodothyronine (T_3) syndrome, characterized by a shift in the deiodination of the thyroxine (T_4) to "reverse" T_3 (Bermudez, Surks, and Oppenheimer 1975; Carter et al. 1974; Chopra and Smith 1975). As a result the metabolic requirements of the chronically ill person are lowered. Additionally, the low-T_3 state alters the kinetics and metabolic clearance of steroid hormones (Boyar et al. 1977; Boyar and Bradlow 1977).

Therefore, in infectious and in chronic disease both specific and general physiological changes occur. It behooves those interested in the relationship of stressful experience to (other than infectious) disease onset to clarify whether specific and general responses take place in response to threats to the survival of the organism.

Evidence for and against the Role of
Stressful Experience in Disease

In the past fifteen years, much effort has been expended in an attempt to document the role of stressful experiences in the inception of illness and disease, and to quantitate them with the aid of the Schedule of Recent Events (SRE). The quantification of stressful life experiences—changes and events—has allowed investigators to predict that high SRE scores—due either to the accumulation of a large number of stressful experiences, or a few profound ones—would be associated with the onset of illness and disease within one year. An inspection of the individual items on the SRE reveals that those with the highest loadings pertain to separation or to the disruption and loss of key personal relationships. These experiences by implication are undesirable.

In a variety of predictive and retrospective studies of many different populations, some confirmation of the role of antecedent life experiences of this kind in the onset of disease and illness has been obtained. Accidents, illness, and disease of a variety of kinds—myocardial infarction, mental illness, infections, the complications of pregnancy, gastric and duodenal ulcer, etc.—are more likely to begin after, or at the time when, scores on the SRE have increased, rather than at times when they are low (Dohrenwend and Dohrenwend 1974; Gunderson and Rahe 1974).

These studies deal with groups of individuals rather than with a single person; they are, therefore, subject to a logical error. It is a fallacy to believe that an association between two characteristics—the increased number of undesirable experiences in a population; illnesses and diseases (or any one of them)—will generalize to the same characteristics when measured across, or in, indivuals (Arthur 1982; Kasl 1979). In fact, some individuals with high scores on the SRE seem impervious to illness and disease, while others with low scores fall sick. Additionally, this line of research overlooks the fact that many risk factors interact to culminate in illness and disease; some persons are more liable to disease than others, some are protected against certain diseases. Furthermore, this line of investigation makes it impossible to predict the nature of the illness and disease from which the person will suffer. The SRE also contains a tautology—illness, injury, and pregnancy are said to be antecedents of illness, accidental injury, disease, and the complications of pregnancy!

The correlations in a large number of studies between the incidence and prevalence of symptoms of illnesses (including psychiatric ones) and disease and SRE scores, although statistically reliable, are in the range of .2 to .3. They would, therefore, account for 4 to 9% of the variance (Arthur 1982). But this may be the wrong way of presenting the association of life events and illnesses. A better way is to calculate the population-attributable-risk percent. Using psychiatric cases only, 32% can be attributed to stressful life events; the figures rise to 41% when only women patients are studied (Cooke and Hole 1983).

Because relatively little of the etiological variance of disease is accounted for by stressful experiences per se, it is not surprising that many authorities have concluded that this line of approach is unpromising (Rabkin and Struening 1976; Thoits 1982). Before coming to such a final conclusion, one might ask whether indeed there is any temporal relationship between stressful life events and experiences and the onset of symptoms. This question arises because many deny the association. Studies of this nature are based on retrospection or are cross-sectional: Subjects are asked to look back one year in time in order to determine what had happened in their lives, but they may be liable to all the familiar infirmities and distortions of human memory. When confirmation of the subject's recall of experiences is sought from spouses or other persons, they are often unable to remember the same set of events (Horowitz et al. 1977; Schless and Mendels 1978). One solution to this problem is to devise a longitudinal and prospective research strategy, such as the one used by Grant and his colleagues (1982). They compared and followed 72 psychiatric outpatients of a variety of diagnostic categories in a VA Mental Health clinic and 94 employees of the same facility (unfortunately not matched for age and socioeconomic status) for a period of three years. The SRE and Symptom Checklist were administered every two months. The data were subjected to Fourier and spectral analyses. The results show that in 42% of the patients and 31% of the control subjects symptoms increased and were time-locked with a rise in the number of undesirable experiences. In another group of patients (8%) and subjects (12%), the categories were 180° out of phase with each—a result that raises the question whether the increases in symptoms preceded life changes or followed them. In another group of patients and subjects, events and symptoms were at times closely coordinated while at other times they were not. Two residual subgroups remained: In one no coherent pattern of association emerged; in another, life events changed but no symptoms were reported, or admitted to, by 9% of the patients.

Despite the limitations of such a numerical assessment, the results of this study were impressive but not surprising. Many patients respond immediately with an increase in symptoms, but some do not; they only become more symptomatic after a time because some systems (e.g., the emotional and the immune ones) may respond after a latent period. Nor should it be surprising that a minority of psychiatric patients do not respond at all to changes in their lives; they seem to be impervious to, or oblivious of, certain categories of experiences.

Stressful life experiences are dramatic occurrences that are recorded as major changes in the lives of people. They are generally not considered to be the straw that breaks a person's back, but a club. But life can also be boring or constantly irritating, frustrating, or distressing. Work or marriage can be chronically demanding, discordant, or troubling. Bosses can be tyrants. For a poor woman, to raise children and have to support them by working can be an unrelieved burden. In fact, most people lead lives of quiet desperation. In such people some relatively minor specific event—of a personal or financial nature, or increasing lack of privacy, another disappointment, or a minor illness—tips the scale, and sickness ensues. A chronic background of distress, irritation, and frustration leads to poor morale, depression, and disease, associations that have only recently been the subject of investigation (Brown and Harris 1978, 1986; DeLongis et al. 1982; Kanner et al. 1981).

Despite the fact that many inconsistencies remain to be resolved, an impressive body of evidence supports the notion that adverse experiences, personal habits and characteristics, certain occupations, social isolation, unemployment, and dissatisfaction are also correlated with excess morbidity and mortality (Berkman 1980; Berkman and Syme 1979; Cassel 1976; House, Landis, and Umberson 1988; Jenkins 1976).

It is likely that the role of these stressful experiences is most evident in populations that are at risk for a particular disease, and not in those who are not "programmed" in this manner. But even in such special populations the yield may be low, and disease may not be the inevitable outcome (Hinkle 1974; Weiner et al. 1957).

The Multifactorial Nature of the Risk Factors for Disease

With the exception of gross physical injury resulting from natural or manmade disasters and leading either to recovery, disability, or death, stressful experiences do not on their own produce disease or ill health. Disease is never unicausal or linearly related to the inciting agent: An environment-host interaction always occurs (Copeland 1977).

Stressful experiences in most instances do not determine the specific disease outcome; they are one of several risk factors that may in interaction with others promote the onset of disease (Haynes et al. 1978; Haynes, Feinleib, and Kannel 1980). They may interact with preexisting, latent, or asymptomatic disease; e.g., the colon of two-thirds of all patients with ulcerative colitis is the seat of permanent mucosal changes, but the patient may be asymptomatic (Dick, Holt, and Dalton 1966). Clinical evidence suggests that any disruption of a relationship antecedes the recurrence of symptoms (Engel 1973). And, as already mentioned, forced unemployment may exacerbate latent, preexisting, or ongoing cardiac or pulmonary disease (chapter 4).

Thus it is not likely, but by no means proven, that the interaction of the same stressful experience with normal bodily function or an anatomically intact organ is different than it is with an abnormally functioning or structurally impaired one.

The Interaction of Stressful Experience with Other Risk Factors

The complexity of this issue is considerable. A risk factor for one disease may be a protective one for another. Two risk factors may cancel each other out or modify each other's expression. Protective factors may override risk factors.

Even in the laboratory, the production of disease in animals is marked by variability—multiple factors are involved (Ader 1980). When persons at risk for a disease are exposed to stressful experiences in their lives, only some develop the disease. To compound the matter further, the factors that are associated with etiology, initiation, and pathophysiology of illness and disease are often, if not always, different from those that sustain them. For example, the maladaptive physiological adjustments to high BP levels sustain them but differ from the physiological factors that initiate them (Weiner 1977).

The multifactorial model of disease attempts to account for all the factors that protect against, and are responsible for the predisposition to, initiation, maintenance, and variable natural history of, illness and disease and their consequences for the ill person, his/her family, the society in which he/she lives and its economy and structure. The multiple, interacting factors are genetic, bacterial, immunological, nutritional, developmental, psychological, behavioral, and social.

The Heterogeneity of Disease

Most diseases, traditionally defined by characteristic changes in organ, tissue, or cell structure, are heterogenous in nature. This realization has only dawned on physicians lately. Had they read Darwin they might have predicted that variation would be present within every "species" of disease!

Variation within a disease is illustrated by the autoimmune diseases: Many of them are genetically heterogeneous. A number of major histocompatibility complex (MHC) genotypes predisposes to, and increase the risk for, one disease phenotype. Nine MHC/HLA-antigens are known to do so for systemic lupus erythematosus, and five for multiple sclerosis. Therefore, genetic susceptibility to a disease is not associated with any one special HLA.

Adult patients with rheumatoid arthritis (RA) can be divided into two groups: Those who are seropositive for rheumatoid factors (RF), and those who are not. The former are significantly more likely also to express the HLA-DR4, -Dw4, and -Dw14 genotypes than the latter (Stastny 1978), especially if they are Caucasion, black American or Asian Indian; Jews with RA preferentially express HLA-DR1.

Therefore, any statement about the role of some set of uniform stressful experience in this (or other) disease(s) must be tempered by the realization that it is (they are) genetically heterogeneous and not homogeneous. Given this conclusion, stressful experience may play a greater or lesser role in the subform of this disease: In fact, the evidence bears out this conclusion, particularly in the case of RA (Baker 1982; Weiner 1990a).

Rimón (1969) divided women patients with RA into two groups based on the presence or absence of a family history for the disease, RF in their sera, the occurrence of adverse stressful experiences, and differences in the onset and course of the disease: (1) In patients without a family history of RA, the disease began acutely in a setting that was discernibly unpleasant for them, and it progressed rapidly. (2) Patients whose disease began insidiously and progressed slowly had a family history of RA. No startling changes in their lives or experiences anteceded its onset. In this second group of women with

RA, Rimón (1973) was again able to sort them into two categories along several dimensions: In the first they were measurably more likely to express anger and irritation, and they were seronegative for RF. Those in the second subgroup were characterized by marked restraint in expressing emotions, and RFs were present in their serum.

These psychological differences have been confirmed independently in other studies. They exist among patients with RA whose serum contains RF and who show erosive joint changes by X-ray; those with neither of these characteristics; and a third group with chronic arthritis of nonrheumatoid origin. Patients in the first set were remarkably uniform psychologically, scoring low on measures of anxiety, hostility, depression, "psychoticism," confusion, and fatigue. The second scored much higher on these measures but lower than the group with mixed arthritis of nonrheumatoid origin (Vollhardt et al. 1982). Differences in seropositive and seronegative patients have also been found in other studies using different psychological measures; the former are like a normal comparison group (Crown, Crown, and Fleming 1975; Gardiner 1980; Moos and Solomon 1965).

The issue of heterogeneity in disease was brought to the fore in the study of duodenal ulcer (Grossman 1979; Rotter and Rimoin 1977). Duodenal ulcer (DU) may be anteceded by gastrinomas, extensive resection of the small intestine, alcoholic cirrhosis of the liver, chronic renal failure, or chronic obstructive lung disease; it may also be associated with a syndrome that occurs in families and consists of limb tremors, congenital nystagmus, and a disturbance of consciousness reminiscent of narcolepsy (Neuhäuser et al. 1976). When these antecedents to DU are not present, one is still faced with the fact that not every patient with this disorder has an elevated serum pepsinogen level, nor does he or she have the same psychological profile (Weiner et al. 1957).

The study of the heterogeneity of peptic DU disease has become complex; at the same time, however, many of the issues that previously confounded this particular field of investigation have been clarified (Ackerman and Weiner 1976; Rotter and Rimoin 1977; Weiner 1977). The new thrust of these investigations derives from the fact that human pepsinogens can be separated immunochemically into two main groups—pepsinogen I (PG-I) and pepsinogen II (PG-II) (Samloff 1971a, 1971b; Samloff and Liebman 1974). Elevated levels of PG-I are found in about two-thirds of all unrelated patients with peptic DU (Samloff, Liebman, and Panitch 1975). The remaining third have normal levels of PG-I. The distribution of PG-I is bimodal in patients but not in control subjects. PG-II levels are also greater in patients with peptic DU (and especially gastric ulcer) whose PG-I levels are elevated than in hospitalized control patients (Samloff 1977). But we still do not know whether PG-II levels are elevated in patients whose PG-I levels are within the normal range. Two groups of patients with peptic DU have, therefore, been identified—those with elevated PG-I (and possibly PG-II) levels and those with normal PG-I levels.

We know that elevations of PG-I levels are inherited as an autosomal dominant trait, because about half of the offspring of parents with such elevations also own the trait (Rotter et al. 1977a, 1979), and no children of parents without the trait manifest it. Yet the enhanced PG-I level is not invariably associated with DU disease; 42% of those with it had the disease, the rest did not. Based on other studies carried out by Rotter and Rimoin (1977c), it is now possible to calculate that in those patients with raised PG-I levels the genetic trait accounts for 25% of the etiologic variance of this form of DU disease, leaving other factors to interact with it. These observations also lay to rest a long-standing doubt that the raised levels of pepsinogens (or PG-I) are inherited and not merely a result of age, gastric mucosal damage, eating meals, or the diminished excretion of the enzyme due to renal damage.

Patients with normal pepsinogen levels also develop DU, as do their siblings, in a small percentage of whom PG-I levels may be elevated. The incidence of DU in siblings of patients with normal PG-I levels is almost as great as in the siblings of patients with raised PG-I levels (Rotter et al. 1977a, 1977c). However, the mode of inheritance in the former has not been worked out, nor is it known how the genes express themselves as markers of risk for this subform of the disease.

In DU disease, additional genetic markers have been found. Individuals who have blood type O and do not secrete the blood group antigens ABH, which are secreted into the saliva and gastric juice, have higher incidences of both gastric ulcer and DU (Hanley 1964; Marcus 1969; Sievers 1959; Vesley, Kubickova, and Dvorakova 1968). The blood group and nonsecretor factors account for about 2.5 to 3% of the etiologic variance of peptic ulcer disease. Stated in other terms, people of blood type O who do not secrete ABH antigens are 25 to 35% more likely to develop peptic ulcer than are individuals of blood type A, B, or AB who do secrete these antigens.

The HLA-B5 antigen also occurs more frequently in patients with DU than in normal controls. White males who possess it are 2.9 times as likely to develop DU than those who do not (Rotter et al. 1977b). By contrast, the relative risk for the same disease in a person with blood group O is 1.3; for one with blood group nonsecretor status, it is 1.5 (Langman 1973; McConnell 1963). When both blood group O and nonsecretor status are combined the risk is 2.5 greater.

Studies on these genetic markers did not take into account the heterogeneity of peptic ulcer disease: We do not know whether they are associated differentially with normal or raised PG-I levels.

The previous discussion might lead to the assumption that peptic DU consists of two forms, one of which is characterized by elevated and the other by normal PG-I levels. However, this conclusion is not fully warranted. A variety of different regulatory disturbances are also found in patients with peptic ulcer disease: Some have an increased proclivity to secrete gastric acid and pepsin;

others produce excessive hydrochloric acid when stimulated by pentagastrin; some have a postprandial hypergastrinemia, an increased rate of gastric emptying, or an impaired feedback inhibition of gastrin secretion by acidification of the gastric antrum; and some patients' capacity to release prostaglandin E (PGE, an inhibitor of gastric acid secretion) is impaired when hydrochloric acid is secreted into the stomach lumen by vagal stimulation (Cheun et al. 1975; Grossman 1978, 1979). In addition, acid-neutralizing bicarbonate secretion may be impaired in the duodenum (Isenberg et al. 1987).

These regulatory disturbances are seen after the onset of disease; therefore, one may not lightly assume that they are present before it. Yet these abnormalities characterize different patients with the disease. They are not present in all patients.

Obvious questions are raised by these observations: Do patients with elevated PG-I levels differ psychologically from those with normal PG-I levels? Why do some persons with elevated PG-I levels develop a peptic DU and others do not? A beginning answer to the first question has been obtained. Psychobiological heterogeneity may be present in the various subforms of peptic DU. Patients with normal PG-I levels scored significantly higher on blindly rated measures of dependency, but not on scores of anxiety, than did patients with elevated PG-I levels (Feldman et al. 1985).

Heterogeneity of this nature also exists in essential hypertension. Admittedly there are no established ways of identifying people at risk for its development, although two strategies have been devised recently. The first is to classify hypertensive patients according to physiological patterns that consist of deviations of CO, plasma renin activity (PRA), or plasma volume (Julius et al. 1975; Laragh et al. 1972; Tarazi et al. 1970). The second is to study patients very early in the disease process, before the appearance of (mal)adaptive changes in response to the raised BP. Many of such patients are said to have borderline or labile essential hypertension.

Only about 25% of all patients with borderline hypertension go on to essential hypertension. Groups of patients with borderline hypertension tend to have some increase in CO as well as increased cardiac contractility and HR. Their plasma catecholamine levels are likely to be elevated, and their urinary excretion of catecholamines is excessive on standing. Stressful experiences are associated with exaggerated catecholamine and BP responses in some. Sympathetic ganglionic blocking agents produce a fall in BP that closely correlates with a fall in plasma NE levels (DeQuattro and Miura 1973; Julius et al. 1975; Kuchel 1977; Lorimer et al. 1971; Louis et al. 1973).

Patients with borderline hypertension differ as a group (but not necessarily as individuals) from normotensive subjects. But the patients also differ from each other. Not all patients with borderline hypertension have an elevated CO; in only 30% CO is two standard deviations beyond the mean for normal, age-matched subjects. In this subgroup of patients, the total peripheral resistance is inappropriately normal at rest; it should be decreased when increased tissue perfusion is brought about by the increased CO. In other patients with borderline hypertension in whom a normal CO and HR are recorded, the total peripheral resistance is increased at rest, possibly owing to increased α-adrenergic vasoconstrictor tone. Blood volume is unevenly distributed in the circulation (mainly in the cardiopulmonary bed) in borderline hypertension, but only in those patients with an increased CO. In about 30% of all patients with borderline hypertension, PRA and plasma NE concentration are elevated; in others they are not. Yet the increased PRA does not seem to maintain the heightened BP levels through its effect on angiotensin II (AT-II) and aldosterone secretion. The increased HR, CO, and PRA can be reduced to normal levels with propranolol, but the plasma NE concentration and BP continue to remain elevated. Therefore, the enhanced PRA is believed to be a result of increased sympathetic activity, not the primary pathogenetic factor in raising BP (Esler et al. 1977; Julius et al. 1975). The obverse sequence is, however, thought to account for the malignant phase of hypertension, when high PRA occurs.

Nonetheless, PRA is normal or low in 70% of borderline hypertensive patients (Esler et al. 1975). Patients whose PRA is normal tend to be those with diminished stroke volume and cardiac index, normal HR, and increased total peripheral resistance. Their plasma NE concentration is higher than normal but lower than in borderline hypertensive patients with high PRA. The increased peripheral resistance and BP in borderline hypertensive patients with low or normal PRA are unaffected by the administration of α-adrenergic, β-adrenergic blocking agents, and atropine. The administration of these drugs causes a fall in BP and peripheral resistance in borderline hypertensive patients with high PRA (Esler et al. 1975; Esler et al. 1977).

These results suggest that borderline hypertension—a harbinger of established hypertension in 25% of all patients—is a heterogeneous disturbance with perhaps three different physiologic and hormonal profiles, which probably reflect different pathogeneses. In fact, endocrine changes in other borderline hypertensive patients are also not completely uniform. (However, these patients may not be the same ones as those who have been studied for their cardiovascular dynamics, responses to sympathetic and parasympathetic blocking agents, and PRA).

In any case, patients with borderline hypertension can be divided into those who, with reassurance and rest, experience a decline in BP to below 140 mm Hg systolic and 90 diastolic, and those who do not (Genest, Koiw, and Kuchel 1977). In both groups of patients there is a significant mean increase in plasma aldosterone concentration, which reverts to normal levels only in those who become normotensive. When recumbent, both groups of patients have a decreased metabolic clearance rate of aldosterone when compared to normal control subjects. Usually an upright posture considerably decreases the metabolic clearance of aldosterone, but not in patients with mild, borderline hypertension. Although other alterations in aldosterone metabolism (binding of the hormone to a specific plasma globulin and responses to stimulation) occur in borderline hypertensive patients, the point of this discussion is that borderline patients with mild hypertension are not all the same: They resemble each other in some ways and differ in others.

The physiologic heterogeneity of patients with essential hypertension is also reflected in their psychological heterogeneity. Esler and his co-workers (1977) have reported on 16 men, 18 to 35 years of age, belonging to that subgroup of borderline hypertensives in whom high PRA and increased plasma NE levels are found. They differ significantly on a number of psychological measures from 15 borderline hypertensive males with normal PRA and from 20 males with normal BP levels. They are found to be controlled, guilt-ridden, and submissive people with relatively high levels of unexpressed or unexpressible anger and resentment. The only characteristic that differentiated the normal control group from the hypertensive patients with normal PRA is that its members appeared to be more resentful but were capable of expressing their resentments. The meaning of these observations is not quite clear. Julius and Esler (1975) and Esler and his co-workers (1977) have argued that the pathogenesis of high-renin borderline hypertension is neurogenic. As mentioned, the high PRA is secondary to increased sympathetically mediated release of renin because the effect of propranolol is to lower PRA but not BP. They have concluded that in this subform of essential hypertension, the activity of the sympathetic nervous system is increased, or, alternatively, that both sympathetic nervous enhancement and diminished parasympathetic inhibition account for their findings. This dual mediating mechanism is ascribed to a disturbance in central autonomic regulation.

Essention hypertension is not only a heterogeneous disorder but, as previously discussed, also a major risk factor in IHD and myocardial infarction. The proximate, initiating mechanisms of myocardial infarction are also heterogeneous; it may come about through coronary artery spasm, occlusion, thrombosis, or embolism, subendothelial hemorrhage, or congenital abnormalities of the coronary arteries.

Multiple forms of diabetes mellitus also exist, and different initiating mechanisms may produce them. In some forms of diabetes mellitus, levels of circulating insulin may be normal or elevated, but the patient fails to respond to the hormone. Such resistance to either circulating or administered insulin takes a number of forms. It may result from either the formation of antibodies to the hormone or to the insulin receptor, or the opposing action of other hormones. Alternatively, the number of insulin receptors may be decreased, the receptor mechanisms may be defective, or the insulin molecule may be genetically altered in structure by the substitution of one amino acid for the usual one in one of the insulin chains (Tager et al. 1979).

Genetic Factors in Disease

The further complexity of genetic factors in disease will be exemplified by a limited number of examples. The literature on genetic factors in disease tends to be oversimplified. Genes do not only code for enzymes and proteins. They also regulate each other and are in turn regulated by enzyme substrates, hormones, growth factors, and various intracellular "messengers." Several genes may cooperate in the production of one immunoglobulin. Two separate genes may code for the same protein (e.g., dystrophin). A protein may come in several forms. One form may be manufactured at one age, and another at another. Proteins are modified after being transcribed and translated, and when they assume their tertiary structure.

In most instances genes do not directly cause a disease, but they increase the risk for it. This principle is exemplified by the role of genetic factors in autoimmune diseases. The MHC (or HLA) complex molecules are cell surface, glycoprotein receptors that endow organs and cells with their antigenicity (Todd et al. 1988). Originally discovered to account for tissue transplant rejection, they also play a major role in binding other foreign antigens and antigen (peptide) fragments initially processed by macrophages. The chromosomal region coding for these receptors is known as the MHC complex and consists of genes on chromosome 6 in 25 loci, which express about 128 different glycoproteins (Schiffenbauer and Schwartz 1987). Three classes (I, II, and III) of genes coding for the cell surface proteins (receptors) are recognized; MHC-I is arranged in an A, B, C series, MHC-II is arranged in a D/DR series, and MHC-III genes are responsible for complement components.

Both class I and II receptors are capable of binding many peptides but not all. They partly determine the specificity of the immune response; nevertheless, they are "polymorphic." Class I MHC receptors present foreign antigenic fragments to antigen-reactive CD8$^+$ cells and some cytotoxic T-cells. They "restrict" cytotoxic specificity and T-cell lympholysis. Class II MHC receptors perform the same functions (including "restriction") for CD4$^+$ cells and activated cytotoxic cells. Class II DR molecules also appear on intestinal epithelial cells. Class II molecules are present in the membrane of macrophages and B-cells. Foreign antigens (or fragments thereof) are only bound by these various (especially CD4$^+$ and CD8$^+$) cells when accompanied by a particular MHC glycoprotein; if they are not presented in this manner they will not be bound by the receptor.

Therefore, the immune response is partly specified by MHC gene products. As the antigen-MHC complexes are bound, each by specific (T-cell) receptors on CD4$^+$ cells, the cells are activated and their clonal expansion occurs. Interleukin-2 and other lymphokines are secreted to stimulate B-cells to produce specific antibody to the antigen. And γ-IF increases the expression of class II MHC (HLA) molecules on T-cells (Wallach, Fellous, and Revel 1982).

Both class I and II HLA-genotypes increase or decrease the risk for, at least, forty different autoimmune diseases. But it is not as yet known whether these genes directly endow susceptibility to a disease or do so (indirectly) by acting on, or in interaction with, different yet closely associated (e.g., immunoglobulin heavy chain) genes. The HLA genotype may also influence the degradation of antigen or the monocyte number (Stobo 1982). Nonetheless, the same genotype (e.g., HLA-B27) may be expressed as four different disease phenotypes (e.g., ankylosing spondylitis, Crohn disease, Reiter and Sjögren syndromes). Yet most persons with the same disease-associated MHC alleles do not develop autoimmune disease. Therefore, susceptibility is not determined by mutant alleles (Nepom, Hansen, and Nepom 1987).

Because there is discordance for autoimmune disease in monozygotic twins, and also because a particular MHC genotype need not be expressed as a specific disease phenotype, other factors, including hormonal and environmental ones, play a role in their etiology.

Other HLA genotypes (B8, B15, DR3, DR4, DRw6) have been linked to an increased risk for, and still others (A11, B5, B7, DR2, DRw2) to decreased susceptibility to juvenile-onset diabetes (Notkins 1979). Paradoxically, the HLA-B5 allele has been associated with increased risk of certain types of peptic duodenal ulcer (Rotter et al. 1966b). Simple links such as this between genetic variation and disease are rare. Most diseases are genetically multifactorial; they are a product of several genetic and a variety of nongenetic risk factors.

Genetically determined defects in protein structure may protect their bearers against a specific disease. Other defects, while they may not be protective, may not be manifest in disease. There are four-hundred different variants of the enzyme glucose-6-phosphate dehydrogenase (G-6-PD) (Beutler 1991). Some lead to deficient levels of G-6-PD especially in erythrocytes. Only twenty-two of these have been correlated with, or expressed in, disease. Each genetic variant is the product of a distinctive change in the structure of the enzyme, in which a single amino acid is substituted for the customary one at one position in its polypeptide chains. The enzyme deficiency is therefore due to the presence of the structurally abnormal enzyme in red blood cells. Some of these enzyme variants only express themselves in certain situations—after birth or infection; when the person ingests specific drugs or eats fava beans. Another set of seven enzyme variants is associated with a chronic nonspherocytic, hemolytic anemia without the apparent intervention of environmental factors. Therefore, structural variations in enzymes—a marker of disease— are not necessarily expressed in disease. Quantitative variations in enzyme levels are also seen in healthy persons.

The expression of a gene is not always invariant: Even in diseases in which genes play a predominant role, genetic variation exists. To exemplify: The chromosomal abnormality Turner syndrome, in both the XO and the XO/XX mosaic variety, may be expressed in primary anorexia nervosa (AN) or in mild mental deficiency (Kron et al. 1977). However, most patients with anorexia nervosa do not have this X-linked genetic defect: Some women, for example, develop the disease after they stop taking the oral contraceptive pill (OCP) (Fries and Nillius 1973), which has been associated with the development of high BP and thromboembolic disease in women with other predispositions. In most diseases, genetic heterogeneity is the rule. A particular disease, defined anatomically, generally is made up of a number of subforms with different genetic and nongenetic predisposing factors, which are acted upon by a variety of initiating factors.

Gender as a Factor in Disease

Many diseases are unevenly distributed between the two sexes. Marked gender differences occur in the incidence and prevalence of some autoimmune diseases. Women and girls are considerably more liable to Graves disease, by a factor of 4 to 9; six times as many women develop autoimmune thyroiditis; and three times as many women of childbearing age have RA (but after the menopause an equal number of men and women fall ill with it). The ratio of women to men with systemic lupus erythematosus (SLE) is 10:1. In some families, however, another form of SLE occurs primarily in men and is transmitted through the fathers (Dixon 1982). Yet only slightly more women have ulcerative colitis than men do (Weiner 1977).

To make the matter even more interesting, alterations in a patient's internal, hormonal environment may precipitate, ameliorate, or aggravate some of these diseases: Graves disease may begin, be attenuated, or remit during pregnancy. The incidence of RA is one-half in women using OCP than in those who are not. Pregnancy may be associated with remission in RA.

Yet two of the autoimmune diseases—ankylosing spondylitis and polyarteritis nodosa—are far more common in men. Furthermore, the incidence and prevalence of RA in men who were exposed to diethylstilbestrol when their mothers were carrying them is the same as in women not exposed to the steroid (Turiel and Wingard 1985).

These observations suggest that sexual dimorphism in the organization of the immune system exists (Grossman 1984). One can only speculate when during maturation and development this dimorphism is established. The organizational effects of development may be influenced by transitory ones produced by pregnancy, the OCP, or treatment with sex steroids. At the present time we know more about the latter than the former. Most of our current knowledge suggests that a complex interaction exists among pituitary hormones, gonadal steroids, thymic hormones, and other immune functions.

Anorexia nervosa almost exclusively occurs in young (adolescent) women. Obviously, breast cancer occurs mainly in women. But it is not a uniform disease either, because it occurs earlier in those with a family history of the disease, and some of its forms are hormone dependent while others are not.

Infectious and Immunological Risk Factors

The model of infectious disease permeates medicine. But the manner in which it is stated is oversimplified, as the previous discussion has already indicated. Factors of age, ethnicity, nutrition, and immune status in part determine the incidence, frequency, and severity of the outcome.

This statement is in part supported by observations on lymphocytic choriomeningitis: It is a viral disease that is, however, characterized by the invasion of the meninges by a profusion of lymphocytes; the virus itself does not appear in the brain or the meninges. The immunological response to the presence of the virus elsewhere in the body produces the inflammatory response in the brain.

Multiple factors are at work in the production of this and other diseases. If the lymphocytic choriomeningitis virus is first injected into a pregnant animal and later into its offspring, lymphocytes do not invade their meninges. When newborn mice are infected with the scrapie virus, a latent period of one year occurs before it manifests itself. However, when the animals reach 18 months of age, high titers of the virus can be found in their brains and spleens. If mice are injected at 4 days or older, the virus replicates immediately and kills 70 to 100% by the time they are 10 months old (Hotchin and Buckley 1977).

These two examples illustrate a developmental principle. The kind of lesion produced by a virus depends on the age at which the animal is injected with it. Developmental factors in part account for the multidetermined nature of these virus diseases.

The role of developmental and experiential factors in the immunological response cannot be overlooked either. Immunological tolerance can be imparted to mammalian embryos by injecting them with antigens from another strain (Ader 1980; Medawar and Medawar 1977). After birth they are tolerant to repeated challenge by the antigens.

Another immunological risk factor is the capacity of the host to form immunoglobulin-E, which is associated with various diseases: atopic dermatitis, allergic rhinitis, and bronchial asthma. Yet bronchial asthma will not develop unless bronchial hyperreactivity is also present. Both of these tendencies are permanent characteristics of asthmatic persons. Yet attacks of the disease are intermittent and are incited by many factors, including infection, exercise, and personal loss and the grief it engenders. To complicate the topic further, bronchial asthma in childhood is a potent risk factor for psychopathology in adulthood (Langer and Michael 1963).

Autoimmune factors play a role in Graves disease and RA. Additionally, exposure to danger and the fear of death are associated with the onset of the acute form of Graves disease, and bereavement is associated with start of RA (Weiner 1977).

Stressful experience and its consequences also alter immune function (Ader 1981). Whether these changes adversely affect health status is a much debated topic. It is likely that bereavement and depression only impair health if immunocompetent cells or their communication signals are already impaired by infection: The correlation between depression and specific changes in immune function appears only to occur if the CD4$^+$ cells carries the HIV-1 virus; if not, nonspecific immunological changes are seen (Kemeny et al. 1990).

Age as One Factor in Disease Onset

We have seen that bereavement, with its consequences, is an experience that has been correlated with the onset of many diseases (chapter 4). Their association is in part age-dependent. (Children and the elderly are especially sensitive to such experiences.) However, the integrated responses to bereavement observed at one age in a particular system are not necessarily the same as those seen in that system at a subsequent age; in fact, our understanding of this difference is still rudimentary. No a priori reason exists for believing that a later integrated response to bereavement should have the same conformation in any one system as an earlier one. One possible explanation for this discrepancy is the transformations with age that occur in the responsiveness of every organ system. For this reason alone bereavement may have particularly adverse effects on the members of one age group and not another—in enhancing, for example, the mortality of widowers of 55–74 years of age (Helsing, Szklo, and Comstock 1981).

Age-related changes have been described affecting several systems.

1. *The endocrine system.* The hypothalamic pituitary ovarian (Boyar et al. 1974) and the hypothalamic pituitary adrenal axis (with a low DHA to cortisol ratio prior to adrenarche) (Rich et al. 1981) go through maturational sequences. After menopause, gonadotropin levels rise. In AN, including that brought on by separation, both gonadotropins and the ratio of the two adrenal hormones revert to premenarchal and preadrenarchal patterns of secretion—retrogressions that depend on their previous maturation. Previous patterns reemerge (Weiner 1989c). Perhaps for that reason, the peak age of incidence of AN is at about puberty, although its onset may occasionally occur earlier or later in life.

As aging proceeds, the initiation of the adrenocortical response in rats to traditional, stressful experimental procedures remains unimpaired, but their ability to terminate it is altered. High levels of corticosterone persist for 3 to 24 hours after the experiment has ended (Sapolsky, Krey, and McEwen 1986).

2. *The immune system.* The thymus increases in size during childhood and then progressively shrinks. Eventually its function as an endocrine organ is

reduced, producing less and less thymopoeitin after the age of 30 to 40 years. After that age, more and more immature lymphocytes appear peripherally, particularly CD4$^+$ cells. Cellular immune responses are impaired, and the responses to a specific antigen are less vigorous. Autoantibodies—RF and antinuclear and antithyroglobulin antibodies—become more prevalent.

Infants who languish in institutions are prone to opportunistic (viral) infections, suggesting that their cellular immune system is impaired. Elderly people are prone to a variety of infections. They are also at increased risk for malignancies, presumably because of diminished immune surveillance over transformed cells. Bereavement has also been cited as an onset condition for malignancy; an interaction between bereavement and impaired immune function in the elderly is, therefore, suggested.

3. *The stomach.* In rats at least, the main control mechanisms of gastric acid secretion—acetylcholine, gastrin, and histamine—go through a maturational sequence. Gastrin levels, for example, rise just before normal weaning occurs. The amount of gastric acid secretion also goes through maturational changes. The development of an acid secretory response partly explains the finding that prematurely separated rats do not begin to develop gastric erosions during the challenge of restraint until they are 22 days of age. Yet up to 90% of them are prone to do so between 30 and 40 days of age. Later in life they become decreasingly susceptible to restraint (Ackerman, Hofer, and Weiner 1975).

4. *The brain.* Both apical and circumferential dendrites in many areas of the brain grow and branch, then fade and eventually disappear altogether (Scheibel, Tomiyasu, and Scheibel 1977). Brain volume begins to shrink, and cognition declines, after the age of 40 years. Despite this, major behavioral changes in older persons may not express themselves until after a separation or bereavement occurs.

5. *Circadian rhythms.* The endocrine, immune, central nervous, gastric, and other systems have their own time (e.g., circadian) periodicities with their own maturational sequences. Rhythmic changes occur in neurotransmitter, enzyme, and hormone levels, receptor binding, B- and T-cell function, the urinary excretion of electrolytes and metabolites, the effects of drugs and antigens, HR, BP, gastric secretion, temperature regulation, attention, motor activity, and dreaming. These processes are under the control of a hierarchy of oscillators and pacemakers, which require daily synchronization by *Zeitgebers* such as light and personal relationships (Moore-Ede, Sulzman, and Fuller 1982).

Circadian rhythms determine hours of maximal or minimal resistance to pathogenetic agents such as infection and restraint. Constraining rats at the height of their activity cycle is a potent factor in gastric ulceration (Ader 1964).

Therefore, the topic of the interaction of time-periodic systems with their own maturational sequences and bereavement experiences at different ages is of potential interest. The relationship between age and the timing of disease onset is complex. It can be understood in part as the result of alterations in rhythmic time-periodic systems, and in part as the result of disrupted personal relationships.

Socioeconomic Factors in Disease

Socioeconomic factors play a role in every aspect of ill health and disease. The poor in many countries have less access to care. Low socioeconomic status has been associated with a shorter life expectancy and an increased risk for mental illness (Brown and Harris 1978). Virtually every disease and a shorter life span are associated with poverty and low socioeconomic status. These conduce to essential hypertension and IHD in the United Kingdom (Marmot et al. 1978), obesity (in women in America), premature delivery, social and nutritional deprivation in children, more birth complications, higher infant mortality, tuberculosis, cancer of the cervix in women, alcoholism, and drug abuse (Syme and Berkman 1976). Single, divorced, and widowed persons are more susceptible to a wide variety of diseases, illnesses, and causes of death than are married persons (National Center for Health Statistics 1970). Persons who are socially or culturally mobile tend to have an increased prevalence rate of IHD unless they preserve their traditional customs in their new country and culture (Marmot and Syme 1976).

Obesity predisposes to a number of diseases including high BP, IHD, diabetes mellitus, cholelithiasis, gout, osteoarthritis, and the Pickwickian and sleep apnea syndromes, as well as carcinoma of the breast and uterine endometrium in women (De Waard 1975; Mirra, Cole, and MacMahon 1971; Wynder, Escher, and Martel 1966). Obesity is also associated with the effects of rapid sociocultural change or with migration, not only with poverty. It may also result from increases in dietary fat intake and lack of exercise in adult life, which may both raise serum cholesterol levels and account for the association between obesity and increase of prevalence of IHD (Marmot, Syme, and Rhoads 1975; Marmot and Syme 1976; Ostfeld 1979; Syme and Berkman 1976). Obesity differs in men and women. The distribution of fat in regions of the body is specific to gender.

However, the effects of a diet high in saturated fats and of being overweight are modified by social stability and living in a community with established traditions. These two known risk factors for IHD and myocardial infarction seem to be modified by a slow rate of social change (Wolf 1969). The members of a community of southern Italian immigrants in Roseto, Pennsylvania, have preserved their traditional patriarchal and religious ways and have trusting, mutually supportive, and cohesive relationships. The rules of the community and the roles of its members are well defined. Their typical diet contains 41%

fat. The average individual is 9.1 kg overweight. By contrast, the population of Bangor, an adjacent town, is of mixed English, German, and Italian stock. Families there are less gregarious and religious, and their social roles are less clearly defined. The death rate from myocardial infarction in Roseto was one-half of that in Bangor. By 1976, as the younger inhabitants were leaving Roseto and entering the mainstream of American life, the incidence of myocardial infarction of this group was increasing to the levels seen in the general population.

Studies contrasting Japanese and Japanese-Americans, American Benedictine priests working in the community and members of the same religious order who remain cloistered, and nomadic Bedouins and Bedouin settlers in villages in Israel have all come to similar conclusions (Caffrey 1966; Marmot and Syme 1976; Matsumoto 1970). A stable social environment is by definition unchanging and predictable. It imposes a minimum of demands, challenges, and tasks on its members. Conversely, social disruption, ethnicity, poverty, discord, and danger conduce to high BP (Harburg et al. 1973) and its complications.

Interactions of Risk Factors

The foregoing account implies that risk factors are dynamically related. It also documents that no one risk factor is associated with any one disease outcome. To take obesity as an example: it is a risk factor for IHD and for sleep apnea and type II diabetes mellitus, both of which in turn predispose to, and are associated with, IHD. This form of heart disease is said to occur in well-nourished people who exercise little and ingest excess calories and saturated fats. Yet the relationship of low levels of exercise and excessive food intake is mainly associated with obesity in women (Goldblatt, Moore, and Stunkard 1965; Stunkard 1975). However, men are more prone to IHD in Western societies because male obesity is mainly abdominal, and not the pelvic variety seen in women.

Saturated fats, cholesterol, and triglycerides raise LDL levels. A low ratio of HDL to LDL is a metabolic risk factor for the disease. In familial (genetic) hypercholesterolemia (type IIA hyperlipoproteinemia) (Brown and Goldstein 1986), LDL levels are high and coronary atherosclerosis and myocardial infarction occur before the age of 30 years in homozygotes (Frederickson, Goldstein, and Brown 1978). Thus genetic factors play a predominant role in one form of IHD leading to fatal myocardial infarction. On the other hand, the HDL:LDL ratio falls in unemployed male workers without their having this genetic trait (Saxena 1980).

There are six genetic forms of hyperlipoproteinemia (Frederickson, Goldstein, and Brown 1978). Type IIA is the best understood. It is a receptor-mediated defect in cholesterol metabolism (Brown and Goldstein 1986). In type III hyperlipoproteinemia a defect in the liver's uptake of LDL occurs due to a deficiency in the apolipoprotein E (III). In homozygotes this rare disorder is also likely to antecede IHD; yet the clinical expression of the genetic defect is enhanced by hypothyroidism, diabetes mellitus, and obesity (Kidd and Morton 1989).

Hypertension is a frequent antecedent of IHD. It in turn interacts with, and is exacerbated by, obesity and excess calories. Additionally, hypertension conduces to myocardial hypertrophy, relative myocardial insufficiency, and myocardial failure, especially in the presence of arteriosclerotic coronary arteries.

Except in the particular instance of hyperlipoproteinemia IIA, IHD is a product of a variety of interactive factors. What is usually overlooked, however, by investigators interested in the role of stressful experience in this disease is that coronary atherosclerosis appears (silently) to develop early in the lives of young persons and evolves over many years (Enos, Holmes, and Beyer 1953)—a datum suggesting that whatever the etiological or pathogenetic roles of stressful experiences for IHD are, they are likely to be synergistic and permissive (Grossarth-Maticek et al. 1988). No one category of stressful experience has invariantly or universally been associated with IHD and its complications. And it does not occur independently of socioeconomic and ethnic status, age, gender, or personal characteristics. Several categories of long-term, predisposing stressful experiences have been identified for IHD: social isolation; bereavement; excessive noise; heavy manual work; shift work; specific work conditions with and without assurance of future employment; and unemployment.

The Role of Stressful Experience in the Initiation (Pathogenesis) of Disease

The mechanisms by which stressful experiences such as bereavement, change, and challenge set off a chain of events leading to bodily disease are largely unknown. Implicit in all past and current theories of pathogenesis is the belief that the brain, which regulates every bodily process, mediates in an undisclosed manner the changes that lead to physiological disturbances in bodily systems or to structural changes in organs and their constituent cells. And, in fact, there is a growing body of experimental evidence suggesting that the brain participates at some stage in diseases as diverse as AN, bronchial asthma, and essential hypertension (Chalmers 1975; Weiner 1977, 1989c; Weiner, Hofer, and Stunkard 1980).

A part of our ignorance stems from the fact that the pathogenesis of most diseases remains unknown. Therefore, we are still unable to describe the chain of events that links the stressful experience with the physiological mechanisms in the brain (and its outflow systems) and, in turn, with the proximate pathogenetic factors that incite disease in the target organ(s). The relationship of stressful experience to disease onset is of both a correlational and retrospective nature. We do not really know what most correlations mean; they may be causal or they may merely be temporal.

The traditional postulate is that the emotional response to the stressful experience is translated in some unknown manner into bodily changes, consisting of altered autonomic nervous system activity or altered hormonal or immunological levels or patterns. But this conceptual approach begs the question, because the problem of the translation of an emotion into bodily changes has not been, and may never be, solved (chapter 8). There is no point in stating that this profound puzzle will at some time in the future be solved if it cannot be. The emotions and the physiological changes may be correlated, but the former do not necessarily cause the latter; they are part and parcel of an integrated response. To put it another way: Emotions do not cause disease.

Alternative ideas have been put forward that attempt to circumvent this time-honored conundrum. A more fruitful approach is to postulate the likelihood that each percept is processed in parallel by the brain (Weiner 1972, 1989b): Visual information is transmitted to the visual cortex, but it also goes more directly by a retinohypothalamic tract to the suprachiasmatic (SCN) and PVN nuclei of the hypothalamus and to the pineal gland (Moore and Lenn 1972). Therefore, the theoretical notion, supported by evidence, is that a visual experience and a physiological response may occur in temporal, but not causal, relationship to each other by virtue of the fact that visual information is processed by two or more parallel pathways. Additionally, different (e.g., nonvisual) aspects of the same experience are processed by different receptors and neuronal circuits.

If we apply this set of ideas to the experience of bereavement as an onset condition of disease we shall not conclude that the resulting depressed mood directly causes physiological changes such as elevated levels of serum cortisol, an increased content of NE or its metabolites in urine, and other changes in many critical bodily functions such as appetite, sleep, elimination, temperature regulation, and patterns of hormonal rhythms (Weiner 1990a, 1990b). A more fruitful approach to the problem is to inquire how the disruption of a relationship could alter the regulation of physiological rhythms (Weiner 1975). The answer may well lie in the fact that human relationships consist of more than the emotional bonds that tie two persons together, as was discussed in chapter 4 (Ehlers, Frank, and Kupfer 1988; Hofer 1984; Moore-Ede, Sulzman, and Fuller 1982).

This line of thought also contradicts the customary approach that seeks to link a stressful experience (such as a task) to changes in the levels of a single variable (such as a neurotransmitter or a hormone). In actuality, we have known since Mason's work (1968) on animals and Brod's on humans (1960, 1970) that such experiences generate a patterned panoply of hormonal or cardiovascular responses respectively, which at that time were measured in terms of changes in their levels rather than in their rhythms. Indeed, in most instances no single hormonal change occurs with most stressful experiences.

Physiological and behavioral response patterns are often anticipatory. They are especially likely to occur when a person is faced with a novel experience (Bruhn 1987). Some physiological changes habituate with repetitive experience: When neurotransmitter or hormone levels remain elevated, their specific receptors may be "down-regulated," become "resistant" to the ligand, or be desensitized.

It is not known how acute or chronic stressful experiences and the distress they generate, or the failure to cope with them, directly contribute to the onset of one disease or illness. Despite decades of research in autonomic psychophysiology, psychoneuroendocrinology, and now psychoneuroimmunology (Ader 1981), progress in answering this question has been slow.

It is one thing to demonstrate that in nature, or in the laboratory, stressful experiences produce physiological changes in bodily systems, but it is quite another matter to demonstrate that such acute changes lead to disease. Thus it may very well be true that the normotensive children of a hypertensive parent have larger and more persistent BP responses (Light 1981; Light and Obrist 1980) but it is quite another matter to demonstrate that this BP hyperreactivity eventuates in hypertension (Weder and Julius 1985); in fact, the evidence is quite to the contrary.

Therefore, physiological correlates of stressful experiences have been neither causally, temporally, nor experimentally linked with the onset of most diseases, with a few possible exceptions and in some animal models of disease (see chapter 7). Until such links are forged we shall continue to rely on correlations. However, new concepts about the mediators of stressful experience are being developed that may lead to new ways of carrying out investigations and analyzing the data they generate (see chapter 9), in the hope that insights about the pathogenesis of specific illnesses and diseases will be gained.

The Pathogenesis of Disease

Much is known about the multiple risk factors in many diseases. And a great amount of knowledge has been accumulated about the pathophysiology and the pathological anatomy of many diseases, but as noted, our knowledge of the pathogenesis of most diseases remains rudimentary, with the exception of the infectious diseases (and the avitaminoses), the immune and acute phase responses to infectious agents leading to inflammation, and the eventual clearing (or not) of antigen-antibody complexes.

Physicians usually do not, or cannot, study disease prior to its inception. Their understanding of disease is based on retrospection. As a result it is almost impossible to infer pathogenesis from pathophysiology. To illustrate the point: The manner in which an autoimmune disease begins is by no means established, except in those instances in which it (e.g., SLE) is precipitated by a drug, or when it is associated with a persistent virus infection (e.g., rubella in children who develop juvenile RA) (Chantler, Tingle, and Petty 1988). Specifically, it is unknown how tolerance to native antigens is broken. Therefore, all speculations about the pathogenetic role of psychosocial factors in autoimmune disease must be tentative; they might contribute to, interact with, or exacerbate an initial infection, add somehow to intolerance to native antigens, or intervene at some stage in the ensuing cascade of immunological changes that follow the onset of disease. But at the same time, no one change in the immune system characterizes any one of the autoimmune diseases; rather, patterns of change are observed.

Our current lack of knowledge about the pathogenesis of diseases, and, therefore, our inability to link stressful experiences to unknown pathogenetic processes, weakens the argument about their contributory role. Nonetheless, it seems likely that most diseases have a multifactorial etiology, in which genetic, gender, hormonal, (possibly) infectious, and immunological factors, socioeconomic status, and stressful experiences interact. But the manner in which they do so remains uncertain. Each of these categories may contribute more or less to the etiological and pathogenetic variance in the different subforms of each disease.

Another reason for the conundrum of relating pathogenesis to pathophysiology has already been alluded to: In the most general sense, disease is the end-product of the interaction of an inciting agent and the host's responses to it. In addition, each disease is heterogeneous, not only in terms of various combinations of risk factors, but also in all likelihood in its pathogenesis. The same anatomically defined lesion may come about by a variety of ways or different combinations of pathogenetic mechanisms. As Grossman (1978) has pointed out, a peptic DU is the product of various admixtures of "protective" and "aggressive" gastroduodenal functions—hydrochloric acid and bicarbonate secretion, gastric contractions, and mucous output. None of these is by itself sufficient, or even necessary, to produce the lesion. Furthermore, each by itself is the end-product of complex regulatory and counterregulatory processes.

Duodenal ulcer is not the only example of the complexity of the pathogenetic riddle. A disease such as diabetes mellitus exists in at least three forms, each characterized by elevated levels of blood sugar and glycosuria. The pathogenesis of the juvenile form is quite different from the adult form's, and each form requires different treatment. However, the emphasis in medicine is to diagnose and define a disease in terms of a change in the level of a single variable: in the case of DU, raised levels of hydrochloric acid secretion; in diabetes mellitus, elevated blood sugar levels.

The blood sugar level is, on the surface, a very simple variable, but it is actually a fluctuating signal—the integration of a large number of other variables. They in turn increase and decrease the level of blood glucose according to the organism's, and a particular organ's, need for it. Insulin lowers glucose levels by diminishing its production and increasing its utilization. Epinephrine, glucagon, and the corticosteroids, each by different means, increase its level in the bloodstream. Insulin secretion by pancreatic islet cells is a rhythmic process, proportional to blood glucose fluctuations (Cryer and Gerich 1985). It is the product of a variety of intrinsic (pancreatic) feedback systems (chapter 8). In addition, exercise, the nature of the diet, food intake, and the state of sleep alter insulin secretion (Molnar, Taylor, and Langworthy 1972). Increases in insulin level indirectly reduce an animal's carbohydrate intake.

Therefore, the study of the level of a single physiological variable at one point in time as a criterion of disease, obscures the complex, dynamic interplay of factors that determine it. The various influences that bring about insulin and glucose fluctuations also include the behavioral activities and state of the organism, mediated by complex regulatory neural and hormonal interactions.

As one studies any physiological system over time, one is struck by the fact that it fluctuates rhythmically. Each system, however, has its own characteristic rhythm (see chapter 2). In disease these rhythms are altered. In supraventricular and ventricular cardiac arrhythmias, the heartbeat changes from a regular to an irregular rhythm, with either increased or decreased frequency. Or the heart may suddenly cease to beat altogether—its normal rhythm is abolished.

The pathogenesis of these two forms of arrhythmias has been extensively studied but is not fully understood. However, the evidence suggests that several interactive influences produce cardiac arrhythmias and arrest. In one such form—the long QT syndrome, which was discussed in chapter 5—a combination of factors antecedes ventricular arrhythmias and death. During the prolonged QT period the cardiac muscle is depolarized longer than usual. At the same time, excessive left cardiac sympathetic activity constitutes a bias in one of the main regulatory systems of the heart, which interacts with its relatively prolonged state of depolarization. As a result a new state of organization is established, consisting of uncoordinated and chaotic cardiac activity reflecting the circus motion of rotating, spiral waves in the heart (Winfree 1983).

The pathogenesis of the consequences of structural cardiovascular disease—angina pectoris, myocardial ischemia and infarction, cardiac arrhythmias, and sudden cardiac death—is also fairly well known. Furthermore, it is recognized that in most instances these sudden events are triggered by stressful experiences, especially challenges, certain tasks, and sudden changes in the lives of patients (Weiner 1991a). They occur after a buildup of atherosclerosis in the coronary arteries, which may take many years (Ross 1986). This form of disease is one of the few in which some insight about its pathogenesis has been obtained.

Stressful Experience, Coronary Vasospasm, and Myocardial Ischemia

Until recently the possibility that a transition may occur between ill health due to the hyperventilation syndrome, and coronary artery disease, myocardial ischemia or infarction, or sudden cardiac death was not entertained (Kruyswijk, Jansen, and Miller 1986). In some hyperventilators the signs of myocardial ischemia may occur due to a reduction in coronary blood flow with or without vasospasm (Yasue et al. 1978; Freeman et al. 1987). Spasm limits coronary blood flow; it may occur at rest with or without pain. In turn, coronary blood flow may be reduced by structural narrowing or occlusion of a coronary artery, which is conducive to spasm and may lead to pain and ischemia when the myocardial oxygen requirement increases, with exercise, and then exceeds the blood supply. And arteries comprised by atherosclerosis, leading to thrombosis and acute myocardial infarction, can still show vasospasm (Hackett et al. 1987). But there is no one to one relationship between the amount of coronary artery narrowing and symptoms, occlusion, or infarction (Freeman 1987).

Vasospasm can occur with or without coronary atherosclerosis and in any phase of IHD. And hyperventilation may be manifested with or without such disease. Vasospasm is not necessarily associated with anginal pain, but myocardial perfusion is diminished, and left ventricular wall motion abnormalities may occur (silent ischemia). When anginal pain is present and cardiac perfusion deficits are produced, the EKG may show no abnormalities. On the other hand, elevations or depressions of the ST-segment of the EKG—as a criterion of myocardial ischemia at rest—are only accompanied by pain in 32% of 6,009 episodes in 33 patients (Maseri et al. 1978). These EKG changes may occur without any or consistent increases in HR or BP.

The question is: How, and under what circumstances, does silent ischemia occur (Schiffer et al. 1980)? It is recognized that it can be incited pharmacologically by histamine, NE, and neuropeptide-Y (NPY) (Gu et al. 1983), which all produce vasospasm. Hyperventilation does so in 25% of patients with proven coronary artery disease (Mortenson, Vilhelmson, and Sande 1981; Rasmussen et al. 1987).

Of greater interest to those investigating the role of stressful experience in the inception of silent ischemic episodes with ST-segment changes is the work of Deanfield and his colleagues (1983, 1984). They showed that in 16 patients with angina pectoris, episodes of transient myocardial ischemia occurred in the absence of physical exertion. During the performance of serial subtraction (100 minus 7, etc.), 12 of the 16 had abnormalities of regional myocardial perfusion measured by positron emission tomography with rubidium-82. While subtracting numbers, only 6 of the 12 showed ST-segment depression,

and a mere 4 complained of angina pectoris. Exercise produced perfusion abnormalities and ST-segment depression in all 16, and angina pectoris in 15
patients. The act of public speaking may induce a fall in ejection fraction in
about one-third of patients with coronary artery disease. Regional wall motion
abnormalities occurred while reading a book, during the Stroop test, or while
doing mental arithmetic in 59% of 23 of these patients. Public speaking and
exercise were equivalent in producing cardiac dysfunction (Rozanski et al.
1988).

The incidence of anginal pain is, therefore, a severe underestimate of the
true prevalence of myocardial ischemia as judged by ST-segment changes or
perfusion deficits. The EKG changes also do not faithfully reflect myocardial
perfusion deficits, which in turn are associated with coronary vasospasm, or
reduced coronary blood flow induced by common, everyday tasks and events.
It is now rather certain that myocardial ischemia occurs during everyday
physical and mental activities in patients with, or people without, coronary
artery disease who are going about their daily lives. Myocardial ischemia, as
judged by ST-segment changes, less frequently occurs during sleep (Barry et
al. 1988). The ischemia is, however, potentially damaging to the myocardium.

Why should a simple task such as mental arithmetic (serial subtraction) produce silent ischemia? Even if it is not experienced as unpleasant, it increases
sympathetic discharge to the heart and lowers baroreceptor activity. Norepinephrine and possibly NPY are secreted. Heart rate and BP levels increase.
The ischemia is subendocardial and not transmural; it is likely to be secondary
to an (unmet) increased demand for oxygen by the myocardium and is not
necessarily due to reduced coronary blood flow or spasm, even if the coronary
arteries are partly blocked. This form of myocardial ischemia is much more
often associated with an elevated than a depressed ST-segment in the EKG.
But in about 40% of patients no such (ST-) segmental changes are observed.
Mental arithmetic is most likely to produce myocardial ischemia in patients
who complain of ischemia (and pain) at rest and/or during exercise (L'Abbate
1990).

Stressful Experience, Coronary Vasospasm, and Cardiac Arrhythmias

Cardiac arrhythmias may accompany coronary vasospasm with or without ischemia. Various forms of supraventricular and ventricular arrhythmias have
been recorded (Tzivoni et al. 1980). In Maseri's series (1978) of 37 patients,
episodes of ischemia with perfusion deficits were accompanied by ventricular
premature beats in 27, ventricular tachycardia in 19, ventricular fibrillation in
9, and atrioventricular block in 9. The various arrhythmias were not associated with pain. Three of the 19 patients had no serious narrowing (by athero-
mata) of their coronary arteries.

Arrhythmias have also been observed in patients with no discernible coronary artery disease who are speaking in public, doing mental arithmetic, driving a racing car, awaking from sleep, confronting danger, or experience an outburst of anger (Russell 1984). During public speaking increased levels of plasma E occur first and are followed by a rise in the plasma content of NE. When NE levels increase, NYP is cosecreted. Beta-adrenergic blocking agents on such occasions prevent the appearance of arrhythmias. On the other hand, FFAs are secreted in anticipation of danger and exercise (Taggart, Gibbons, and Somerville 1969). A role has been assigned to FFAs in inciting arrhythmia formation and prognosis during and after myocardial infarction (Oliver, Kurien, and Greenwood 1968). However, the role of stressful experiences or tasks in inciting arrhythmias requires much further study, using advanced monitoring techniques (Orth-Gomer et al. 1986).

The observations of Deanfield et al. (1983, 1984), Rozanski et al. (1988), and Russell (1984) raise serious questions about the usual definition of stressful experience with its traditional dire implications. They describe everyday activities, tasks, challenges, and perturbations (that are not necessarily distressing) that are associated with silent myocardial ischemia, perfusion deficits, possible coronary artery flow reduction, and arrhythmias. The fact remains that common-or-garden tasks and challenges perturb the functions of the (damaged) heart to produce potentially lethal effects. Exercise-induced silent ischemia, on the other hand, predicts angina pectoris and a small number of nonfatal myocardial infarctions—a conclusion based on 50 patients followed over a period of 13.5 years (Erikssen 1987).

Stressful Experience, Sudden Cardiac Death, Myocardial Infarction, and Angina Pectoris

The literature on the pathogenesis of angina pectoris, myocardial infarction, and sudden cardiac death remains unsettled. Endicott (1989) summarized six major papers on the topic and concluded that 90% or more of the hearts of patients dying of acute myocardial infarction showed at least one coronary artery with more than 75% narrowing by atherosclerosis. By contrast Epstein, Quyyumi, and Bonow (1989) concluded that most patients who die of an acute fatal myocardial infarction or sudden cardiac death, have mild to moderate coronary stenosis—defined as less than 50%, or at most 70%, occlusion of an artery (especially the proximal left anterior descending artery)—which must be combined with a thrombus. Patients with severe stenosis (70–80% or more) develop a collateral coronary circulation, which averts acute death and is associated with angina pectoris. Factors other than mild stenosis and thrombosis may be involved in myocardial infarction or sudden death: An atherosclerotic plaque may rupture, or a thrombus may form. Spasm may occur with stenosis due to platelet releasing factor. Platelet-fibrin emboli pass into arterioles. The atherosclerotic plaque may depress the release of endothelial relaxing factors. Another important variable is the threshold for pain in each patient; in 15% it may be so high that ischemia may be silent even with severe stenosis.

But Baroldi, Falzi, and Mariani (1979) have come to other conclusions, based on studying 208 patients who died suddenly: 25% of them had coronary artery stenosis of less than 70%—a number that was less than in the control subjects dying accidentally from other causes. There was, therefore, no proof that sudden death is due to stenosis or thrombotic occlusion. They concluded that no linear causal relation exists between stenosis and sudden death. In fact, acute thrombosis occurred in only 15% of those who died suddenly. What they did find was that in 75% of all the patients who died suddenly, a cardiac necrosis was present. This disease was first described by Raab (1970) and has been ascribed to excessive NE secretion (Baroldi 1975). Thus sudden cardiac death cannot be used as a synonym for myocardial infarction; it may occur with or without infarction, stenosis, or thrombosis.

Neither coronary atherosclerosis nor thrombosis is necessary, or sufficient, to induce sudden death of this kind. Other processes contribute, such as fatal ventricular arrhythmias, a cardiomyopathy induced either by NE excess or by as yet unknown processes. The antecedents of various ventricular arrhythmias are not uniform either; they may be triggered by early or late after-potentials, periods of repolarization, or electrical instability, or they may occur in the Wolfe-Parkinson-White syndrome, which may antecede ventricular tachycardia (Chung 1989).

Sudden Cardiac Death

Every year about 4×10^5 persons die suddenly in the United States. Just exactly how many of these die with the heart in ventricular fibrillation is unknown. This arrhythmia may occur at a slow or rapid rate. Initially regular, these new rhythms undergo a transition to low-amplitude irregularity. Such patients die with or without coronary atherosclerosis or valvular lesions.

Determining the role of stressful experience in sudden cardiac death is problematic for at least three reasons: (1) Based on the previous discussion, there is no uniform set of its pathogenetic antecedents. (2) Attempts to identify the experience once the patient is dead are unreliable. (3) Given the heterogeneity of the sources of dying suddenly, there is no reason why an invariant set of stressful experiences, their mediators, and the terminal pathogenetic process should exist.

Two exceptions to these axioms may be made: First, resuscitated patients who have had cardiac arrests may be able to remember what they were doing, thinking, and feeling and where they were prior to losing consciousness. Second, the catecholamine cardiomyopathy—when it is not associated with a phaeochromocytoma—has been described in patients who have experienced great personal danger (accidents, rapes, etc.) accompanied by terror.

The current belief about sudden cardiac death occurring in most patients is that the usual long-term risk factors for coronary atherosclerosis obtain (Kannel et al. 1975), but that transient perturbations are superimposed on them (Lown 1982). They are generated by reciprocal imbalances between vagal and sympathetic efferent cardiac discharge (Lown, Verrier, and Corbalar 1973). Sudden cardiac death is especially seen in depressed individuals (Lown 1977).

Stressful Experience and Myocardial Infarction

Unexplained to date are the observations that the onset of myocardial infarction occurs with excess frequency in the morning hours when the person is alert and active. However, it is also known that in some persons infarction may occur during sleep. During abrupt experiences—exercise, arguments (often about "who is right" or issues of power), excitement, or the elimination of feces or urine—infarction may take place. Bereavement also antecedes myocardial infarction.

These everyday events, or bereavements, are imposed on long-standing risk factors, including social factors, and adverse work conditions. But none of these observations fully explains why infarction should then occur at a particular hour after years of adverse, pressured, uncertain, or prolonged work conditions (Siegrist, Matschinger, and Siegrist 1987), disappointment about success, and unsatisfactory and boring marriages. It has been suggested that mounting dejection, demoralization, and fatigue to the point of exhaustion antecede an episode of infarction (Groen 1976). In turn, demoralization has been associated with increased variability in plasma fibrinogen, clotting time, and BP values (Wolf 1969). And some demoralized patients hyperventilate (Freeman 1987).

Much more information is required to sort out the various factors that lead to myocardial infarction in identified subgroups. They in turn need to be related to various antecedent experiences. The determinants of recurrences of infarction with or without death also need further study (Brackett and Powell 1988).

Stressful Experience and Angina Pectoris

Very few prospective studies relating stressful experience and uncomplicated angina pectoris have been carried out in the light of the contention that such a pure form of IHD occurs more frequently with extensive stenosis and a collateral circulation. Two studies have been published (Groen et al. 1968; Medalie et al. 1973) on 10,000 male Israeli workers followed over a five-year period. The usual risk factors for atherosclerosis were present. Two additional factors were associated with pure angina pectoris: The men had poor marital relationships—the wives were perceived as cold, indifferent, and unsupportive by their husbands—and they felt chronically anxious and tense and slept poorly all of the time.

To summarize: There is evidence that certain kinds of stressful experiences may trigger myocardial ischemia and arrhythmias and antecede sudden death. However, in the past the pathogenesis of these cardiac events has on the whole been discussed in terms of single variables—an increase in sympathetic discharge to the heart, vasospasm, or a diminished myocardial oxygen supply. But the matter is more complex. All of these factors may interact; they do not operate in isolation. Some experience may trigger increased sympathetic efferent discharge, which may arrive during a phase of partial depolarization of the muscle and trigger a cardiac arrhythmia or an arrest. Sudden cardiac death is the final outcome of changes in hemodynamic status, myocardial ischemia, and an arrhythmia. Ischemia, in turn, is usually a compound result of oxygen supply and demand and vasospasm; but it may occur with or without coronary artery spasm. Finally, it is clear that each of these factors may modulate the other, and that the interactions of stressful experiences, challenges, tasks, and changes in state are different when the heart is damaged than when it is not.

Factors That Sustain Disease and Alter Its Prognosis

We know less about the factors that sustain disease than we do about its pathophysiology. Yet in the case of experimental high BP the factors inciting it differ from those that sustain it: The brain stem and hypothalamic mechanisms that participate in the maintenance of experimental BP elevations have been shown to be separate (Chalmers 1975; Ganten, Schelling, and Ganten 1977; Weiner 1977) from the brain mechanisms that initiate them (chapter 8).

In some cases of human hypertension, secondary physiological adaptations to the elevation of BP include a diminution in the sensitivity of the arterial baroreceptors (Korner et al. 1974), an increase in peripheral resistance in response to an increase in cardiac output, structurally increased resistance to regional blood flow (Folkow and Hallbäck 1977), and changes in cardiac performance (Frohlich, Tarazi, and Dustan 1971).

Other changes in many systems are also found in abiding essential hypertension. To mention just two: (1) Significant increases in the plasma concentration of aldosterone occur with age in essential hypertension—in contrast to a decline with age of plasma aldosterone levels in normotensive subjects (Genest, Koiw, and Kuchel 1977). (2) Plasma renin activity is markedly increased during the development of the malignant phase of hypertensive disease and renal failure. Complex changes also occur in renal dynamics. They are believed to be the consequences of a subform of the borderline hypertensive state, in which there is increased activity of the sympathetic nervous system. Renal blood flow is reduced by reversible intrarenal vasoconstriction and by increases in circulating NE and in sympathetic drive, both of which reduce the urinary excretion of sodium and water (Brown et al. 1977; Hollenberg and Adams 1976). But the rise in BP should cause an increased excretion of sodium and water, which at first does and later does not occur. Therefore, a progressive resetting of the relationships of BP to sodium and water excretion—a regulatory disturbance—is produced. Progressive renal changes ensue, accounting for the change from borderline labile hypertension to essential hypertension. In short, by a fall in renal blood flow and a rise in total and renal vascular resistance, the kidney maintains the BP increases that were initiated elsewhere (Brown et al. 1977).

Not only do secondary physiological (mal)adaptations occur in essential hypertension, but the psychology of patients with this disease also changes during its course. Safar and his colleagues (1978) have shown that patients in the borderline phase of essential hypertension demonstrate aggressive tendencies that engender anxiety in them. Such individuals have few fantasies but a variety of bodily symptoms. In the later phase of sustained hypertension, these symptoms and signs vanish as anxiety disappears. The hostility is still inferable, but it is neither apperceived nor recognized by the patients.

The course and prognosis of many diseases are influenced not only by the doctor-patient relationship and the personal characteristics of patients (Moos and Solomon 1964), but by the help and advice of many others: For example, the prognosis after myocardial infarction is considerably worse in widowers than in age-matched married men (Chandra et al. 1983).

Patients who have successfully been treated with antithyroid medication or thyroid surgery for Graves disease may show persistent metabolic alterations and psychological deficits and maladaptations (Ruesch et al. 1947), which impair their capacity for work and for relationships. Noncompliance to medical regimens may endanger the patient. Improper or inadequate medical care may lead him or her to eschew all further help, resort to inexpert treatment, or seek help from untrained people.

Failure to appreciate adequately a patient's psychological responses to an illness may lead to his or her chronic invalidism; indeed, chronic symptomatology is the rule in the case of injuries sustained at work, which are compensated by insurance payments. Society, therefore, contributes to the maintenance of symptoms that are only indirectly related to the industrial accident or illness. On the other hand, some societies stigmatize the helpless or socially incompetent—especially the mentally ill or defective, the handicapped, and the elderly—providing inadequate care or insufficient funds for their education, rehabilitation, nutrition, and housing.

These examples are selective; they do justice to only a small number of the factors that sustain disease or influence its course and that may need correction before adequate treatment results can be achieved. In practice, however, the physician is in a position to help patients to achieve optimal functioning despite being ill and to live with their illness; he or she is often able to relive suffering and help patients to die with dignity.

The Potentially Stressful Effect of Illness and Disease

The meanings and effects of illness and disease on patients, their families, and their social group have been studied and written about at great length (Bibring and Kahana 1968; Binger 1945; Engel 1962; Karasu and Steinmuller 1978; Pasnau 1975; Strain and Grossman 1975; von Uexküll 1979). Suffice it to say that illness and disease constitute a threat and a change in people's lives. Additional tasks are imposed on the sick person by the specific nature of the illness and its symptoms: whether the illness comes on abruptly or gradually; whether it is treatable or not; whether it carries a special meaning or stigma; and whether it will require hospitalization, special technical procedures, or surgery. A vital factor in the patient's successful adaptation to illness is the role and response of the caring professional person; much has been written about the positive and negative therapeutic effects of the doctor-patient relationship.

The successful adaptation of patients to illness and disease is partly a function of their experience of, and ability to cope with, previous illnesses and of their relationships with those who provided care during them. However, additional factors must be considered in the patient's responses to illness: For example, the illness or its symptoms may acquire a very individual meaning (chapter 3).

The metabolic and physiological alterations caused by the illness or the drugs used to treat it may impair cerebral metabolism and function, thereby altering the patient's perception, memory, or problem-solving ability and thus his or her ability to cope with experiences. Elderly people and children have fewer coping abilities and strategies than those in other stages of their lives; they require very special care in the strange environment of the hospital as well as help in adapting to illness and disease. Many people other than physicians are involved in the care of the chronically ill, disabled, or handicapped.

Summary

A selective review has been carried out on the relationship of stressful experience (which can include illness and disease) to the etiology, pathogenesis, and course of disease. The emphasis has been that such experiences are but one of several interactive factors in predisposing to disease, precipitating it, or altering its course.

The relationship of stressful experiences to disease in humans is complex and recursive. Only a relatively small proportion of persons develop disease unless they are exposed to certain epidemics; that low number is presumably accounted for by those who are predisposed to it. The general predisposition to disease is in part a function of the age and gender of the subject. But there are also very specific risk factors that result from genetic variation, intra-uterine or postnatal experience, or nutritional or structural factors.

Until recently, the assumption was made that the onset of disease was a direct, or linear, outcome of stressful experience: In Selye's rats the structural changes in the stomach, lymph nodes, and thymus were presumed to be the direct consequence of the action of the corticosteroids. But the matter seems much more complicated. The predisposition to, and the "choice" of, a disease is to be found in organ-specific, (local) regulatory disturbances. This axiomatic statement is supported by the fact that bronchial hyper-reactivity is the sine qua non for bronchial asthma; it is due to an excessive responsiveness to acetylcholine of the postganglionic, muscarinic receptor of bronchial smooth muscle. A number of regulatory disturbances have also been described in human peptic duodenal ulcer: the failure of gastric hydrochloric acid to suppress gastrin production by the antrum, an excessive acid secretory response to histamine and amino acids, an accelerated transit time, etc. In Cushing's disease cortisol has a positive (rather than a negative) feedback effect on ACTH secretion. The predisposition to some infections lies at times with an incapacity to produce antibodies (in the agammaglobulinemias); at other times T-helper (CD4$^+$) cells die and cannot "aid" B-cells to secrete them (as in AIDS). Even benign infectious agents become pathogenetic in AIDS when no immune response is mounted.

These few examples of local disturbances in the control and regulation of a particular system (many other instances exist) support the contention that disease comes about in complex ways. The local disturbances may also be structural. The interaction of coronary artery disease with mental arithmetic produces ST-segment changes on the EKG, ventricular wall motion abnormalities, and defective myocardial perfusion. And the arterial disease predisposes to the instability of spasm. In patients without coronary artery disease no such changes usually occur.

So far, nothing has been said that would allow one to understand how a subsystem of the organism is regulated or that would explain its form of operation. The formal properties of every function subserved by each subsystem are rhythmic. The manner by which these rhythms are generated requires discussion (chapter 10).

Nonetheless, changes in rhythmic functions occur in every one of the illnesses and diseases described in the last two chapters. In the syndromes of ill-health the usual patterns of gut motility are altered; in the hyperventilation syndrome respiratory rhythms change; and in fibromyositis a new rhythm is interspersed during slow-wave sleep. As we have seen, hyperventilation can produce coronary vasospasm and arrhythmias. It can also complicate coronary artery disease.

The study of disease has been obscured by measuring only single variables, rather than patterns of change. However, the latter were described in borderline hypertension. That disturbed rhythms are associated with changes in structure is exemplified by the cardiac (ventricular) arrhythmias.

The tentative conclusion is that ill health results from a change in the normal rhythms of a subsystem incited by stressful experience. Disease, by contrast, occurs when stressful experience interacts with a preexisting regulatory disturbance or with structural change.

The interaction of the organ-specific, regulatory disturbances or the structural defects, with the outputs that emanate from the brain, that mediate stressful experiences to produce or enhance disease is poorly understood. Stressful experiences that occasion specific and integrated alterations in behavioral and physiological systems, which are mediated by the brain and its neuronal and hormonal outputs, do not linearly produce disease. They only do so in a nonlinear manner in interaction with organ-specific disturbances, which are either genetically programmed or are the product of early experience or slowly progressing structural changes (e.g., in arteries).

The relationship of stressful experience to disease occurs with a low probability in humans and animals except under certain conditions: Action to avoid the stressful experience is impossible, prevented, or punished; the experience is overwhelming; genetic predispositions to disease are present; prior experience acts as a risk factor; or stressful experience is chronically sustained.

7 The Experimental Study of Stressful Experience in Animals

In the years following Cannon's and Selye's work a vast body of literature on the experimental study of stressful experience has accumulated, despite the fact that no consensus could be reached about its definition and classification.

To add to the confusion and the complexity of the topic, individual responses to the same experience were observed in animals of the same species. In part, the individual differences could be understood on the basis of genetic species and strain differences; in part, investigators who neglected their subject's individual histories and gender—thus contravening a fundamental tenet of biology—did so at the price of not being able to understand the results of their studies. Other investigators neglected to take into account the context in which their experiments were carried out, or the behavior of their animals.

Much of the research on the effects of stressful experience on animals has been limited to the study of its immediate (not the long-term) outcomes, in the tradition begun by Cannon and Selye. Until recently, little was known about the effects of sustained, or of intermittent but repetitive, experiences, or of applying acute experiences upon a background of ongoing ones.

The controlled study of stressful experience in animals has employed many of the techniques Selye used—injury, cold, heat, restraint, painful stimuli, and frightening situations. To these have been added enforced activity (running and swimming), electric shock (avoidable or unavoidable, continuous or intermittent), handling, novel environments, conditioning exercises (both classical and operant, avoidance and "emotional"), crowding animals together, or socially isolating them.

Only recently have investigators studied stressful experiences that are more akin to those found in nature: how the process or the attainment of a particular social status, which is fraught with strife, affects the behavior and physiology of animals and places them at risk for disease; how territorial and other conflicts produce integrated responses; how crucial affiliative bonds are formed, and how their disruption has immediate and subsequent effects on the behavior and physiology of young animals.

In nature, injury and infection do befall animals, but they are not paradigmatic of conditions encountered in their everyday lives. Stress research has recently become a study of some characteristic selective pressures. Furthermore, the relationship of stressful experiences to the induction of disease in animals is not as clear-cut or linear as Selye believed: Disease is not their inevitable outcome. However, their effect in initiating, ameliorating or worsening disease in animals, which model their effect in humans, has considerable heuristic power.

The ultimate aim of this line of research would seem to be to provide a complete description of the response of the organism to stressful experiences. In turn, these responses are individual, in the same manner as the individual is unique. The sources of such individual differences must be identified before we can truly understand how one organism rises to challenge and remains in good health, and another fails and succumbs to disease.

Despite some intrinsic limitations, the experimental study of stressful experience in animals has partly substantiated, refined, modified, and extended many of the observations and claims made, and conclusions arrived at, in the previous chapters of this book. Investigations carried out in animals have many advantages: Critical variables can be controlled for; pure strains of animals can be bred; the mechanisms in the brain and the body that mediate the effects of the stressful experiences or perturbations can be analyzed; reliable observations may be made, but their validity and meaning must still be demonstrated by comparing the results of patently artefactual, stressful experiences with naturally occurring ones. Because behavioral and physiological differences in response patterns occur within and between species, caution must be exercised in overgeneralizing the results obtained in members of one genus or species to those obtained in others.

The limitation of many of the experimental procedures used in stress research must be cited; many are artefacts (see chapter 1). Social animals are frequently housed by themselves prior to subjecting them to experiments. Little attention is paid to their nutritional status or previous reproductive experience. Nocturnal animals are subjected to experimental procedures during the day when they customarily sleep.

Investigators do not regularly study the behaviors of their animal subjects during experiments especially if they are prevented (by restraint) from acting. The psychological responses (e.g., pain, fear, anger) cannot be studied directly in animals; they must be inferred from behavior.

Despite these cautionary statements, much progress continues to be made in understanding the mediators of integrated responses to stressful experience, and the ensuing pathogenesis of disease when it occurs. The instructive value of experimental stress research in this regard has been considerable.

It is not the intention of this chapter to review the vast literature on experimental stress research in animals; a selective account of it will be given. The focus of this chapter will be on new insights into the consequences of stressful experiences that illuminate the exquisite specificity of the responses. It will describe the long-range effects of acute experiences—especially if they occur early in the lives of animals. It will summarize recently discovered phenomena, such as stress analgesia and "learned helplessness." It will emphasize that stressful experiences affect rhythmic functions and that their behavioral and physiological consequences are patterned. And it will illuminate the complexity and heterogeneity of the pathogenesis of the disease produced in animals by these experiences.

Genetic Factors in the Response to Stressful Experiences

The genetic makeup of animals is a source of variability in their responses to stressful experiences. Rats sensitive or resistant to stressful experimental procedures have been bred. Naturally occurring strain differences in corticosterone responses to the same procedure were first described thirty years ago (Levine and Treiman 1964). Mutant forms of the liver enzyme cytochrome P450, involved in the synthesis of corticosteroids, exist in rats (Rapp and Dahl 1976), as do variations in the rate of catecholamine biosynthesis and receptor binding (Ciaranello 1979). However, many other factors, including early experience (Henry et al. 1971) and salt intake, alter catecholamine function, and they may modify or interact in an unknown or unpredictable manner with strain differences in the synthesis secretion or disposition of the mediators of stressful experiences.

Rats differ in their abilities to learn to prevent or avoid electric shocks to their feet. Some rats of the same strain are rapid learners; others are deficient in their learning ability. Both good and bad learners can be bred so that their offspring increase or diminish their capacities (Henn, Edwards, and Johnson 1988).

One pure mouse strain (CXBK) is deficient in the usual number of opiate receptors. Its members do not develop analgesia when they are injected with morphine (Baran et al. 1975), when they are subjected to intermittent and unavoidable foot shocks (Moskowitz, Terman, and Liebeskind 1985), or when they are defeated in a fight with another mouse (Miczek, Thompson, and Schuster 1982). Laboratory rats of various strains also vary in their ability to develop analgesia when subjected to such circumstances. Wild field mice manifest a much more profound analgesia by standard tests than do laboratory mice (Marek and Szacki 1991 in press). Therefore, the conclusions reached by the use of domesticated mice in experiments cannot be generalized to their untamed peers.

The Role of Intrauterine and Early Stressful Experience and Its Long-Term Consequences

Almost all experimental stress research in the past fifty years has focused upon the acute effects of stressful experience on adult animals to produce (phasic) changes in bodily function and structure, and in behavior. Two examples of the long-range effects of an acute experience on immature animals will now be cited. Ward and Ward (1989) have shown that pregnant rats exposed to light and restrained during the last week of gestation produce male offspring who, when sexually mature, do not copulate or ejaculate when in the company of receptive females. They also display the female copulatory pattern ("lordosis" behavior) to ardent male rats.

Anatomical and hormonal differences occur in the sons of stressed mothers: Their sexually dimorphic, hypothalamic preoptic area is smaller than it normally is. This anatomical discrepancy is correlated with a failure of the normal sharp increase in serum T levels to occur at 18 to 19 days of gestation in these fetuses. The male fetus also has reduced plasma levels of LH, a reduction in the hypothalamic content of the enzyme aromatase, which converts androgens to estrogens in the brain, and of δ-3-β-hydroxy-steriod dehydrogenase activity in the Leydig cells of the testis.

The effects on the behavior and physiology of the offspring can be prevented by pretreatment of the dams with naloxone prior to exposure to light and restraint. But the offspring still manifest feminized sexual behavior if they are treated with the same opioid-blocking agent after birth.

The second example of the long-term effects of stressful experience is provided by studies on the effects of separation (premature weaning) at 10 to 15 days of age in rats, and in infant monkeys. The technique is simple: The infant rat is removed from the presence of the mother. For the next 48 hours it does not eat chow or drink water. It is also poikilothermic. It shows immediate increases in motor activity after separation; it rears up, grooms itself in excess, and emits high-frequency sounds. (These cries also are produced in young separated birds and mammals of various species. They are said to be signals of distress, designed to be heard by the departed mother). When 10-day-old rats are removed from the mother, litter mates, or nest for as brief a period as 5 minutes, they respond with a marked increase in these emitted signals. They are also analgesic during this period. The administration of naltrexone (0.5 mg/kg) diminishes the analgesia and increases the frequency of the squeals. The injection of morphine sulphate (0.5 mg/kg has exactly the opposite effect (Kehoe and Blass 1986). The validity of these observations is enhanced because the opioid systems in the brain mature on about the 16th day of gestation (Bayon et al. 1979; Coyle and Pert 1976; Khachaturian et al. 1983).

Separated rats survive, so the long-term changes in their behavior and physiology may be followed. Such studies have led to an analysis of the articulation between mother and infant (Hofer 1984). Based on an extensive series of Hofer's and other investigators' studies, which have systematically examined the short-term effects of separation on the behavior and physiology of infant rats (and monkeys) while varying separate aspects of the mother-infant interaction, these investigators have concluded that the mother's milk regulates her

Table 1. Infant Systems and Maternal Regulators

Infant Systems		Maternal Regulators
Behavioral		
Activity level	↑	Body warmth
Novelty	↓	Tactile and olfactory
Sucking		
Nutritive	↓	Milk (distension)
Nonnutritive	↓	Tactile (perioral)
Neurochemical		
CNS: NE, DA	↑	Body warmth
CNS: ODC	↑	Tactile (dorsal)
Metabolic		
O_2 consumption	↑	Milk (sugar)
Sleep-wake cycles		
REM	↑	Periodicity: milk and tactile
Arousals	↓	Periodicity: milk and tactile
Cardiovascular		
Heart Rate (β-adrenergic)	↑	Milk (interoceptors)
Resistance (α-adrenergic)	↓	Milk (interoceptors)
Endocrine		
Growth hormone	↑	Tactile (dorsal)

Note: On the right are listed the influences supplied by the mother rat that increase (↑) or decrease (↓) specific behaviors and physiological systems in her infant offspring (Hofer 1982, 1984).

infant's HR; her body heat maintains its body temperature; her licking its neck sustains the infant's growth hormone (GH) and ornithine decarboxylase (ODC) levels; a pheromone secreted by the mother's areolae produces attachment to her nipple; and her touch controls its activity. The vital role of these interactions is attested to by the profound consequences of a 48-hour separation at 14 days of age that alters physiological functions and also places the young animal at risk for later disease.

Hofer's conclusion is solidly based in data: Prior to weaning, the mother acts as an external regulator of the behavior and physiology of her infant, affects the normal maturation of its brain and bodily rhythms, and even influences gene expression. Additionally, the effects of separation on young rats are permanent and affect every organ system studied to date.

The physiological consequences of premature separation of rats at 15 days of age include a fall of 40% in HR despite a marked increase in motor activity—an effect that is observable 4 hours after separation (Hofer and Weiner 1972, 1975). Starting at 20 days, the average HR of normally weaned rats at rest falls from a level of about 420 to about 300 beats per minute. The prematurely separated animal's HR, having initially fallen, begins to climb and by 28 days is significantly higher (350 beats per minute) than in its normally weaned peer (Hofer 1981). Yet the acute effects of separation on HR are not associated with a fall in BP; it is maintained by an increase in peripheral resistance (Hofer 1984).

Motor activity in infant monkeys is also increased upon separation from their mothers (Mason and Berkson 1974). Both in the 15-day-old rat and in 6-month-old monkeys, separation produces a sleep disturbance (Hofer 1976; Reite and Short 1978; Reite et al. 1974). Sleep onset is delayed, activated (REM) sleep is lost, rapid transitions occur between the two sleep stages, sleep is fragmented, awakenings are more frequent, and overall sleep time is decreased. The sleep disturbance does not depend on a fall in body temperature; it occurs even when the animal's body temperature is artificially maintained within the normal range. Recovery of normal sleep patterns occurs by 30 days of age in rats; they are indistinguishable from those of normally weaned rats of the same age. When prematurely separated animals are next food-deprived or restrained at 30 days of age, they initially fall asleep. They demonstrate an increase in sleep, mainly due to more slow-wave sleep— changes that are not seen in normally weaned animals and are also independent of alterations in body temperature. But subsequently they become progressively sleepless, due to decreasing amounts of slow-wave sleep (Ackerman, Hofer, and Weiner 1978; Weiner 1982).

Prematurely separated rats, therefore, initially respond to separation and not eating with one kind of sleep disturbance. At 30 days a different change in sleep patterns occurs when they are not fed or are restrained. These two experiences also elicit a latent disturbance in temperature regulation, not present before challenge. Therefore, challenging separated rats at two different ages produces different sleep disturbances, and also elicits a disturbance in temperature regulation that had previously been latent (Ackerman, Hofer, and Weiner 1978). The prematurely separated rat at 30 days of age reverts to its previous poikilothermic state.

Both sleep and temperature regulation are rhythmic functions. They show circadian variation. They are under the control of at least two oscillators in the brain, which are in turn regulated in part by the environment. Hofer (1984) has analyzed the maternal regulator of REM sleep in his young rats; it is initially under the control of the periodic supply of milk provided by the mother, and also of her intermittent touch. Withdrawal of both influences leads to the disruption of REM sleep in separated rat pups.

Other circadian-clock functions are already evident in fetal rats at 19 days of gestation. The pregnant dam entrains the light-dark cycle of the fetus; she mediates its circadian rhythm. The oscillators resident in the SCN of both the mother and the fetus are coordinated. The mother's influence on the offspring's light-dark rhythms continues in an unknown manner until 3 to 4 days after parturition. After that age, the direct retino-SCN neuronal pathway develops. Light falling upon the retina entrains the circadian rhythms controlled by the SCN (Reppert, Duncan, and Weaver 1987).

One of the immediate consequences of the premature separation of young rats is a change in serum levels of GH and in the content of ODC in several organs. The enzyme ODC is crucial to polyamine and, therefore, to protein and nucleic acid synthesis, and ultimately to growth and maturation of organs such as the heart, kidney, liver, and brain. Growth hormone is one of several regulators of ODC expression. Premature separation of rats for 1 hour at 10 days of age lowers levels of both GH in serum and ODC (Butler, Suskind, and Schanberg 1978) in the heart, cerebellum, kidney, and liver (but not the lung) by 50–60%. After 2 hours of separation, and unless the infant is then returned to the mother, ODC becomes permanently unresponsive to the stimulatory effects of administered GH (Kuhn and Schanberg 1979). But the enzyme continues to be expressed with cyclic AMP (cAMP), dexamethasone, or insulin administration (Schanberg, Evoniuk, and Kuhn 1984). The levels of both GH and ODC can be restored by vigorous stroking of the separated infant's fur with a stiff brush, especially if brushing is administered to the back of the neck (Evoniuk, Kuhn, and Schanberg 1979; Schanberg and Field 1987). The response to brushing can be blocked by cyproheptadine and a diazepam.

Beginning at 20 days of age, separation produces an increase in PRL levels. When fluoxetine (a 5-HT reuptake inhibitor) or 5-hydroxy-tryptophane (a 5-HT precursor) is administered, GH alone is released in the normal 10-day-old animal. At 25 days of age they additionally stimulate GH and PRL secretion. Thus 5-HT, but also α-adrenergic and dopamine (DA) agonists, acting through peptides and the GH-releasing hormone, promote GH secretion only at an early age and stimulate the release of both GH and PRL (which in utero and in infancy is tonically inhibited by DA) at a later age (Schanberg, Evoniuk, and Kuhn 1984; Schanberg and Field 1987).

Fifteen-day-old rats do not usually feed themselves laboratory chow during the 48 hours following separation. They lose weight, and body temperature decreases. These animals remain underweight and have less brown body fat at 30 and 40 days of age (Ackerman 1981). Their body weight continues to be lower than their normally weaned peers' for the remainder of their lives. The failure to put on body weight during maturation may in part be accounted for by the initial fall in GH and ODC levels.

After 3 days of separation the brains of 15-day-old rat pups raised at room temperature contain lower amounts of catecholamines, protein, DNA, and RNA. When the pups are maintained at ambient temperatures of about 35°C, the levels of NE and DA in the brain are actually increased, but those of protein, DNA, and RNA continue to be depressed in the cerebrum and cerebellum. Their body weights are also uninfluenced by these warmer ambient temperatures (Stone, Bonnet, and Hofer 1975).

These observations demonstrate that separation has immediate and permanent behavioral, physiological, and biochemical effects. It also alters the response of the previously separated animal to later challenges.

This experimental model has made it possible further to analyze the mother-infant interaction: The behavioral and physiological effects of separation are precisely replicated when the infant rat's olfactory epithelium is destroyed by cautery or by the application of zinc sulfate. The areolar glands of the mother's breasts produce a pheromone that is secreted under the control of OT. This chemically unidentified substance activates a patch of neurons in the accessory olfactory nucleus during nipple-attachment and suckling (Teicher et al. 1980). The subsequent neuronal pathways involved in the altered behaviors and physiological changes remain to be traced. Nevertheless, the separation-stress model has the potential of providing us with an analysis of the brain mechanisms that mediate a specific experience with a variety of bodily effects, some of which culminate in disease.

These studies on separation have only been instructive because of the precision with which the analysis of the mother-infant interaction was carried out. Disrupting the interaction has revealed that it was made up of separate components, each with its own effects, and has led to a determination of the receiving site of the sensory input on the infant's body at which it takes place (Hofer 1984; Weiner 1982).

When rhesus and squirrel monkey infants are removed from their mother's side and placed into a novel environment, a marked increase in plasma cortisol levels is detectable. The critical variable in this hormonal response is not their new surroundings, but the disruption of the infant's interaction with its mother. This conclusion is based on the fact that plasma cortisol levels remain unchanged if both the mother and her infant are placed in the same novel environment. But the level of plasma cortisol attained in the separated infant is also a product of the status of the mother in the social hierarchy; the more dominant she is, the higher are the plasma cortisol levels of her infant.

Interesting also is the observation that the plasma cortisol levels of the mother, without regard to her social status, increase when she is removed from her social group. They remain significantly elevated for 24 hours, but then they fall back to remain about 10% above their usual baseline levels as long as she is alone.

The infant's behavioral and hormonal responses are determined by the presence or absence of the mother, but not necessarily in the same way. The infant's cortisol responses recur following separation for several days; they remain higher especially in the mornings of each successive day. The morning elevations do not occur if the infant can see the mother through a transparent partition. By contrast, the amount and quality of its vocalizations are maximal and different under two conditions: If the mother is out of sight the infant cries out less and less, and the quality of its cry is different. But if the infant continues to see the mother, its plaintive cries persist unabated.

Various biogenic amine levels have also been measured under these two conditions. The major influences of separation appeared to be on cerebrospinal NE levels. They are significantly increased when the infant is completely isolated from the other and remains so for 4 days (Coe, Wiener, and Levine 1983; Levine 1987).

The Role of the Age of the Animal in the Response to Stressful Experience

The effects of a specific stressful experience in part depend on the age of the animal. Each bodily system has its own maturational timetable. This principle is implicit in the observations made on the effects of separation on young animals. Weaning cannot occur until the organism can manage on its own; until then, the mother regulates its behavior and physiology. The retino-hypothalamic pathway becomes functional at 3–4 days; until then, the infant's light-dark rhythms are regulated by the mother. Until weaning, however, she continues to influence the infant's sleep patterns. Restraining rats prior to weaning, even after premature separation, does not produce gastric erosions. Their unresponsiveness to restraint is presumably related to the fact that the regulation of acid secretion by acetylcholine, gastrin, and histamine has not matured (Ackerman 1981).

In the first two to three weeks of a rat's life, separation, exposure to cold, or electric shock does not release ACTH. High levels of corticosterone are present in immature rats and appear tonically to inhibit ACTH secretion. This conclusion is based on the fact that adrenalectomy raises ACTH levels when young rats are exposed to these stressful experiences. The unresponsiveness of ACTH in the normal young animal does not result from a hypothalamic-pituitary-adrenal system that is not functioning, because the administration of CRF to the baby rat elicits an ACTH response (Rivier 1989).

Long-Term Effects of Acutely Stressful Experiences in Adult Animals

One of the contentions of this book is that both young and adult organisms are permanently changed by an acutely stressful experience. This assertion has already been supported. Stressful experiences alter animals in many different ways: They may learn from the experience; they may habituate with its repetition; or their reaction patterns may never again be the same.

A particular elegant example of this last thesis has been provided by Kelly and Silverman (1988). They simultaneously studied the subacute and long-term effects of an ambiguous stressful experience on rat behavior and the anatomy of specific regions of the rat's brain. They chose to present the rat with a white noise that was followed by electrical shocks administered randomly only 50% of the time for 72 hours. The initial effect of this procedure on their rats was to reduce their food and water intake and to produce a slowly developing analgesia. After its conclusion, the animals startled whenever they heard a noise—a response that persisted long after the end of the experiment. The 72-hour exposure to noise and shocks also increased by 15% (to 27%) the number of CRF-OT secreting cells in the medial parvocellular portion of the PVN of the hypothalamus. The enhancement of the cells persisted. But no such increases occurred in neurons in the rostral PVN. When exposure to noise and shocks was extended for 10 days, the absolute number and the size of detectable CRF-OT neurons increased further but solely in the medial parvocellular part of the PVN.

The Acute Effects of Unavoidable Shock: The Response Is Specified by Its Parameters

Intermittent and unavoidable electric shocks (120 of 2mA intensity given every 5 seconds for 10 minutes) applied to the feet of rats produces a naloxone-reversible analgesia. The analgesia is cross-tolerant with morphine sulphate (MS) (Lewis, Sherman, and Liebeskind 1978). It is abolished by adrenalectomy or adrenal ganglionectomy, suggesting that this procedure releases met-enkephalin from the adrenal medulla. Pentobarbital also blocks the analgesia (Lewis, Cannon, and Liebeskind 1980). One hundred and twenty electric shocks of the same amperage given for 2 minutes produces another form of analgesia. It is not blocked by naloxone or pentobarbital, nor does it show cross-tolerance with MS (Terman, Lewis, and Liebeskind 1983). However, histamine-2 receptor antagonists do reverse the second form of analgesia (Terman et al. 1984). The two different forms of analgesia are, therefore, determined by a subtle change in the shock parameters. Yet both of these forms of electric shock raise corticosterone levels in rats, suggesting that this response is not determined by the specific nature of the shock stimulus.

Intermittent but not continuous electrical shock suppresses NK-cell cytotoxic activity in rats (Shavit et al. 1984). The suppression of NK-cell cytotoxic activity is mimicked by the peripheral or the intraventricular administration of MS, and it can be prevented in shocked animals by the prior administration of naloxone. Although the analgesia produced by intermittent shock manifests cross-tolerance with MS, the suppression of NK-cell activity does not.

Intermittent electrical shock or the administration of MS accelerates the death of rats injected with a PRL-sensitive, mammary cell, ascites-producing tumor—an effect that can also be averted by naloxone (Shavit et al. 1985). The assumption is that intermittent shock releases either met-enkephalin from the adrenal medulla, or β-endorphin from the intermediate lobe of the pituitary gland, to suppress NK-cell cytolytic activity and enhance tumor progression.

However, the matter may be even more complex. The various endorphins have different effects on immune function. Furthermore, NK-cells are not the only cytotoxic cells; CD8$^+$ cells and certain classes of macrophages also are. Alpha- and β-endorphins have different effects on immune function—the former inhibit antibody formation to ovalbumen, and the latter enhance it while also modulating CD4$^+$ cell function (Heijnen, deFouw, and Ballieux 1986).

Intermittent foot shock presumably is associated with the secretion of PRL. The mammary ascites tumor cells are PRL-sensitive. Tumoricidal macrophages are activated by PRL. The hormone also stimulates the release of lymphokines from T-cells. T-cells in turn contain PRL receptors (Bernton, Meltzer, and Holaday 1987).

One important variable in tumor rejection or growth is the specific parameters of the administered electric shocks. In Shavit's and his colleagues' studies (1984, 1985) the electric shocks are regularly applied but the animal has no means of avoiding them—they are uncontrollable. Thus the intermittent, regularly applied form of uncontrollable shock enhances tumor growth. And unpredictable, irregularly applied shock from which the animal cannot escape is associated with one-half the rate of tumor rejection than is the same escapable shock (Henry and Stephens-Larson 1985; Shavit et al. 1985).

Other effects of intermittent electric shock on immune function have been demonstrated (Keller et al. 1983). Rats were subjected to two levels of electrical shock applied to their tails. (Low shock was 0.8 mA for 8 hours, 1.0 mA for another 8 hours, and 1.2 mA for 4 hours; each shock lasted 2 seconds at an average rate of 1 per minute. High shock was 1.6, 2.4, 3.0 mA for the same duration and intervals.) The procedure was followed by lymphopenia that depended on the integrity of the adrenal gland. But the suppression of 5-iododeoxyuridine incorporation into isolated peripheral blood lymphocytes in fixed numbers after stimulation by the mitogen PHA was unaffected by adrenalectomy. By contrast, diminished splenic lymphocyte responses to PHA did not occur under any conditions. Thus the suppression of T-cell function (mitogenic stimultion by PHA), but not lymphopenia, is independent of corticosterone and may depend on the integrity of the pituitary gland.

Another set of shock parameters has also been studied to determine its effect on hormonal function. Randomly administered, unavoidable, intermittent electric shock (2 mA, 2 sec. duration) abolishes the pulsatile release of LH but not FSH in the castrated male rat (Rivier, Rivier, and Vale 1986). When the CRF antagonist α-helical ovine CRF (9-41) is instilled into the lateral ventricle of such rats, the suppressive effects of electric shock are prevented. The intraventricular administration of CRF by itself lowers LH levels, inhibits ovulation, and prevents the proestrous LH surge in female rats (Rivier and Vale 1984).

A considerable body of literature suggests that the unpredictability of a stressful experience has much more profound, different, and even longerlasting behavioral effects (such as "learned helplessness") than does a predictable one. The time course of corticosterone responses differs according to whether the electric shocks are predictable or not (Bassett and Cairncross 1975). The largest increases in plasma corticosterone levels in rats occur with unpredictable shocks randomly applied six times in an hour. These large hormonal responses are greater than those associated with other stressful experiences, such as predictable shocks, restraint, or exposure of rats to an ambient temperature of 2.5–5.5°C.

Increases in FFA levels also occur when rats are exposed to the cold, restrained, or shocked; they reach their height at the end of the shock procedure (Odio and Maickel 1985). The same procedures, and enforced swimming, cause OT but not aVP to be released in the rat. But induced pain, hypoglycemia, and hypoxia antecede the secretion of aVP. Bleeding rats is followed by increases in both aVP and OT levels. Thus certain life-threatening metabolic changes and pain preferentially incite the secretion of one over another hormone, and cold or exercise has the opposite effects. The secretion of the two hormones is specific to each class of stressful experience.

But one may not generalize about the ensuing actions of these two hormones across species: In the rat both aVP and OT interact with, and modulate, the release of ACTH by CRF. In primates aVP also potentiates the action of CRF; but OT inhibits it. In stressed primates, OT and ACTH seem to be secreted in inverse, rather than in positively correlated, amounts (Gibbs 1986). Therefore, hormonal response patterns appear to covary with specific categories of stressful experience, but they also differ in their nature in different species.

Repetitive Stressful Experiences: The Importance of Novelty

When an animal is repeatedly exposed to the same experience—cold or heat, predictable electric shocks, conditioned avoidance or "emotional" procedures—the physiological response, determined by various hormonal, autonomically mediated or catecholaminergic measures, is much higher on the first than on subsequent exposure. The novelty of the experience is critical. Some form of habituation occurs, whose intrinsic physiology is not yet fully understood (Kant et al. 1983; Mason 1968). Only recently has the question been asked whether "habituation" occurs when the same animal is exposed seriatim to different stressors—foot shock, forced treadmill running, or restraint. The results of such studies confirm previous ones: Habituation occurs to the same repeated stressful experience; when a novel one is next applied, it provokes a new round of maximal corticosterone responses. But PRL, or pituitary cAMP, responses decline on repetition and with novelty: They habituate. The conclusion of such studies is that the animal adapts readily to ("learns" strategies for) every new contingency. This adaptation occurs at the behavioral but not at the corticosterone level (Kant et al. 1985).

New Phenomena Related to Stressful Experience

Unpredictable Shock and the Phenomenon of
"Learned Helplessness"

It is now a well-established fact, judged by several different criteria and in a variety of species (cats, dogs, and rats), that unpredictable and random, and in all likelihood painful, electrical shock produces profound and rather specific changes in an animal's behavior and physiology. The ensuing condition has been called "learned helplessness" (Maier and Seligman 1976; Seligman 1974, 1975). This anthropomorphic label does not do full justice to the phenomenon that follows: Some animals, once having been exposed to these conditions, do not attempt to escape; they "sit and take it." They later fail to learn a (shuttlebox) escape-avoidance task (Overmier and Seligman 1967). After the experience of unpredictable shocks, rats show diminished motor activity. Their sleep, grooming behavior, food intake, and weight are reduced (Weiss, Simson, and Simson 1989). Some rats become more fearful than others after the initial experience (Osborne et al. 1975).

If the onset of the electric shocks is signaled by a tone (Dess et al. 1983), or dogs, rats, and cats (Seward and Humphrey 1967) are taught to escape prior to being exposed to them (Henn, Edwards, and Johnson 1988), the learning deficit is markedly attenuated. Dogs trained to expect the shock show an increase in glucocorticoid levels, which attain only one-third the levels measured in untrained dogs (Dess et al. 1983). Dogs that had not been forewarned are later likely to startle with every novel stimulus and have repetitive and correlated large increases in glucocorticoid levels (Levine et al. 1973). The hormonal response does not habituate.

The outcome of unpredictable, unavoidable shocks is influenced by a number of other factors—the strength of the current used (Rossellini and Seligman 1978), the number of shocks administered, the opportunity, or lack of it, for escape, and the strain of the animals (Weiss and Glazer 1975; Weiss, Stone, and Harrell 1970). Individual differences in the duration of the learning deficit after unavoidable shock have also been reported.

Insights into the chemical changes in the rat brain following unavoidable shock have been obtained (Weiss et al. 1976, 1979, 1980, 1981, 1985). Large diminutions in the content of NE within the locus coeruleus (LC) occur. The release of large amounts of NE by the presynaptic terminals of the LC eventually leads to its diminished secretion (Stone 1976; Tanaka et al. 1982). In this nucleus, NE usually acts as an inhibitory neurotransmitter, whose effects are mediated by α_2-adrenergic receptors on its cell bodies and dendrites. A reduction of NE release would disinhibit them to increase their firing rates.

By a series of analytic studies, using agonists (e.g., clonidine) and antagonists (e.g., yohimbine) infused into the fourth ventricle of the brain of normal rats, the conclusion was reached that stimulating or blocking the α_2-adrenergic receptor is respectively associated with opposite behavioral changes. Deficits similar to those produced by unavoidable shock have been produced by antagonists (Weiss et al. 1982). And α_2-agonists reverse the behavioral effects of unavoidable shock (Simson et al. 1986b); the administration of inhibitors (e.g., pargyline) of the enzyme, monoamine oxidase (MAO), that degrades NE (Simpson et al. 1986a), or drugs (e.g., meprotiline) that retard its reuptake by presynaptic neurons, also do (Weiss et al. 1975).

The disinhibition of LC neurons, which are widely distributed in the cerebellum, hypothalamus, limbic system, and forebrain, should result in increased noradrenergic activity "at a distance." In fact, intraventricular administration of an α_1- or a β-adrenergic agonist both simulate the effects of unavoidable shock (Weiss, Simson, and Simson 1989).

But the matter is again more complex. The LC contains receptors for CRF, which modulate α_2-adrenergic receptors. In all likelihood, CRF is secreted after unavoidable shock applied to dogs. Receptors for SP, NPY, OT, aVP, met-enkephalin, acetylcholine, and 5-HT have also been identified on LC neurons (Foote, Bloom, and Aston-Jones 1983; Guyenet and Aghajanian 1979; Segal 1979; Vizi 1980), but their involvement in unavoidable shock has not as yet been comprehensively studied.

Depletion of NE throughout the brain occurs with other stressful experiences—forcing rats to swim in cold water (Barchas and Freedman 1963), or applying unavoidable electrical shock to their feet (Anisman, Pizzino, and Sklar 1980; Anisman, Remington, and Sklar 1979; Zigmond and Harvey 1970), a form of shock that also decreases the release of gamma-aminobutyric acid (GABA) from corticol neurons (Perry and Sherman 1981). The net reduction of NE in the brain is thought to be due to an imbalance between the rates of its synthesis and release (Bliss and Zwaniger 1966; Weiss, Simson, and Simson 1989).

Much less work has been done on changes in E content in the brain. Restraining rats seem to diminish E more than NE or DA levels in the brain stem (Saavedra, Kvetnansky, and Kopin 1979)—a reduction that is mainly localized to the brain stem and the hypothalamus. The E content of the nucleus of the tractus solitarius (NTS), the LC, the PVN, and the arcuate nucleus (NA) of the hypothalamus falls less. But NE release is also reduced in the periventricular and ventromedial hypothalamic nuclei under conditions of restraint.

The content of one or another neurotransmitter in the whole brain, and in a particular region or nucleus, is probably not a good measure of its activity; a more dynamic measure—such as its turnover rate (Glowinski 1975)—is needed. Furthermore, measures need to be done recurrently if animals are exposed to repeated stressful experiences; once NE levels in the brains of rats have been lowered by one trial of foot shock, they show no further changes even when the procedure is repeated daily for two weeks (Zigmond and Harvey 1970).

Modifiers of Unavoidable Shock

In most experiments, an animal cannot predict, prevent, avoid, or escape intermittent or continuous electric shock, regularly or randomly administered. But the effects on an animal that can predict the onset of signaled shocks differ from those on an animal that cannot do so: The extent of the gastric erosions produced is six times greater in rats receiving shocks to the tail that are not regularly paired with a warning tone than in those exposed to shocks that are signaled. The first group also loses more weight. When a rat can learn to avoid receiving shocks by turning a wheel that switches off the current, the number and extent of gastric erosions is smaller than in experimental animals not provided with one. Corticosterone blood levels are much higher in the rats unable to prevent the electric shocks (Weiss 1972).

The turning-off of the current can be made to coincide with another brief electric shock. In this manner, the animal is punished for its attempts to avoid the shock. Rats subjected to this procedure develop even more extensive gastric erosions than a yoked partner that regularly and only receives shocks. Conversely, animals that cannot prevent receiving shocks but are allowed to maul a neighboring rat have fewer gastric erosions (Weiss et al. 1976). If the rat is allowed a choice between predictable and unpredictable shock, it "elects" the former and develops fewer gastric erosions (Gliner 1972). These experiments illustrate important principles. Preventing or avoiding a painful, stressful experience reduces its damage; punishing attempts to do so maximizes its effects.

Rats vary in their abilities to learn, and to remember, how to avoid electric shocks. Relatively resistant rats may selectively be bred. Those most sensitive to the procedure become even more so in each later generation—their capacity to learn to avoid shocks becomes less and less (Henn, Edwards, and Johnson 1988).

Some rats are deficient in their responses to signaled, preventable shocks. They initially differ neurochemically from those who are not so; the content of 5-HT is increased, and of NE is decreased in the hippocampus of those lacking the capacity to respond. During the three weeks following exposure to shocks, the response of cAMP of neurons to NE in hippocampal slices of rats is exaggerated. The β-adrenergic receptors of these cells develop a greater binding capacity for their specific agonists. After 23 days these changes vanish. Avoidance-learning can also be restored after shocking rats by treating them with imipramine—a catecholamine reuptake inhibitor—and fluroxamine—an inhibitor of 5-HT reuptake (Johnson et al. 1982).

The increase of 5-HT content in the hippocampus may be a factor in deficient escape behavior after unavoidable shock. Prior depletion of 5-HT with parachlorphenyalanine averts the defect in avoiding shocks (Henn, Edwards, and Johnson 1988).

Other forms of stressful experience seem to have different effects on the brain of rats. Exposure to cold reduces the NE content of the NTS, the NA, the ventromedial nucleus (VMN), and the PVN of the hypothalamus of rats. Restraining them additionally depletes the LC and the PVN of NE.

The Analgesias Produced by Experimentally Induced Stressful Experience

The phenomenon, now called "stress-induced analgesia" was first described in 1976 (Akil, Mayer, and Liebeskind 1976; Akil et al. 1976; Hayes et al. 1976). In retrospect, these two groups of investigators had discovered two different forms of analgesia: One was incited by intermittent foot shock, applied for 30 to 60 minutes, and was abolished by naloxone (Akil et al. 1976; Cannon et al. 1982); and the other was produced by shorter foot shocks, but it could not be reversed by antagonists of the opioid peptides.

These two different forms of analgesia are also critically dependent on the parameters, not only on the duration, of the shock current employed. As previously discussed in this chapter, intermittent shock produces a naloxone-reversible analgesia in rats, but continuous shock does not (Lewis, Cannon, and Liebeskind 1980). However, the analgesic phenomenon is even subtler: At low current intensity (1–2 mA), or at higher current intensity (2.5–3.5 mA) of brief duration (1–2 mins.), continuous shocks delivered one per second produce the analgesia that is abolished by naloxone; but at higher current intensity, or low current intensity of longer duration (4–5 mins.), the irreversible (by naloxone) form of analgesia is observed (Terman et al. 1984). Both forms of analgesia can also be produced by shocks in rats previously anesthetized with pentobarbital (Terman et al. 1984). Furthermore, shocks of low current intensity applied to the forepaws of rats produce the naloxone-reversible form of analgesia, whereas the nonreversible variety follows the same shocks to the hindpaws (Cannon et al. 1984; Watkins and Mayer 1982).

The phenomenon of stress analgesia is not a global one; it is highly discriminated. It depends not only on the strain of the animal used and the body region stimulated, but on the parameters of the (painful) stimulus applied. It also manifests itself in rats that intrude into the home cage of another (male) rat, rats defeated in a fight, 10-day-old rats separated from their mothers (Kehoe and Blass 1986), and rats made to swim in cold water (Ben-Eliyahu et al. 1990; Bodnar et al. 1979). When the temperature of the water is low, or when the rat is repeatedly made to swim in warm water, the analgesia is refractory to naloxone or naltrexone. When the water temperature is close to the rat's body temperature and the rat is only immersed once, the analgesia is abolished by both opioid antagonists (Terman 1985).

The mechanism of the analgesia is complex (Akil et al. 1986). By implication, it depends on the central release from the pituitary gland of opioid peptides (Amir and Amit 1979), which may be mediated by acetylcholine (Watkins et al. 1984). The integrity of the dorsolateral funiculus of the spinal cord must be preserved for analgesia to be instituted (Lewis et al. 1983). It can also be partly reversed by scopolamine, an antagonist of the muscarinic receptor for acetylcholine. Acetylcholine is believed to mediate the release of (some) opioid peptides in the brain (Lewis, Cannon, and Liebeskind 1983).

Unavoidable shocks regularly release corticosterone in rats. Originally, it was believed that analgesia was the outcome of the secretion of CRF and ACTH. At the same time CRF would stimulate the secretion of β-endorphin, an endogenous opioid peptide. In fact, hypophysectomy does attenuate the naloxone-sensitive form of analgesia, but it enhances the resistant form produced by intermittent foot shock (Lewis et al. 1981). The opioid-dependent form of analgesia is also increased by low doses, and diminished by high doses, of corticosterone (Terman et al. 1984). The inevitable implication of these observations is that the corticosterones "feed back" to regulate the release or action of opioid peptides within the brain (MacLennan et al. 1982; Millan, Przewlocki, and Herz 1980). The feedback is positive at low doses and negative at higher doses.

The discussion of stress analgesia does not end here. Only the opioid-dependent form of analgesia is reversed by denervation or removal of the adrenal glands (Lewis et al. 1982a). Both direct and indirect evidence suggest that enkephalinlike peptides are released by these glands after intermittent, but not after continuous, electric shocks (Lewis et al. 1928b). The receptors in the brain for the opioid peptides have been identified as belonging to the μ, κ and δ types—predominantly the μ form (Lewis et al. 1984). The most likely location for the receptors is subcortical, especially in the brain stem, because decortication of rats does not abolish opioid-dependent analgesia.

Several sites in the brain stem have been implicated in stress analgesia; the periaqueductal grey matter of the mid-brain, belonging to the "nonspecific" reticular system, and the NTS are likely ones. Their electrical stimulation produces analgesia (Lewis et al. 1975; Mayer et al. 1971; Reynolds 1969). These systems are known to receive afferent fibers from every specific sensory (afferent) pathway, including the "somesthetic" tracts and those that transmit the sensation of pain. Visceral afferent fibers also pass to this region of the midbrain; they seem important because bilateral vagotomy attenuates the analgesia that follows intermittent foot shock (Maixner and Randich 1984; Randich and Maixner 1986). Stimulation of the proximal end of the cut vagus nerve also induces analgesia. But it is not known in what way intermittent foot shock activates vagal afferent fibers. They are known to pass to the NTS, a nucleus that also receives spinal afferent inputs. Injection of MS and glutamate into the NTS produces analgesia (Morgan, Sohn, and Liebeskind 1987; Oley et al. 1982). Ascending fibers from the NTS pass to the reticular system and its nuclei, including the periaqueductal grey matter (Loewy and Burton 1978), whose cells contain opioid receptors (Khachaturian et al. 1985).

However, these generalizations do not hold for all forms of stress analgesia. The form produced by application of shock to the forepaws of a rat is mediated by the raphé nuclei of the ventromedial brain stem, from which fibers return to the dorsal horn of the spinal cord where opioid peptides and 5-HT exert their effects. The action of the peptides is abolished by CCK. The other form of analgesia, produced by shock to the hindpaws, uses a different circuit, ascending first by neurons to the parabrachial nucleus, which are subserved by acetylcholine. Ascending pathways then travel to the periaqueductal grey matter, but also descend to the dorsal horn from the parabrachial nuclei.

To summarize: The development of one of several forms of analgesia produced by intermittent, unavoidable electric shock is complex. It involves spinal, possibly vagal, adrenal, and brain stem mechanisms in interaction with each other. However, the experience of pain, as judged by behavioral criteria, such as squealing, appears to depend on an intact thalamocortical system and the cerebral cortex.

Naturalistic Situations as Stressful Experiences: Fighting, Victory, and Defeat

Animals fight each other for territory, food, and mates, and to determine their status in the social hierarchy. They fight predators and defend their young. Fighting behavior is a process that emerges from certain specific situations essential to survival and reproduction. It may end in victory, defeat, injury, or death.

Fighting behavior has mainly been studied in vertebrates. Some representative examples from three species follow in order to illustrate the thesis that at various stages of the fight and its outcome, both the behavior and the physiology differ but are still integrated, coordinated, and specific.

Fighting behavior is more apparent in certain species of fish (*Tilapia*, and rainbow trout) or eels than in other species during the establishment of social hierarchies. The outcome of the encounter between two fish determines their respective dominant or subordinate status. Defeated (subordinate) rainbow trout are more susceptible to infection with *A. hydrophila* and have elevated levels of circulating corticosteroids, catecholamines, glucose, and lactate (Peters and Hong 1985; Peters et al. 1988).

Members of the species *Tilapia* when confronted with each other initially remain in their own territory, but soon venture into each other's domain. They swim around each other in ever-diminishing circles. As the distance between them narrows, they engage in vigorous combat, pushing with their tails and biting each other. When the fight is won, the victor prevents the loser from escaping. The defeated fish stops swimming, goes belly-up, fails to respond to further threats, and loses its tail reflex that customarily aligns the tail fins with the body.

Significant immunosuppression occurs in the loser, consisting of a suppression both of the proliferative responses of its (pronephric) leukocytes to mitogens and of nonspecific cytotoxic activity. The serum of the defeated fish contains a soluble factor that suppresses these two immunological activities not found in leukocytes obtained from a normal and from the victorious fish. Naltrexone reverses the suppression of the nonspecific cytotoxic functions of the loser's leukocytes. But it has no effect on the diminished responses of immunocompetent cells to lipopolysaccharide mitogens, nor does it restore the normal behavior of the defeated fish. Therefore, one may infer that unspecified opioid peptides mediate the suppression of nonspecific cytotoxicity and may be contained in the soluble factor (Faisal et al. 1989a, 1989b).

Cannon (1929) described that fighting between animals was associated with activation of the sympathoadrenal medullary system (i.e., the secretion of E). Since his time, it has become obvious that anticipatory behavioral and physiological responses occur prior to the actual fight. Integrated cardiovascular and hormonal patterns are also observed during a fight and its outcome—different responses occur in the victorious than in the defeated animal (Henry, Stephens, and Ely 1986).

The "defense" reaction (first described by Hess 1957) occurs even when an animal, such as a cat, is slightly alerted (Abrahams, Hilton, and Zbrozña 1964; Folkow 1987), in anticipation of, and at the start of vigorous physical activity to meet some challenge—attacking an intruder, enemy, or rival, or fleeing from the scene of battle. The reaction consists of HR, BP, CO, and peripheral resistance increases. Beta-adrenergic antagonists prevent the rise in HR and BP. Levels of E, NE, ACTH in serum, and the content of the enzyme tyrosine hydroxylase (TH) in the adrenal medulla also increase. Enhanced plasma renin activity is blocked by captopril (an inhibitor of the activity of the angiotensin-I and -II converting enzymes). Skeletal blood flow increases, but renal blood flow decreases. The gut absorbs more sodium and water, but their excretion by the kidney diminishes (Henry, Stephens, and Ely 1986). The appetite for salt is enhanced.

Patterned physiological responses are even more discrete than the initial work on the "defense" reaction had suggested. The anticipation of exercise in animals elicits an increase in HR and systolic and diastolic BP; stroke volume and CO rise; blood flow through the skin and muscles is greater, but is reduced in the mesenteric bed; and the peripheral resistance falls. Parasympathetic (vagal) constraint on the circulation is reduced.

A cat confronted by another cat's attack that does not terminate in a fight shows a specific pattern of cardiovascular changes that differs from the one observed when a fight takes place. The HR and CO rise, while splanchnic and resistance vessels constrict (due to increased sympathetic discharge) but blood flow through skeletal muscles increases (due to cholinergic sympathetic activation); thus on balance, only a minimal BP increase occurs. This pattern

(Parati, Casadei, and Mancia 1989) differs from the classical "defense" reaction. The cardiovascular pattern is also somewhat different (i.e., iliac flow is increased) if the cat is attacked by a dog but does not fight it.

The cat about to fight another one manifests a circulatory pattern different than that seen during the actual fight. While the cat is preparing to fight (during which it may paw the air), BP does not change, HR and CO fluctuate, and blood flow in the mesenteric, renal, and iliac arteries is reduced. During the actual fight—especially when prolonged and intense—BP, CO, and HR increase, vasoconstriction in the renal and mesenteric arteries is intense, but dilatation of the iliac arteries occurs and total peripheral resistance is reduced (Zanchetti, Baccelli, and Mancia 1976).

The defeated mouse, rat, or monkey, or one prevented from acting (e.g., by restraint) or "coping," shows an increase in BP and peripheral resistance that is not averted by β-adrenergic antagonists. The defeated rodent manifests a deep analgesia. The HR remains unchanged. ACTH, corticosteroid, β-endorphin, and PRL blood levels are increased. But the serum content of T falls. Plasma catecholamine levels do not change (Henry, Stephens, and Ely 1986).

Thus the behavioral and physiological responses of the organism are exquisitely related to the preparation for, and the actuality of, a fight. The behavior and the patterns of cardiovascular changes in cats confronted with an opponent constitute an integrated whole. They are both under the control of identifiable circuits within the brain (chapter 8), which are activated in an as yet unknown manner by the threatening signal of a dog or another cat.

Naturally occurring stressful experiences, in contrast to artificial ones, seem to have a quite different effect in mice when they are housed together and engage in combat daily for 14 days; high levels of whole brain E, NE, and 5-HT are sustained throughout this period (B. Welch and A. Welch 1965; A. Welch and B. Welch, 1971). With few exceptions, experiments of this nature do not take into account the prior experience or the strain of animals; when they do, new and interesting findings emerge. Socially isolating young animals alters the mean brain levels of catecholamines, indoleamines, aminoacids, and their biosynthetic and degradative enzymes (A. Welch and B. Welch 1968b, 1971). Rearing young rodents in social isolation alters their reaction to changes in their environment, their dominance and submission patterns in the social group, and their proclivity to fight. When previously isolated mice are introduced to group living, marked changed occur in levels and turnover rates of these substrates and enzyme levels in their brains.

Not all members of an animal genus, species, or strain are temperamentally inclined to fight (Bourgault, Karczmar, and Scudder 1963; Karczmar and Scudder 1967). The brains of fighting mice contain lower levels of 5-HT and NE than those of mice that are peaceful. The content of biogenic amines in the brains of mice of different fighting strains also differs. In some aggressive strains, low levels of 5-HT are found in the brain stem (Maas 1962). In other strains, brain stem levels of 5-HT are normal, but forebrain levels are low (Lagerspetz, Tirri, and Lagerspetz 1968). When 5-HT synthesis is inhibited by parachlorphenylalanine (PCPA), peaceful mice kill members of their own species (Karli, Vergnes, and Didiergeorges 1969; A. Welch and B. Welch 1968a). Other mice of the same strain become killers when NE biosynthesis is inhibited by α-methylparatyrosine (Leaf, Lerner, and Horovitz 1969). Inhibiting the synthesis of 5-HT and NE by PCPA and α-methylparatyrosine respectively is followed by increased exploratory behavior in addition to muricide. Therefore, the depletion of both 5-HT and NE may cause members of some strains of mice to become killers and explorers.

However, this effect cannot be the final answer to the problem of muricide, because reserpine, which also depletes the brain of 5-HT and NE, sedates mice. (Sedated mice do not kill members of their species). So far, we have no explanation for such observations, because it is difficult to understand how a change in the level of a single neurotransmitter alters a number of complex behaviors such as muricide, exploration, or even escape and avoidance (Glaser et al. 1975).

It is easier to understand that certain kinds of early experience may lower the levels of an enzyme in the brain. They are associated with low levels of neuronal discharge in the brain, which in turn produce low levels of neurotransmitter biosynthesis and release (A. Welch and B. Welch 1971). When mice are placed in a new and unfamiliar environment, both fighting and BP levels increase, because novel and excessive signals need suddenly to be processed. As a consequence, a precipitous rise in the biosynthesis and secretion of neurotransmitter substances takes place. This conclusion is supported by the observation that male mice that had previously been isolated fight when they are individually paired with another mouse in an unfamiliar environment. The speed with which the fighting begins, and the duration and intensity of the fight, are directly related to the length of prior isolation (A. Welch and B. Welch 1971). Being reared alone leads mice to assume a dominant role in the social hierarchy to which they have been introduced. Previously isolated animals even defeat a dominant animal that had been raised in a social group (A. Welch and B. Welch 1971). Mice raised together in groups take a much longer time to start a fight; the latent period before the onset of fighting depends on the number of peers in the group in which they had been previously raised (B. Welch and A. Welch 1966; A. Welch and B. Welch, 1971).

In conclusion: Marked differences in fighting occur between and within different strains of rodents. The prior experience of a rodent determines its proclivity to fight; rodents isolated when young fight more and achieve the dominant role upon rejoining their group. Their fighting behavior is in some way functionally related to marked changes in the levels of enzymes involved in the biosynthesis of catecholamines in the brain. Levels of the enzymes in the brain are initially lower in animals isolated from the time of weaning but increase dramatically and excessively when the animals rejoin their group. Even when the animals have not previously been isolated, fighting changes levels of brain catecholamines. Furthermore, animals that are mere spectators to a fight, not participants, show changes in NE levels in the brain stem (A. Welch and B. Welch 1986b; B. Welch and A. Welch, 1969).

Creating Conflict between Dogs

When food is taken away from a dog while it is eating and given to another dog, the former may either show an angry or a fearful response: In the first instance, the deprived dog growls, snarls, bares its teeth, and prepares to attack the other; in the second, it cowers, lowers it forepaws, or retreats, and its pupils dilate.

The angry dog has an increase in HR and BP and a doubling of the NE:E ratio in blood serum, mainly by virtue of increased NE secretion. At the same time, a progressive decrease in coronary blood flow occurs, which continues well after the conflict has terminated and the angry response has ceased. During the recovery phase, coronary vascular resistance is increased and the ST-segment of the EKG is elevated. The delayed dilatation of the coronary arteries incites myocardial ischemia that is mediated by α_1 receptors and averted by stellate sympathectomy. It results from increased levels of NE in the great cardiac vein, which persist as BP levels return to normal levels and produce persistent coronary artery vasoconstriction and reduction in flow. By contrast, the fearful dog shows a fall in the NE:E ratio by virtue of a marked increase in E secretion, but it does not show any coronary artery vasoconstriction (Verrier 1991).

Such encounters between two dogs are frequently seen in nature. They are instructive on several counts: The specificity of the integrated behavioral and physiological responses is exquisite; and the regional vascular aftereffects of the conflict persist. In fact, in certain situations in human beings, a short delay occurs between a behavioral response, such as hyperventilation, and later manifestations of myocardial ischemia (Magarian 1989). Verrier's observations of a delay in coronary dilatation may provide a model for such observations in human beings.

Exposure to Predators

When six different species of wild rodents are exposed to snakes and the silhouette of a hawk—their natural predators—members of four of the species—chipmunks, ground squirrels, wood rats, and grasshopper mice—become tonically immobile (Hofer 1970). (Immobility has obvious survival value for the rodent-prey because the cells of the hawk's retina respond mainly to moving objects.) During the state of tonic immobility the rodent's breathing rate is increased fivefold. Little change in HR occurs, but 56% of the animals have a variety of cardiac arrhythmias—sinus, different degrees of atrioventricular block, and ventricular ectopic beats—that are individual- and species-specific. In the two other species—the deer mouse and kangaroo rat—the HR rises 33 to 100%, but no arrhythmias are recorded. Therefore, marked inter- and intra-species individual differences characterize these fearful encounters between rodent and predator.

Wild rabbits, on the other hand, develop "fright" hyperthyroidism after initially being trapped by ferrets, and it persists when they are repeatedly exposed to these predators, or to dogs. Initially they also become tonically immobile and tremulous, have marked increases in HR and respiratory rates, and develop exophthalmos. One reexposure to their predators the wild rabbits begin to lose weight, show increases in the uptake of radioiodine, and eventually die. Antithyroid drugs or thyroidectomy averts weight loss and death (Kracht 1954).

Intrusion of One Animal into the Home Territory of Another

When a male rat is introduced into the entrance of the home cage of a resident male, it generally manifests immobility. As the second rat makes a movement toward it, the intruder rolls on its back and becomes insensitive to pain. If the intruding animal is sacrificed and the content of NE is measured in various regions of its brain, elevations of the catecholamine are found, specifically in the nucleus accumbens. However, if the animal does not freeze, but instead fights and is defeated by the home-cage rat, no such regional changes in NE content are measurable (Cools 1987).

The hormonal patterns of the two animals also differ. The intruding animal that has gone belly-up secretes increased amounts of PRL, α-MSH, β-endorphin, ACTH, and corticosterone, but T levels change very little. A very different change in hormone patterns is seen in the resident animal: Corticosterone and T levels increase, but insignificant changes in other hormone levels occur (Smelik 1985, 1987).

In the rat, α-MSH and β-endorphin are products of the intermediate lobe of the pituitary gland; they are released by E and can be blocked by β-adrenergic antagonists (Smelik 1987). A reduction in cellular immune responses is also observed, but only in the intruder (Raab et al. 1985).

Dominance Status and Its Consequences

The dominant male mouse or rat is more active than the subordinate one: It patrols its territory, fights its rivals, and is the first to mate and to eat. It initiates and displays more of these spontaneous behaviors than do subordinate males. The spontaneity of such behavior is enhanced by DA agonists and diminished by the bilateral destruction of nigrostriatal pathways. When DA neurons are injured, or the GABA content of the substantia nigra is reduced, the motor behaviors are only initiated by the appropriate visual and proprioceptive clues (Cools 1987); they cease being spontaneous.

A male mouse that is isolated following weaning and later placed back in a colony becomes the dominant animal. It manifests the behaviors just described (Henry, Stephens, and Ely 1986). During the period of isolation, levels of TH and phenyl-ethanolamine-N-methyl transferase (PNMT) in the adrenal medulla are lower than in nonisolated peers of the same age. When he is returned to the colony, and while he is establishing his dominant position, his levels of these two enzymes become excessive (compared to his subordinate peers'); NE and E levels are also greater in the adrenal medulla, but serum levels of ACTH and corticosterone are not increased.

The increased synthesis of the catecholamines is transsynaptically induced by increased presynaptic sympathetic activity. The establishment of dominant status is associated with increased levels of nerve growth factor (NGF) in the blood; its source is the salivary glands, and its production is regulated by T (Aloe et al. 1986). The NGF induces a slow proliferation of sympathetic neurons. When dominance is on the way to being attained, T levels in mouse serum are high. (Castrated males do not achieve dominance).

As the social hierarchy becomes stable, the changes in hormone and transmitter levels in the dominant mouse vanish. During the establishment of the hierarchy, subordinate males by contrast have elevated levels of ACTH and corticosterone (but not TH, PNMT, or T). When a subordinate male mouse is placed in a dominant position, the "defense" reaction is activated, and TH and PNMT levels in the adrenal medulla increase, NE blood levels rise, and corticosterone levels fall. But when this animal is housed with another dominant, TH and PNMT levels again fall.

Rats show similar patterns. The dominant rat in a stable colony has persistently higher T levels than the subordinates. But a defeated or chronically submissive rat has consistently high serum corticosterone levels. The dominant rat's splenic lymphocytes incorporate the greatest amount of thymidine after mitogenic stimulation, the subordinate animal's a lesser amount, and those of the once-dominant animal cast out of the colony the least of all. The largest number of cytotoxic $CD8^+$ cells is found in the outcast animal, and the smallest in the dominant. A linear (and inverse) relationship exists between the number of these cells and the status of the animal in the social hierarchy (Ballieux and Heijnen 1987). (Because a change in status of an animal produces an alteration of these two immune parameters, the animal's social status cannot be a product of changes in its immune system.)

Consistently high serum cortisol levels over a six-year period also characterize subordinate, compared to dominant, male olive baboons living in stable social hierarchies in the wilds of East Africa. Hypercortisolemia in the subordinates is not a product of either diminished metabolic clearance of the hormone, or increased sensitivity of the adrenal cortex to ACTH. Actually, in the subordinate baboons the ACTH response to an injection of CRF is diminished, even when cortisol secretion by the adrenal cortex is inhibited by metyrapone. Therefore, the decreased responsiveness to CRF is not a product of feedback inhibition of ACTH secretion by cortisol, but is due to the decreased responsiveness of corticotrophs to CRF (Sapolsky 1982, 1989).

The behavioral physiology of dominance status in male vervet monkeys has also been studied. It is positively correlated with whole blood 5-HT levels and 5-HT uptake by blood platelets. The dominant's 5-HT blood levels are 1000 ng/ml, while the subordinates' are 650 ng/ml. However, the subordinate animals have persistently greater levels in blood serum of NE and the enzyme tryptophane pyrrolase. And if a subordinate male becomes the dominant one, his whole blood 5-HT and serum cortisol levels rise.

When both kinds of animals are fed tryptophane (20 mg/kg daily), 5-HT blood levels increase significantly more in the dominant male than in the subordinates. On the other hand, the elevated levels of 5-HT are not sustained in dominant animals that are removed from the colony. If isolation is so arranged that the dominant male can keep the other male monkeys in sight through a one-way screen, the 5-HT levels diminish except when the other males display their usual submissive postures before the dominant male. When male monkeys aspiring to the dominant position are fed serotonin agonists (e.g., tryptophane or quipazine), they achieve dominance (McGuire and Raleigh 1985; Raleigh et al. 1984).

In stable societies of marmoset monkeys, the female animal's background levels or patterns of LH and progesterone depend on her status in the social hierarchy: They differ markedly in the dominant and subordinate female. Subdominant marmosets are constantly harassed by the dominant female. They are excluded from food resources and male partners. They do not ovulate. Their mean levels of LH and progesterone are low. When they are removed from the colony, oscillatory LH patterns resume and mean levels of LH and progesterone rise. A preovulatory LH surge occurs. When they are returned to the colony, the hormone levels and patterns are again suppressed. Yet when LHRH (1 μg every 2 hours) is infused into subordinates living in the colony, LH pulses, a preovulatory LH surge, and raised progesterone levels are generated (Abbott 1987). In the subordinate female monkey living with a dominant one, LH secretion is under tonic inhibitory control, possibly by β-endorphin, which is known to be released by CRF.

The hormonal correlates of dominant and subordinate status in squirrel monkeys have also been studied. The dominant male monkey shows the greatest increases in T and cortisol, when three males are housed together. As soon as a female is put into this group the dominant male achieves peak T levels, which continue to increase over time; in subordinates they fall. Mating is not a prerequisite for these changes in T levels; it does not by itself account for them (Mendoza et al. 1979).

One might well ask what it is that is stressful about the experience of being in the subordinate position in a stable social group. In part this question has already been answered (Sapolsky 1988). Subordinate males of a variety of vertebrate genera and species are repeatedly, randomly, and unpredictably intimidated by the dominant one. They are cowed to the point of infrequent courtship of, or mating with, receptive females; when they do attempt to mate they are chased off by the dominant. They are also interrupted while feeding. But the picture is quite different for a male who presumes to become the dominant when no fixed hierarchy has been established, or when he falls from his exalted position. As the previous account has told, a wide-ranging pattern of physiological changes is associated with subordinate rank. This characteristic pattern is conserved on the whole in different vertebrate species. It entails the adrenal-cortical and gonadal steroids, levels of adrenal catecholamine-synthesizing enzymes, indoleamines, raised LDL to HDL ratios (Sapolsky and Mott 1987), the progression of atherosclerosis (Shively and Kaplan 1984), and some measures of immune function (Coe, Rosenberg, and Levine 1988). These physiological patterns change as the social status of the animal is altered: They are a "function of rank" (Sapolsky 1989).

The Integration of Behavior and Physiology

Ever since Darwin, we have known that challenges and threats by predators, enemies, or (dominant) conspecifics are followed by a sequence of patterned responses in their subjects. For heuristic reasons, one may separate these integrated responses into an anticipatory phase (often called orienting, alerting, or preparatory responses), and a response phase, which may consist either of diverting or fighting the adversary. The fight in turn may end in victory, defeat, submission, death, or flight (Cannon 1929).

Each phase is characterized by integrated behavioral and physiological responses, which are well exemplified by studying the circulation in fighting cats. As already mentioned, they are highly discriminated (Zanchetti, Baccelli, and Mancia 1976). Anticipatory cardiovascular responses to exercise are also seen in animals: They consist of increases in HR, systolic and diastolic BP, stroke volume, and CO; blood flow through the skin and large muscles rises, but it falls in the mesenteric bed to result in a net decrease in peripheral resistance. During the anticipation of exercise parasympathetic (inhibitory) constraint on the circulation is reduced.

So far the emphasis has been placed on some of the cardiovascular and hormonal changes that occur during the anticipatory and fighting phases and before exercise. It should not be forgotten that they are integrated with specific behaviors: The cat about to fight assumes a posture preparing it to spring; it claws and bites; its pupils are dilated; its hair stands up. The question of the integration of these behaviors and the physiological patterns remains to be answered (see chapter 8).

Even molecular changes specific to stressful experiences occur at a receptor. When rats are group-housed, an increase in binding of the flunitrazepam ligand to the benzodiazepine receptor in the brain is seen. Foot shock, however, reduces binding to the same receptor, which regulates the passage of chloride ions into cerebral cortical and hippocampal cells (Drugan et al. 1989).

Thus the physiological responses of the organism are exquisitely attuned to the stressful experience.

A Perspective on the Role of Stressful Experience in the Etiology and Pathogenesis of Disease in Animals

Ethical and logistical considerations prevent or limit the planning and execution of prospective and longitudinal studies on the development of disease in human beings. Therefore, it is traditional in medicine to develop animal models of disease. Thanks to great scientists such as Ehrlich, Koch, and Pasteur, this strategy has been carried forward with great benefit to humankind. Koch established criteria by which later investigators could judge the validity of the pathogenesis of infectious disease; they have never been improved upon. However, he also biased future generations of scientists toward a linear, exogenous, and unicausal, rather than a multifactorial, model of pathogenesis (Copeland 1977). There is no room in the unicausal model for other factors, such as stressful experiences, to interact with an infectious or other pathogenetic agent. It has taken many years to correct the traditional impression of single causes for diseases, and the battle to do so is by no means over. The multifactorial model of the etiology and pathogenesis of human disease and ill health has already been presented (chapter 6). It is supported by the ensuing and selective review of some animal models of disease.

Selye pointed the way to the study of the role of unavoidable damage in producing disease. Throughout this chapter the role of stressful experience in producing disease (e.g., high BP, infections, and gastric erosions) has been alluded to. But the outcome—a disease—after stressful experience is by no means inevitable: Many factors combine to prevent or promote it.

Evidence for the Genetic Heterogeneity of Risk Factors and of the Pathogenesis of Disease

Animal Models of High Blood Pressure

Genetic strain differences in experimental high BP

For many years, human essential hypertension was modeled by constricting the renal artery of various animal species, or injecting a mixture of deoxycorticosterone acetate and salt into rats. But these two models did not veridically mirror the human disease. Over the last thirty-five years in Italy, Japan, New Zealand, and the United States, a variety of rat strains that develop high BP by different pathogenetic pathways have been bred. Among the most interesting of these is the spontaneously hypertensive rat (SHR); subforms of this strain also develop complications, such as "strokes." The stroke-prone variant (SHRSP) develops systolic BP levels of over 200 mm Hg at 10 to 15 weeks of age. Its members go on to die of cerebral hemorrhage or thrombosis. The stroke-resistant strain develops equally high BP levels but does not succumb to "strokes" (Okamoto and Aoki 1963; Yamori et al. 1979; Yen et al. 1974). Three other substrains of the SHRSP have been bred: They either develop atherosclerosis when fed diets high in cholesterol, thrombose blood vessels, or infarct their myocardium.

Rats of the genetically hypertensive Münster or Lyon strains may also develop BP levels that equal those achieved in the SHR. Although their hearts become enlarged, none of the vascular complications that characterize rats of the SHRSP substrains are seen. Rats of a fourth—the Milan—strain (MHS) develop mild high BP levels after 2 months of age, which do not increase much further as they become older. The Brookhaven rat strain depends on a high-salt diet for the development of its high BP (Dahl, Heine, and Tassinari 1962). (Salt-resistant strains have also been bred.)

Heterogeneity of the Pathogenesis and Pathophysiology of High BP in Members of Two Rat Strains

Experiments in rats underscore the fact that high BP may be initiated and maintained in a variety of ways. In one rat model—the Kyoto Wistar SHR—the brain plays a primary role in initiating the rise in BP; in other related animal strains it plays a secondary one. This conclusion is documented by comparing two closely related strains. In the MHS the kidney is the site of origin of the high BP (Bianchi et al. 1973; Folkow and Hallbäck 1977). By contrast, the primary pathogenetic factors in the SHR strain are mediated both by enhanced sympathetic outflow from the brain, and by increased release of several pituitary hormones—PRL, ACTH, TSH (Okamoto 1972), and aVP (Möhring, Kinz, and Schoun 1978). Subsequent changes in resistance vessels, the kidney, and the chemical composition of the heart occur to sustain the high BP (Folkow and Hallbäck 1977). However, environmental influences interact with genetic predisposition in such animals: The development of high BP may be slowed by socially isolating very young animals of this strain (Hallbäck 1975) and accelerated by shocking them with electricity (Yamori 1981; Yamori et al. 1969). The SHR also avidly eats salt if given the opportunity to do so.

The inheritance of high BP in the SHR is under the control of three or more autosomal genes. In the MHS two genes appear to suffice (Rapp and Iwai 1976; Yamori et al. 1980). The mode of inheritance is multifactorial in both strains. The inheritance is additive—the more genes the SHR offspring inherit, the greater is the likelihood that high BP will develop. What it is that is inherited is not known: Some believe that it may entail a defect of the transport of the sodium ion across, or the exchange of sodium and potassium ions through, cell membranes.

The problem in the rat, as in humans, is to differentiate the nature of the physiological changes before, and at the inception of, the disease from the later compensatory, or complicating, ones. At the start of high BP in the SHR, the HR, CO, peripheral resistance, and renal vascular resistance are raised. Later CO and stroke volume fall. In the MHS and the HR and CO are not increased at any time. In fact, in this second strain the HR may be lower at all times, but the peripheral resistance may be heightened at a later stage of the disease. Early in the development of high BP in the SHR, NE levels are elevated both in the plasma and in the adrenal medulla (Yamori 1976). At the same time, the activity of the enzyme DA β-hydroxylase in plasma is raised. Postganglionic sympathetic activity in splanchnic and renal nerves, recorded in the steady state, is greater than usual (Okamoto et al. 1967). The heightened sympathetic outflow can be reversed, and the BP can be lowered by α-adrenergic blocking agents.

The body of the SHR contains more water than usual, even in the early stage of the disease, but its kidneys handle the excretion of excessive body water normally. However, in order to excrete a standard amount of salt and water, the kidneys in these rats require a higher perfusion pressure. Later in the course of the disease their renal vascular resistance is high. Aldosterone and 18-hydroxy-desoxycorticosterone acetate levels may be raised; their increase may, however, be a result of the high BP, not its antecedent. Angiotensin-II activity in arteries and arterioles is elevated. There are more receptors for this peptide in the rat's renal tubules after high BP levels have been established (Yamori 1983).

The current view of the pathogenesis of SHR is that the brain first enhances sympathetic nervous system activity and NE secretion. The changes in the kidney follow. However, the matter may not be so simple. As mentioned, TSH levels are high in the SHR, yet T_3 and T_4 levels are decreased. Thyroidectomy lowers the elevated BP in the SHR for unknown reasons.

Furthermore, the role of renal PGs in the process of the disease is problematic: They have pressor effects in normal rats, but the SHR excretes greater quantities of them (Dunn 1978; Okuma et al. 1979). However, when the synthesis of PGs is inhibited, the BP of SHR rats paradoxically increases further (Chrysant 1979). Therefore, it has been assumed that the increased excretion of PGs was compensatory, once the BP was high. But this assumption may not be correct. Increased renal production of thromboxane A_2 has been described during the inception of high BP in young, but not in adult, SHR rats. When renal cytochrome P-450 monooxygenase (which metabolizes arachidonic acid) is inhibited by tin salts, normal BP levels are restored; its administration is followed by a natriuresis, but only in young SHRs (Sacerdoti et al. 1989). Thus the role of the kidney and of PGs in the pathogenesis of high BP in the SHR is currently being reassessed.

Research on the SHR also supports the thesis that the initiation and maintenance of high BP is a two-step process, mediated by different brain mechanisms. Injections of 6-hydroxydopamine (6-OHDA) (which causes degeneration of NE and DA nerve endings in the brain, and depletion of their transmitter stores) into the lateral ventricles of young rats of this strain prevents the development of elevated BP levels (Folkow and Hallbäck 1977). But the intraventricular injection of 6-OHDA does not lower high BP levels once established (Haeusler, Finch, and Thoenen 1972; Haeusler, Gerold, and Thoenen 1972). Therefore, NE and DA neurons in the brain play a role at the onset but not in the maintenance of high BP (Saavedra, Grobecker, and Axelrod 1978). Once instituted, the high BP levels are maintained by 5-HT neurons in the brain since PCPA, which depresses 5-HT synthesis, reduces established high systolic BP in this rat strain (Jarrott et al. 1975).

Additional factors in other regions of the brain sustain high BP in the SHR. The intraventricular injection of a competitive antagonist of angiotensin-II lowers BP levels in SHRs after bilateral nephrectomy. The isorenin-angiotensin systems in the hypothalamus apparently maintain high BP. In addition, angiotensin levels are high in the cerebrospinal fluid of these rats before they develop BP (Scroop and Lowe 1968). Angiotensin-II excites neurosecretory neurons in the rat's brain and stimulates the release of catecholamines (Ganten et al. 1971; Nicholl and Barker 1971; Phillips et al. 1977).

The formulation that high BP in the SHR is due to the unfolding of a genetic program is correct. But the belief that the disease is "spontaneous" is wrong. In the SHR an interaction between stressful experience, social isolation, salt, and BP levels has been observed. In the MHS no such interactive effects are believed to occur. The current belief is that the MHS rats are avid water drinkers, and that from inception these rats have smaller kidneys with a reduced ability to excrete water. The urine osmolality is high. When salt is administered, their kidneys excrete more salt and a greater volume of urine. Their renal resistance is normal. Plasma and blood volume are raised. Low levels of PRA, angiotensin-II, and aVP are present in these rats. The actions of these hormones on the kidney are reduced. Yet no serum electrolyte disturbances occur. But α-adrenergic sympathetic blocking agents given peripherally, or centrally administered NE agonists, lower the BP of the MHS rat. Therefore, a pathogenetic role for increased sympathetic activity in the MHS animal is inferred, even though the kidney is believed to play a primary pathogenetic role.

In still other models of experimental high BP, a wide variety of smells, sounds, and social behaviors play roles in altering BP levels. When angiotensin-II is infused into the vertebral arteries of dogs (McCubbin 1967), or when the NTS in a cat's brain is lesioned (Reis 1981), mean BP levels are raised and

BP lability is much enhanced, especially during the day. Everyday sounds are particularly prone to produce such BP fluctuations, as are the acts of eating and grooming, the sight and smell of food, touch, and novel and conditioning stimuli. Brain stem baroreceptor mechanisms of the NTS in normal animals buffer sympathetically mediated vasoconstrictor discharge, and thus phasic BP increases against sensory and conditioning stimuli and aroused emotions. The source of the vasoconstrictor discharge lies rostral to the NTS and other medullary systems, in the anterior basal hypothalamus (Reis 1981).

Thus these experimental procedures not only alter the regulation of tonic levels and phasic increases of BP levels, but also alter the response of the BP to sensory input of various kinds. They change the animal's behavior and circulatory responses to the environment.

Genetic Strain Differences in Gastric Pepsinogen: Role in Gastric Erosion Formation

Pepsinogen is the precursor of the main proteolytic enzyme, pepsin, in the stomach. In humans, elevated levels of one isoenzymatic form of pepsinogen is a risk factor for peptic duodenal ulcer. Being an enzyme precursor, it is under genetic control. The distribution of values for serum pepsinogen levels in populations of rats and humans is similar. Considerable differences in its mean values occur between and within various strains of rats: Male rats of the Osborne-Mendel strain have the highest, and those of the Wistar strain the lowest, values. Female rats of each of four different strains tend to have higher values of serum pepsinogen than male rats of the same strain, but differences between strains are less apparent in females (Ader 1963a).

The role of variations in pepsinogen levels is only revealed when rats are restrained, because the location of the erosions in the stomach depends in part on the nature of the stressful experimental procedure: When rats are subjected to unavoidable electric shock on their way to feeding and drinking, they develop erosions in the rumen, but when they are restrained after food deprivation, the lesions are largely confined to the body of the stomach (Conger, Sawrey, and Turrell 1958; Sawrey and Weisz 1956). No relationship can be found between serum pepsinogen levels and erosion formation in the rumen of the rat's stomach. The body of the rat's stomach secretes acid and pepsin. About 29% of restrained animals, whose serum pepsinogen levels fall into the highest 15% of the distribution, are more susceptible to erosion formation in the body of the stomach than those whose levels are in the lower 15% (Ader 1963b; Ader, Beels, and Tatum 1960).

A critical variable in these experiments is the duration of the restraint; the longer it lasts, the less do variations in serum pepsinogen levels play a role in determining the outcome. Even rats with very low levels eventually develop erosions if restrained for a long enough period. Therefore, the variations in levels are neither necessary, nor are they sufficient, in determining erosion formation; the effects of prolonged restraint override the subtle etiological role of variations in the enzyme precursor levels.

The values for serum pepsinogen are not fixed. Restraint lowers high basal pepsinogen levels and increases low ones. Circadian variations in levels also occur, corresponding with the activity cycle of the animal; they are higher at the beginning of the night and lower during the day, when rats usually sleep.

Restraining rats for six hours at the peak of the activity cycle is associated with gastric erosions, which do not occur when restraint is applied at the nadir of the cycle. But the circadian variation in pepsinogen levels does not seem to account for the results of this second procedure. Corticosterone levels rise before nightfall, and then fall. Despite the fact that restraint increases corticosterone levels in the rat, their circadian variations also do not seem to play a role in the formation of erosions (Ader 1967).

One may conclude that genetic differences play a subtle role in the formation of gastric erosions in rats that is obscured by prolonged restraint. The time of restraint during the circadian activity cycle is another factor determining the outcome of restraint.

This second group of studies reopened the question of the part played by the corticosteroids in the formation of gastric erosions. In fact, the role of the corticosteroids in gastric erosion formation remains unsettled. The fact that procedures such as prolonged restraint (with or without exposure to cold) or unavoidable electrical shocks are both followed by their release, and by the formation of erosions, does not mean that their positive correlation is a causal one. Murphy, Wideman, and Brown (1979) and Weiss (1968, 1970, 1971) believed that it was. But erosions occur even when adrenalectomy is followed by restraint (Brodie and Hanson 1960). No correlation can be found in less prolonged experiments using restraint; in fact, an inverse relationship between corticosteroid levels and erosion formation exists when a "backward" form of Pavlovian conditioning is employed (Murison and Isaksen 1982).

Therefore, one must conclude that the original idea that corticosterone plays a primary pathogenetic role in erosion formation is likely to be incorrect. In part, it was predicated on the fact that in large doses the corticosteroids may be ulcerogenic in the rat (Robert and Nezamis 1964) and in humans. They are known to inhibit gastric PG secretion, which protects the gastric mucosa against erosions (Allen and Garner 1980).

But the corticosteriod response to stressful experiences is but one facet of a broad response pattern. Some of them do release CRF and thus corticosteroids, but CRF release within the brain actually counteracts gastric contractions, hydrochloric acid secretion, and prevents erosions (see this chapter). Furthermore, intermittent electric shocks promote stress analgesia of the "opioid" form. And the severity of gastric erosions after five hours of restraint is attenuated by morphine and increased by naloxone (Arrigo-Reina and Ferri 1980; Glavin 1985).

Genetic Strain Differences in Animal Models of Systemic Lupus Erythematosus

Genetic heterogeneity exists for animal models of SLE (Dixon 1982). Three different mouse strains express the disease phenotype; the pathogenesis of SLE differs in each of these.

The New Zealand Black heterozygote (NZB/NZW) female mouse begins to develop an SLE-like syndrome at about 20 weeks and dies by the age of 54 weeks. The male succumbs to the disease at 42 weeks and lives to be about 86 weeks old. Hormonal factors play an important role in SLE in this strain of mice. Estrogen treatment accelerates the onset of the disease, and androgens administered to female mice retard it.

In a second strain—the MRL/l mouse—both sexes develop an acute form of SLE at 8–12 weeks and are dead by 54 weeks. The genome of these animals contains a recessive lymphoproliferative (lpr) gene that results from a spontaneous mutation. Homozygotes manifest a massive "expansion" of their T-cells. About 20% of older MRL/l mice instead develop an RA-like disease, which is associated with the appearance of RFs in the serum and the characteristic joint lesions (Dixon 1982). Therefore, the gene is expressed in two different diseases.

The lpr gene is absent in the congenic MRL/n mouse, in which both sexes develop SLE at 42 weeks, the death occurring at 90 weeks. The two strains are identical for the MHC (H-2) gene.

A third mouse strain—the BXSB—shows marked gender differences in the age of onset of SLE. Males contract it at 12 weeks of age and die when 40 weeks old. In females the disease begins at about 54 weeks and may last until they are 96 weeks of age. This form of the disease is associated with the Y-chromosome. Because castration of male mice of the BXSB strain does not influence the onset or course of the disease, hormonal factors seem to play no role in its pathogenesis. Yet when bone marrow cells are transferred from male to female BXSB mice (whose marrow has been destroyed by X-rays), SLE develops earlier in life, not later, and its course is accelerated.

Of major importance for any theory of the pathogenesis of SLE is the fact that each of these strains has a different H-2 (MHC) genotype, with quite distinctive lymphocyte surface alloantigens and immunoglobulin-G (IgG) allotypes. Therefore, differing genotypes may express themselves in the same SLE phenotype. The time of development and course of the disease are, however, determined by separate factors present in each strain: estrogens in the NZB mouse; the lpr gene in the MRL/l strain; and gene(s) on the Y-chromosome of the BXSB animal. (This conclusion is based on cross-breeding experiments.) However, these three additional factors do not promote SLE in mice not genetically prone to SLE.

Normal mice infected with lymphocytic choriomeningitis (LCM) virus at birth eventually develop an autoimmune glomerulonephritis, but members of the three lupus-prone strains infected in a similar manner with LCM rapidly succumb to an early onset of SLE-like disease. Therefore, an interaction between LCM infection and a genetic predisposition to it occurs.

Murine SLE is characterized by the formation of antigen-antibody complexes deposited in blood vessels of the kidney, and elsewhere. The native antigens are nuclear ones, IgG, complement, and the normally present gp70 serum protein. Only in the MRL/l strain is CD4$^+$ activity increased. CD8$^+$ cell and cytolytic activities seem to be normal in all three mouse strains. Even before the disease develops, B-lymphocyte activity is enhanced in lupus-prone animals, manifested by increased antibody production to bacterial lipopolysaccharides, elevated resting immunoglobulin-M (IgM) levels, and polyclonal activation. Furthermore, B-cell maturation appears to be accelerated in these animals, possibly because these cells have not acquired tolerance to native antigens (Dixon 1982).

These mouse models illustrate that SLE can come about in a variety of ways: No single genotype is responsible. A variety of factors interact with the various genotypes to determine when the disease expresses itself. Furthermore, the immunopathology is different in one (MRL/l) strain than in the other two. Curiously enough, the MRL/l mouse can also develop RA, not only SLE.

Additional Factors in the Development of Disease

A multifactorial concept incorporates more than the roles of genetic factors and stressful experiences in the etiology and pathogenesis of diseases. The reproductive history of animals and the manner in which they are perennially housed are also antecedents of disease. Mature, virgin rats of either gender housed in communities of fifty or in pairs, but segregated according to sex, weighed less and had smaller hearts, adrenal glands, testes or ovaries, and kidneys, but larger thymus glands, than rats allowed to breed in communities or in pairs. All these organs except the thymus gland (which was smaller) were heavier in rats that bred. All the breeders, but not the virgins, became obese and developed fatty livers. Free fatty acid, triglyceride, cholesterol, blood sugar, and urea nitrogen levels were elevated when compared to the levels in virgin rats of the same gender. All the breeders had elevated systolic BP levels, which rose linearly and progressively as each breeding cycle passed.

Male rats living in a breeding community have the highest BP levels of all; they increased as soon as breeding began. Grossly visible arteriosclerosis occurred in all breeders, especially in the communal ones. The lesions in the aorta were visible to the naked eye in females and microscopic in males. Nineteen percent of the males in the large cages died of myocardial infarction after six months. A variety of muscle, liver, and cardiac enzyme levels increased in breeders. Corticosterone levels increased especially in male communal animals, but decreased in female breeders after four reproductive cycles. The adrenal cortices of these females were the site of hemorrhage and venous thrombosis (Wexler and Greenberg 1978).

The burden of these effects is placed on repeated breeding, which is believed to be associated with continuous activation of the hypothalamic-pituitary-gonadal (HPG) and -adrenal (HPA) axes. However, it should be noted that the greatest damage occurred to the males in the community cages. This situation is bound to engender fighting among males for the dominant role in breeding. No attempt was made in these experiments to determine whether the dominant males bred more frequently and had the highest BP levels, while the subordinates had the high corticosterone and blood sugar levels.

Therefore, the housing conditions and the reproductive histories of mature animals must be taken into account as a factor in the development of high BP and arteriosclerosis.

Models of Disease Following Stressful Experience

Pathogenetic Mechanisms: The Immune System

The long-term physiological consequences of premature separation of young rats has previously been reviewed. Nothing, however, was mentioned about the fact that this experience is a risk factor for subsequent diseases, with or without later challenge.

The T-cells of 40-day-old rats prematurely separated at 15 days of age from their mothers were less able to incorporate thymidine after a mitogenic (PHA) stimulus. The ultimate outcome of separation was that by 100 days of age, 50% (80% of the males and 20% of the female rats) of the animals had died of opportunistic—apparently viral—infections of the lungs (Ackerman et al. 1988).

Effects on immune function have also been studied in separated squirrel monkeys (Coe, Rosenberg, and Levine 1988). The animals were 6 to 12 months of age, older than those previously used in studies on the effects of separation. They had been weaned and were largely functioning independently of the mother. A panoply of immune functions and serum cortisol were measured sequentially, both before and after removing the young animal from its mother. By measuring not one but several functions, new insights have been obtained: A change in one part of the humoral immune system that potentially could have deleterious consequences (e.g., diminished resistance to infection) for the organism may be compensated for by an increase in the protective activity in another set (cellular) of functions.

A 24-hour separation of young monkeys led to a redistribution of phagocytes (e.g., eosinophiles); a relative fall in lymphocyte numbers, presumably due to their relocation in the bone marrow and lymph nodes; and a greater percentage of circulating neutrophilic cells. When the separation was prolonged for a week, both the neutrophilia and the lymphocytopenia continued to increase.

The redistribution of these three cell types is considered to have adaptive significance, preparing the organism for a possible invasion by an infectious agent. On the other hand, young monkeys have lower IgG levels after seven days of being on their own—a response that is ascribed to the prolonged elevation of serum cortisol levels in these animals. (The hypercortisolemia may also, however, explain the redistribution of the three classes of cells, especially of the lymphocytes). The validity of the decline in immunoglobulin levels is supported by the fact that separated animals mount smaller primary antibody (IgM), and secondary antibody (IgG), responses to challenge by a virus, bacteriophage X174. The reduced antibody responses to the viral antigen are ascribable to the diminished ability of accessory cells to initiate an antibody response, rather than a failure of immunoglobulin synthesis. Thus separated animals seem to have a reduced capacity to mount a humoral immune response against a specific antigen.

They also show impaired release of one class (α-thymosin) of thymic hormones, and two critical components of the complement system (C3 and C4)—a deficit that implies that these animals may be less capable of warding off bacteria by lysing them, or of binding bacterial antigen to antibody. However, the hemolytic activity of complement is increased in these monkeys, indicating a compensatory increase of the functional capacity of another component of the system to lyse foreign cells. The ability of intracellular digestion of foreign matter (e.g., bacteria) was also raised, as inferred from enhanced macrophage activity (Coe, Rosenberg, and Levine 1988).

However, the prolonged restraint of mice reduces the nonspecific tumoricidal activity of peritoneal macrophages after activation by partially purified L-cell interferon, and by bacterial lipopolysaccharide (Pavlidis and Chirigos 1980). On the surface, the two results seem to contradict each other. But they are not comparable, either in terms of the species used, the nature of the stressful experiences, or the sources of, or assays for, macrophage function.

Separated monkeys demonstrate an apparent decline in humoral immune function but an increase in cellular immune responses (to dinitrochlorobenzene). Other (squirrel) monkeys, prematurely separated and weaned from their mothers, have enhanced proliferative responses to both B- and T-cell mitogens at 1 year of age (Coe, Rosenberg, and Levine 1988).

Effects on Gastrointenstinal Function and Disease

Prematurely separated rats restrained, or not fed, or both, at 22, 30, and 40 days of age develop gastric erosions with an incidence of 80–95% (Ackerman 1981). (The incidence in normally weaned animals of the same age is 10%.) This effect is mediated by the (aforementioned) fall in body temperature during restraint (Ackerman, Hofer, and Weiner 1978). The animals do not ulcerate when restrained at 17 days of age. After 40 days of age the incidence of gastric erosions progressively declines in separated animals on restraint; by 200 days of age it is 20%. The effects of a challenge in prematurely separated animals is, therefore, age-dependent. The initial separation does not produce erosions but places animals at profound risk for the lesions on subsequent challenge at a later age (of 22–40 days), but not at all ages. The excessive susceptibility of prematurely separated rats to challenge is inherited by maternal transmission to her offspring, which develop gastric erosions on challenge at 30 days with a probability of 65%. In cross-fostering experiments, it can be shown that the susceptibility to erosions is passed on in utero (Skolnick et al. 1980).

A defect in thermoregulation after separation is only manifested on challenge, and is not observed when the animal is left to its own devices in an environment whose temperature is about 20°C. It is originally brought about by depriving the animal of its mother's milk. If young rats are able to lap up milk following separation, they are able later to maintain their body temperature when restrained (Ackerman 1981).

Usually, prematurely separated rats are permanently underweight. They also store less brown fat; when restrained it "melts" off much more rapidly than in their normal peers. As a consequence their usual body temperature is not sustained for any prolonged period of time (Ackerman 1989).

Cooling normal rats artificially in order to produce a fall in body temperature linearly induces increased gastric acid secretion. But when 30-day-old, prematurely separated rats are cooled so that their body temperature falls to 29°C, they actually secrete less hydrochloric acid into the lumen of their stomach than nonseparated rats do (Ackerman 1981).

This insight, and other recent developments in our understanding of the role of stressful experience in gastric erosion formation, in the normal regulation of gastric physiology, and in the central role of the brain in inducing gastric erosions, has led to a major conceptual revision. Increases in gastric acid secretion and in plasma corticosterone levels were initially believed to play the central roles in the formation of gastric erosions. But it is now fairly certain that other factors are primary, and that increased acid secretion and corticosterone levels are neither necessary nor sufficient. Changes in body temperature, diminished mucosal resistance (including bicarbonate secretion), the back diffusion of protons into mucosal cells, and/or reduction in blood flow interact with altered gastric motility to erode the mucosa of the stomach.

Many experimental models have been devised to produce such erosions (Paré and Glavin 1986). They may be divided into two separate categories: those that induce or promote a fall in body temperature—e.g., cold-restraint, continuous motor activity induced by feeding the rat once daily, or premature separation followed by restraint; and those that produce an increase in body temperature—e.g., lateral hypothalamic lesions (Grijalva and Roland 1989), prolonged unavoidable shock, or the intracisternal injection of thyrotropin releasing hormone (TRH).

By the use of miniature pressure transducers attached to the stomach wall, high amplitude, slow (1 every 2 mins.) contractions can be recorded in rats restrained in the cold, 40-day-old prematurely separated animals, and those subjected to intermittent, unavoidable shock. This new pattern of contractions is quite different from the normal feeding one (Garrick, Buack, and Bass 1986). Papaverine pretreatment averts these slow gastric contractions and also the formation of erosions in cold-restrained rats. Yet gastric acid secretion actually diminishes initially in these animals. It merely plays a permissive role in erosion formation; only by completely suppressing it (with cimetidine) are erosions prevented from occurring.

The fact that a fall in body temperature is a critical intervening variable inevitably has led to a number of investigators to examine the role of TRH in altering gastric secretion, motility, and erosion formation. This hypothesis has been supported by the demonstration that exposing rats to an ambient temperature of 4°C increases the TRH content of the median eminence and of third ventricular fluid (Arancibia and Assenmacher 1987; Arancibia et al. 1983). Furthermore, 12% of the total TRH content of the brain is contained in the brain stem, particularly in the dorsomotor nucleus of the vagus (DMV), NA, and NTS (Kubek et al. 1983).

Intracisternal (IC) or intracerebroventricular (ICV) TRH or its stable analog (RX 77368) increase gastric acid and pepsin secretion and vagal efferent discharge (Taché 1985; Taché, Vale, and Brown 1980). Such injections also enhance gastric contractions in a dose-dependent manner—an effect that is averted by atropine or vagotomy (Garrick et al. 1987)—and produce gastric erosions in the gastric body and antrum (Goto and Taché 1985).

The site of action of IC or ICV injections of TRH or its analog is the DMV (Rogers and Herrmann 1985; Okuma et al. 1987). When this nucleus is injected with TRH a gastric secretory response is elicited, whereas injections into the area postrema or various other hypothalamic nuclei have no such effect. Ten to 100 ng of RX 77368 produce a dose-dependent acid secretory response that peaks at 40 min. when injected into the DMV and NTS, but not when injected into the N. reticularis or N. cuneatus (Stephens et al. 1988). The gastric secretory response to TRH is abolished by vagotomy.

While stimulating gastric acid secretion, RX 77368 (100 ng) IC simultaneously enhances the content of 5-HT in the gastric lumen—an effect that peaks at 45 min. The secretion of 5-HT is also abolished by the injection of atropine. When the gastric content of 5-HT is reduced by 66% following pretreatment with PCPA (300 mg/kg), a reduction (57%) of gastric 5-HT secretion occurs on injection of RX 77368. At the same time, pretreatment with PCPA markedly increases the gastric *acid* secretory response to RX 77368. Therefore, TRH, or its analog, releases 5-HT, which counterregulates maximal gastric acid secretion (Stephens et al. 1989). Intraarterial 5-HT (3–10 mg/kg), however, produces a biphasic change in intragastric pressure and increases the amplitude of gastric contractions.

At the level of the stomach, a counterregulatory system modulates acid secretion. But in the brain stem, the action of TRH is opposed by CRF, which is also released by a fall in body temperature. The CRF by itself delays gastric emptying and acid secretion and prevents gastric erosion formation induced by cold-restraint (Taché 1985; Taché, Maeda-Hagiwara, and Turkelson 1987). The role of IC and ICV CRF and gastric contractions stimulated by IC RX 77368, IC 2-deoxy-D-glucose (2-DG), and IV carbachol has also been studied. Intracisternal CRF (6-210 pmol) significantly reduces the contractions induced by the two former, but not those promoted by IV carbachol (200 mg/kg/hr). Intravenous CRF in very large doses (10 × the above) inhibits increased contractions produced by RX 77368, but not those produced by 2-DG or IV carbachol (Garrick et al. 1988). We have as yet no idea at what exact location in the brain CRF functions to inhibit the TRH-analog- or 2-DG-induced contractions, acid secretion stimulated by secretogogues, or a low ambient temperature and restraint.

These observations do not directly prove or disprove the roles of TRH, 5-HT, or CRF in gastric erosion formation when body temperature falls as rats are cold-restrained, or restrained after premature separation. In fact, many other peptides and neurotransmitters in the brain and in the gut are involved in the regulation of the gastric functions and have been implicated in gastric erosion formation. But their physiological and pathogenetic status is not as fully established as their pharmacological actions are.

Furthermore, it has never been quite clear what human disease gastric erosions in the rat are supposed to model. Gastric ulceration occurs in humans after bodily injury, burns, surgery, and brain lesions. But originally the intent of investigators of stressful experiences was to understand the pathogenesis of human peptic duodenal ulcer. Only recently has the aim of producing duodenal ulcers in rats been achieved: Combined histamine and indomethacin injections, or injections of cysteamine, an inhibitor of somatostatin (STS), produce antral and duodenal ulcers in the rat, as does restraint in water at 23°C combined with injections of histamine (Takeuchi, Furukawa, and Okabe 1986). Without the injection of histamine but with the same stressful experience, only gastric erosions form.

At least three factors are involved in producing duodenal ulceration in rats: a normal level of gastric acid secretion, an increase of gastric contractions, and a marked diminution of duodenal bicarbonate secretion. All three are necessary but not sufficient to produce lesions. Presumably the acid is rapidly emptied by the stomach into a duodenum left unprotected by the lack of the neutralizing bicarbonate ion. Restraint and immersion are additive in reducing duodenal bicarbonate secretion. Duodenal bicarbonate secretion is under the control of both branches of the autonomic nervous system and is not only secondary to a fall in duodenal pH (Flemström and Turnberg 1984). Vagal efferent activity stimulates it, and increased sympathetic discharge, mediated by α_2 receptors, inhibits it (Jönson and Fändriks 1989; Jönson, Tunbäck-Hansson, and Fändriks 1989). An increase of sympathetic activity to the duodenum may be induced reflexly when activity in afferent mesenteric neurons increases (Jönson and Fändriks 1988) or, more directly, when the perifornical region of the lateral hypothalamus is electrically stimulated in rats. The effects of hypothalamic stimulation can be blocked by guanethidine (Fändriks, Jönson, and Lisander 1989), suggesting that it is mediated by sympathetic neurons.

Stressful Experiences Designed to Produce Experimentally High BP in Animals

In addition to breeding rat strains specifically for the purpose of inciting high BP, investigators have devised many experimental techniques for the same purpose (Weiner 1979b). They include conditioning procedures designed to produce elevations of BP by classical, operant, avoidant, and "emotional" means. Auditory stimulation by blasting animals with jets of air, brain stimulation and lesions, crowding, and intermittent restraint for prolonged periods also raise a rat's BP. The lessons to be learned from these procedures are mainly heuristic: High BP may come about by a variety of different physiological pathways. It has no single "cause" and no one pathogenesis. It is a multifactorial, interactive process entailing an altered regulation of BP and the factors that determine it.

When rhesus monkeys are trained on a Sidman avoidance schedule, they first show increases in CO, HR, and blood flow through the heart, skeletal muscle, and liver. Eventually peripheral resistance increases. However, the training schedule does not produce high BP levels in monkeys immediately; it takes six or more months to do so. When training sessions are discontinued the monkeys' BPs return to normal levels (Forsyth 1969, 1971). In dogs aversive conditioning has to be combined with the infusion of salt solution to produce sustained BP increases (Anderson 1982). And in rats foot shock and salt-eating together, but not separately, produce the same result (Friedman and Iwai 1977).

The animal model of high BP that has been most instructive is a complex and naturalistic one (Henry, Meehan, and Stephens 1967). For example, the effects on a mouse of social confrontation with members of its own species differ depending on its previous experiences. When male, but not female, mice from different rearing boxes are mixed, or aggregated, in small boxes, exposed to a cat for many months, or involved in territorial conflict, they develop sustained elevations of systolic BP, arteriosclerosis, and an interstitial nephritis. Female mice subjected to such conditions fail to reproduce.

The experience of living together from birth attenuates the effects on BP and reproduction of experimentally induced aggregation and territorial conflict. On the other hand, separating animals from each other after weaning and before maturity exacerbates the effects of later crowding in raising systolic BP levels (Henry, Meehan, and Stephens 1967; Henry and Stephens-Larson 1985). The adrenal glands contain TH and PNMT. Later crowding has the effect of increasing the activity of these two enzymes—an increase significantly greater than in those animals previously accustomed to crowding. In addition, the activity of the enzyme MAO and the concentrations of NE in the adrenal medulla are greater in the experimental group (Axelrod et al. 1970; Henry et al. 1971; Henry and Stephens 1977). The crowded male mouse, or one that establishes its dominance, eventually develops elevated systolic BP and an interstitial nephritis, the former being closely correlated with raised levels of adrenal catecholamine content and PRA, and the latter with urinary reflux. The subordinate animal placed in a dominant position also develops nephritis.

When a dominant mouse is removed from his colony and placed in a new and different one (i.e., he becomes an intruder), a further rise in BP occurs (from a mean systolic BP of 155 mm Hg to 200 mm Hg). His position in the hierarchy is constantly challenged by the other dominants. But subordinate males in this situation show no rise in BP (Henry, Stephens, and Ely 1986).

Experimental Production of Atherosclerosis

Colonies of another strain (CBA) of mice can experimentally be prevented from ever establishing a stable social hierarchy. Confrontations between males may continue for six months. They develop severe fibrotic-stenotic changes in their intramural coronary arteries.

The same results have been obtained in dominant *Cynomolgus* monkeys, regardless of the composition of the diet they eat, subjected to a similar experimental procedure (Clarkson et al. 1987; Manuck, Kaplan, and Clarkson 1983a). The experiments on the monkey are of considerable interest, demonstrating once again that naturalistic experiments seem in particular to advance our knowledge of the role of stressful experience in the production of disease. The *Cynomolgus* monkey is prone to atherosclerosis and myocardial infarction. It lives in a stable social group characterized by very specific hierarchies and relationships. Each group resists the intrusion of newcomers and the disruption of the social order.

The formation of hierarchies can be prevented by reorganizing an established group and redistributing its members every three months for the first year and monthly thereafter for ten subsequent months. The once-dominant male monkey—the victor in all fights—whose status is constantly being challenged and disrupted is the one who develops the greatest degree of coronary atherosclerosis. During this process he is engaged in fights more often than dominant monkeys in a stable group usually are. But subordinate monkeys subjected to unstable social conditions do not develop more atherosclerosis than do animals living in a stable social group.

The results of these experiments may be understood to be the outcome of increased cardiovascular reactivity to experimentally produced threats; *Cynomolgus* monkeys, whose HR responses are the most exaggerated in response to them, are also the ones who after twenty-two months of being on a moderately atherogenic diet have the greatest degree of coronary artery (but not aortic) atherosclerosis. The more reactive animals also have lower HDL:LDL ratios (Manuck, Kaplan, and Clarkson 1983b).

The Role of Stressful Experience in Animal Models of Autoimmune Disease

The role of stressful experience in animal models of autoimmune disease is fraught with controversy. A part of the disagreement derives from the question of whether adjuvant arthritis (AA) is the appropriate model for human RA. It is argued that in the former the role of the T-cell is particularly important pathogenetically, but that in the latter the B-cells carry the main burden.

It is debated whether type II collagen arthritis or streptococcal cell wall arthritis in animals is not a better model for the human disease. Adjuvant arthritis in rats does mimic the joint lesions of the human disease, but no RFs appear in the animal's serum.

The AA model has been used to study the role of overcrowding on the severity of the disease. Overcrowded male Fisher rats seem to recover more rapidly following the injection of the adjuvant (Sofia 1980). Yet in other experiments overcrowded animals develop the disease more rapidly and suffer more severe impairment (Amkraut, Solomon, and Kraemer 1971). Conflicting results have been obtained in these two sets of experiments, and every recent attempt to resolve the issue has been unsuccessful.

Members of different rat strains seem to respond differently to repeated restraint following injection of adjuvant. In male Long-Evans rats swelling in the injected hindpaw is reduced, while in male Wistar rats it is enhanced. Restraint also reduces swelling in the uninjected paw in male Long-Evans rats. If the animals are restrained after reversing their light-dark cycle, no effect of restraint on the course of AA is observed (Klosterhalfen and Klosterhalfen 1987).

Collagen arthritis in rats is a better analog of human RA than is AA. Exposure to a predator cat, transportation, or handling suppresses the symptomatic and histological manifestations of collagen arthritis (Rogers et al. 1980a, 1980b). Transportation and handling have beneficial effects on the disease, but exposure to noise has deleterious ones (Rogers et al. 1984).

To summarize: The sex and strain of the animal are critical variables in all experiments designed to examine the role of stressful stimuli in modifying experimental arthritis. The dose of adjuvant or collagen antigens must be carefully adjusted in the experiments in order not to overwhelm the animals with them. If such precautions are not taken, any interaction between the stressful experience and the antigen is likely to be obscured.

A new chapter in this experimental problem has recently been opened. The female members of an inbred rat of the Lewis strain develop an erosive and proliferative arthritis after one injection of a group A streptococcal cell wall polysaccharide. Rats of the Fischer strain do not. When injected with IL-1α or CRF, Lewis rats do not secrete ACTH and corticosterone. The inability to respond appears to be due to a failure of parvocellular PVN neurons to produce, or to secrete, CRF. In Lewis rats, the enkephalin gene product is also not expressed. Both defects seem to be due to inappropriately regulated, rather than defective, genes (Sternberg et al. 1989). Therefore, one may provisionally conclude that the onset of arthritis in this model is due not to a direct immunological response to the antigen, but a failure to regulate it by corticosteroids.

New insights have also been obtained into the manner in which the nervous system might participate in the antigen-induced inflammatory response and mediate stressful experience. It has been observed that AA in the rat is delayed in onset, and is less extensive, in the joints of a hind limb previously paralyzed by cutting the ipsilateral sciatic nerve (Courtright and Kuzell 1965). Missing from these observations was a tangible hypothesis of the mechanisms by which the nervous system could initiate or contribute to inflammation. Three recent discoveries have corrected this situation: Unmyelinated (nociceptive) afferent neurons and axon reflexes release SP, which is a potent vasodilator that increases vascular permeability and also recruits polymorphonuclear phagocytes. Substance P stimulates phagocytic activity and degranulates mast cells (Payan, Levine, and Goetzl 1984).

Lotz, Carson, and Vaughan (1987) have reported that SP is also released by synovial cells in joints rendered experimentally arthritic. Substance P stimulates excessive secretion of collagenase and PGE into the arthritic joint space. An efferent pathway of unmyelinated fibers passing through the dorsal root ganglion also uses SP as its transmitter agent (Mantyh et al. 1988). Increased numbers of SP receptors are found in the joints of rats with AA.

Thus both primary afferent and efferent neurons release SP. This peptide produces the relevant conditions for inflammation, the release of the enzyme collagenase and PGE, believed to be involved in producing erosions, inflammation, and pain in arthritis. Other peptides—VIP, STS, and the calcitonin gene–related peptide (CGRP) are vasodilators, affect leukocyte function, and influence smooth muscle activity. They have all been implicated in AA (Levine, Moskowitz, and Basbaum 1988).

Further substance to this line of reasoning is added by the observation that depletion of SP (and other mediators of inflammation) in peripheral nerves by capsaicin reduces the signs of inflammation and joint damage in AA (Colpaert, Donnerer, and Lembeck 1983). Sympathetic efferent neurons may play additional roles, because destruction of sympathetic postganglionic neurons by prolonged pretreatment with injections of guanethidine, or two days of reserpine administration, markedly reduces joint damage in rats with AA (Levine et al. 1986).

But it is unclear at what point in this model disease nociceptive afferent, dorsal root, and sympathetic efferent activity come into play: Are these neural pathways involved at the onset of AA, or at the point when inflammation and pain first begin? It must be argued that joint inflammation sets up reflex activity that enhances and perpetuates joint inflammation and damage. Increased sympathetic efferent discharge increases sensory afferent activity (Wall and Gutnick 1974), and painful (nociceptive) afferent activity reflexly generates sympathetic efferent impulses (Beacham and Perl 1964). The sympathetic antagonist guanethedine increases muscle strength and decreases joint tenderness, pain, and daytime and morning stiffness, at least in patients with RA (Levine, Moskowitz, and Basbaum 1988)—a result that suggests that reduction in sympathetic efferent activity reduces symptoms, but is not necessarily involved in the pathogenesis, of RA.

Summary

This chapter has documented that many factors determine the integrated behavioral and physiological response patterns to stressful experiences. Genetic strain differences in the ability to avoid and feel pain have been described; they are correlated with specific neurochemical variations. Intrauterine experiences permanently alter the mating behavior of male rats; they are one of a number of stressful experiences that have long-term consequences on behavior and physiology. Premature separation of rats and monkeys has immediate and long-term effects. Every bodily and behavioral subsystem so far studied is immediately and permanently altered. These observations underscore the critical role of the animal's mother in regulating the behavior and physiology of her offspring so that it undergoes normal growth and maturation and has the usual responses to later experience. Their relationship is articulated in a complex manner; each facet serves a different function in regulating and maintaining the subsystems of which the young rat is composed. On separation an unfolding series of altered behavior and physiology is seen, including disrupted circadian rhythms of sleep and thermoregulation; even enzyme expression is altered by separation. No system is uniquely altered. The experience of premature separation is a risk factor for disease when the rat is later challenged; yet the subsequent disease consequences depend on the age at which the animal is tested.

Experimentally induced short-term experiences are specific: Merely changing the parameters of unavoidable electric shock has different consequences. No one system is affected. Levels of several hormones, of immune function, and of neurotransmitters are altered in the brain and in the body, but the quantity and duration of the changes depend on the animal's ability to avoid or escape from the painful trial. The most dire consequences occur when pain is unavoidable, unpredictable, and novel, or when an avoidant response is punished. Analgesia occurs in many experimental and naturally occurring circumstances. Its physiology is complex. Habituation to repeated experiences occurs, except in corticosteroid responses.

Naturally occurring experiences are particularly instructive for any theory of stress. The process of establishing and maintaining social hierarchies has organismic consequences. One source of individual differences is the dominant or subordinate status of animals. Both ongoing behavior and physiology differ with status, but they are also species-specific.

The patterned cardiovascular changes in cats before, during, and after a fight are exquisitely discriminated; their generation is under different circuits in the brain (chapter 8). Attacking, defending against, and submitting to an opponent are set off by different signals and depend on the context of the combat. The three behaviors are also subserved separately by the brain. The pattern of hormonal changes is not the same in an intruding male rat as it is in the one resident in its home cage.

The price of developing arteriosclerosis is paid by certain monkeys if the social hierarchy is constantly disrupted. The subordinate females of another species of monkeys do not ovulate. The dominant mouse develops a renin-dependent elevation of BP levels and a chronic nephritis.

Experiments in animals document the genetic heterogeneity and multifactorial nature of disease. The pathogenesis of high BP in different rat strains is both complex and distinct in the various models of the disease. In some strains the "genetic program" is modified by experience and salt in the diet.

The ability to determine some of the pathogenetic mechanisms of disease in animals has led to new insights into their complexity, nonlinearity, and multifactorial nature. The question of how the brain and its outflow mediate them, and also generate coordinated physiological patterns, is the subject of the next two chapters.

8 The Mediators of Stressful Experience: The Autonomic Nervous, Adrenal, and Gonadal Systems

The autonomic nervous, adrenal, and gonadal subsystems mediating the physiological patterns during stressful experiences interact with each other. They are multifunctional—neurotransmitters have hormonal properties, and many peptide hormones are colocalized with them or modulate their effects (chapter 9). Hormones and neurotransmitters alter immune function. Monokines and lymphokines of the immune system have several functions: They act as communication signals; they also promote cell growth and differentiation, and some regulate hormone secretion. Immunocompetent cells have receptors for, and produce some, hormones. Thus classical neurotransmitters, hormones, monokines, and lymphokines have broad-ranging functional properties. They also all affect behavior. They act locally or at a distance (Munck, Guyre, and Holbrook 1984; Sporn and Roberts 1988).

These various categories of communication signals regulate and counter-regulate each other by a system of negative, positive, or mixed (negative-positive) feedback systems. They are frequency-, not amplitude-modulated, signals (see chapter 10). They are arranged in parallel; even at the receptor and the intracellular levels of organization they act in this manner. They may induce, repress, or regulate gene expression both directly and indirectly.

Neither neurotransmitters nor hormones act in isolation. They do not produce only one bodily change. They mediate discrete patterns of changes in function, associated with a specific stressful experience, challenge, or task. Individual differences in patterned functional changes are also the rule.

The Physiology of the Autonomic Nervous System

The catecholamine neurotransmitters were once believed to belong to a select category of stress hormones. The tendency is still to write about them accordingly. But this line of thought is wrong because any (secretory) product of the pituitary and other endocrine glands, the autonomic nervous system, the heart, pancreas, and kidneys, and the immune system may change with stressful experiences. Therefore, no special class of such "stress" hormones exists. All the various chemical products of these systems—catecholamines, indoleamines, amino acids, steroid and peptide hormones, glucose, electrolytes, fatty acids, etc.—form an interconnected communication system. They all subserve autocrine, paracrine, and hormonal regulatory and signaling functions.

In the past twenty years, three major developments in catecholamine research have occurred. They had their start when it was realized that the main catecholamines (E and NE) are not elevated in plasma equally under the same circumstances and that regional differences in each of their plasma levels are detectable. Their sources within the body are different. Furthermore, NE is colocalized with NPY, but E is not.

Urinary and plasma E levels increase in association with the anticipation of threat, novel experiences, fear, excitement, and certain intellectual challenges (Baum et al. 1985; Dimsdale and Moss 1980). Distressing experiences are particularly likely to be associated with their enhancement. But changes in E levels also occur when a challenge or stimulus is reduced (Frankenhaeuser et al. 1971). Men respond with greater E (urinary) excretion than women do under increases or decrements in tasks or challenges, despite the fact that the resting levels in the two sexes are the same (Frankenhaeuser 1983).

Assuming the upright posture increases NE plasma levels two- to threefold, but no change in E levels occurs. Mental arithmetic and exercise double plasma NE levels, but E levels increase considerably less. Public speaking, on the other hand, may raise plasma E levels by a factor of 2, and plasma NE content does not rise as much. The time courses of the increases differ: E levels mount right after the start of the talk; the NE increments are much slower to develop (Dimsdale and Moss 1980). Marked individual differences occur in speakers in the degree of change in catecholamine levels. Individual variation is also manifested in soldiers, but only in those who find training for parachute jumping exciting or thrilling, rather than frightening; excited parachutists demonstrate increases mainly in plasma E levels (Ursin, Baade, and Levine 1978).

Some of the determinants of such individual response differences have been identified: Caffeine, alcohol, amphetamines, nicotine, and excessive salt intake all stimulate catecholamine secretion into the bloodstream; age influences it. Production varies with the phase of the menstrual cycle. Circadian rhythms of E and NE levels occur. Personal characteristics also determine catecholamine release. When subjects who demonstrate the so-called type A behavior pattern (Friedman and Rosenman 1959) are made to solve a difficult puzzle, their plasma NE levels achieve greater heights than those who show the type B pattern (Friedman et al. 1979). And when the former are pressured to complete a competitive task, plasma E levels increase much more than in nonharassed subjects of this type, or type B subjects (Glass et al. 1980).

Changes in plasma catecholamine levels vary in different parts of the bloodstream; they depend on the blood vessel from which the sample is taken. Plasma levels of NE are the product of a complex process entailing its release rate from storage granules situated in the terminals of sympathetic neurons; its escape from, and reuptake by these terminals; its diffusion and degradation; and its final clearance by the kidney. Each organ in the body has its own uptake rate of E and NE from the bloodstream. The lungs and the large muscles of the body are particularly avid in capturing them (Esler et al. 1984). Secretion levels of E (whose main source is the adrenal medulla, and to a lesser extent the kidney) are higher in the brachial artery than in the antecubital vein, because E is extracted by muscles in the forearm during challenging cognitive tasks (Jorgensen, Bonlokke, and Christensen 1985). Norepinephrine levels are also higher in the brachial artery than the antecubital vein (Steptoe 1987); NE is preferentially extracted by sympathetic terminals in muscles of the arm, but only when the sympathetic innervation to their vasculature is activated. Regional levels of NE may be high in one vein that drains muscle; but these elevations may not be reflected in other segments of the venous circulation. These facts alter any interpretation of (plasma) catecholamine levels obtained from a brachial vein—the usual procedure. Regional differences in E or NE levels influence changes in the function of end-organs such as the heart, kidney, and liver and are not reliably reflected in a local blood sample.

The different physiological effects of the two catecholamines are also mediated by separate receptors on target organs. These new insights have changed our understanding of the functioning of the sympathetic nervous system: Its activity is not global and nonspecific, but regional and discriminated. Furthermore, BP fluctuations mediated by carotid baroreceptors may occur without discernible alterations in plasma NE levels (Wallin and Fagins 1986). Therefore, one cannot use changes in such levels as the sole criterion of sympathetically mediated responses. The highest correlation between significant HR, BP, and CO changes and total body NE spillover levels—the rate of its release into arterial blood—accounts for but one-half of the variance in the cardiac measures during a challenging task. In fact, the increases in systolic BP and CO are completely unrelated to the content of NE in the antecubital vein. The extraction of NE by sympathetic fibers to blood vessels in muscle is inversely related to blood flow through the forearm, which increases significantly during challenge (Goldstein et al. 1987). Therefore, measurement of plasma E and NE, or even the kinetics of NE, are not valid measures of the activation of the sympathetic nervous system.

Under some dire, life-threatening conditions, however, a generalized activation of both the sympathetic and the adrenomedullary system occurs (Goldstein 1987). When the organism loses large amounts of its blood volume or suffers severe bodily injury, or its blood sugar levels or oxygen supply fall below a critical threshold level, global responses of both systems have been observed. With less dire conditions, such as mild to moderate hemorrhage, E may be secreted in considerable amounts, but sympathetic nerve discharge to the kidney may decrease (Morita and Vatner 1985). Many other hormones (aVP, atriopeptin, AT-II, corticosteroids, β-endorphins) are also mobilized during hemorrhage. Only on recovery from hemorrhage, or during oxygen deprivation, do prolonged increases in sympathetic neuronal discharge occur (Johnson, Young, and Landsberg 1983). They are probably mediated by the release of NPY from sympathetic storage granules.

When experiences are not life-threatening, regional changes in sympathetic nerve activity and NE secretion take place: On assuming the upright position vasoconstriction in the legs is due to reflex increases in sympathetic activity, without any change in mean arterial BP; the increase in peripheral resistance in the legs compensates for a moderate fall in pressure. The orthostasis response is centrally generated by a vestibular-cerebellar-medullary circuit. No change in E secretion occurs during it. But in salt-deprived subjects who stand up, plasma AT-II and aldosterone levels rise to sustain BP levels (Oparil et al. 1970).

On standing up without walking, the blood tends to pool in the veins of the legs. The venous return to the heart falls and, therefore, its stroke volume (SV) diminishes. Tonic inhibitory baroreceptor activity declines reflexly to increase sympathetic vasomotor tone. Blood flow in the skin of the legs falls due to sympathetic spinal vasoconstrictor reflexes. Local axon reflexes constrict arterioles; they are set off as the leg veins distend (Henriksen and Skagen 1986).

Under conditions of zero gravity regional changes in sympathetic nervous system activity, and in associated hormonal secretion, occur. Mild exercise induces mainly cardiovascular changes mediated by the sympathetic nervous system, but little E secretion occurs. The voluntary start of exercise is preceded by anticipatory changes in HR and BP. As exercise begins, reflex changes in cardiovascular hemodynamics are initiated by chemoreceptors in muscles. Muscles pump blood to increase venous return to the heart, and blood flow to muscle is hastened by local vasodilatation, chemically induced. As the body temperature rises with exercise, vagal efferent discharge to sweat glands and the skin increases heat loss. Vasodilatation in skin and muscle, reflexly mediated by baroreceptors, induces increased sympathetic discharge (Goldstein 1987).

Many other examples of regional changes in the autonomic nervous system exist in many states (after meals, with hypothermia, during diving in water, etc.) and during other challenges. Each local change in turn sets off both regional and more widely distributed multiple feedback adjustments.

The activities of the autonomic nervous system and the catecholamines have received thorough study. But only recently has it been realized that they produce clearly defined patterns of response, and that regional changes occur, which are closely tied to the specific nature of the challenges to, tasks of, and perturbations induced in the organism. The generation of these patterns is only partly understood: They are not only the product of the brain's ability to produce them; they are brought about by local and also by baroreceptor, chemoreceptor, and spinal feedback mechanisms.

Epinephrine

The effect of E is not uniform because it acts on effector systems through a dual receptor system. While diminishing cutaneous, mucosal, and renal blood flow by producing vasoconstriction through α-receptors, it increases muscle, splanchnic, and cerebral blood flow by vasodilatation mediated by β-receptors. Thus on balance, E usually decreases total peripheral resistance; in contrast, NE increases it.

Epinephrine directly stimulates the myocardium, strengthens the force of ventricular contraction, and raises the HR, venous return to the heart, and CO. By these means—especially by a rise in CO—systolic BP is increased. The increase in HR is counterregulated by increased vagal inhibitory discharge: In fact, in very small doses given to human subjects, E may actually produce a fall in BP. Diastolic BP, however, may not change at all, or may fluctuate.

Epinephrine also promotes coronary blood flow. It can incite arrhythmias. It accelerates atrioventricular conduction and reduces the refractory period of cardiac muscle cells. The stimulatory effects of E on the heart, and on its pacemaker cells and electrical conducting system, is correlated with, but independent of, increases in venous return or its dual effects on the regional vasculature. Epinephrine enhances the oxygen requirements of the myocardium. The heart works harder under its influence.

When the heart is damaged by disease, the release of E may produce ventricular premature beats and tachycardia. However, this effect may additionally require a lengthening of atrioventricular conduction time brought about by increased vagal activity; and its action can in some instances be blocked by α- and β-adrenergic blocking agents, working through different receptor mechanisms. Epinephrine can produce all the changes associated with myocardial ischemia, because the coronary blood flow, though increased, is unable to supply sufficient oxygen to a myocardium whose requirements are heightened.

Epinephrine stimulates respiration. It relaxes the smooth muscle of the bronchial tree, thus increasing the lung's vital capacity and tidal volume. The smooth muscle of other organs—the pregnant uterus and the gut—are also relaxed by E. By contrast, it contracts the muscle of a nonpregnant woman's uterus. Epinephrine not only reduces the gut's motility but also relaxes its various sphincters. It reduces duodenal bicarbonate secretion. However, much of the effect of E on the gut depends on the state of its ongoing rhythmic muscular activity: If it is high, E reduces it; if low, E enhances it.

The action of E on the brain and behavior is variable. When given experimentally it may produce fear, tremulousness, and apprehension, but only in some persons. It may cause tears to flow, sweating, a dry mouth, and the dilatation of the pupils of the eye.

The metabolic actions of E are of particular interest. It induces enzymes. It counterregulates, in concert with glucagon and the corticosteroids, the action of insulin (Cryer and Gerich 1985). The enzyme PNMT, which converts NE to E in the adrenal medulla (and elsewhere), is also under the control of, and its activity is increased by glucagon, insulin, ACTH, and CRF (Axelrod 1971; Brown et al. 1985; Yuwiler 1976). Thus insulin may stimulate E synthesis in the adrenal medulla, but it is in turn counterregulated by E. Epinephrine promotes the release of glucose into the bloodstream. It diminishes glucose utilization, which insulin increases.

Epinephrine acts through two specific receptors. By a complex intracellular process it promotes the conversion of glycogen into glucose in the liver and in striated muscle. The β-receptor in the cell membrane is coupled to, and then interacts with, a membrane-bound G-protein (Gilman 1987) to displace guanosine diphosphate (GDP), and to bind guanosine triphosphate (GTP), thereby freeing the enzyme adenylate cyclase. Adenylate cyclase increases the synthesis of cAMP, which activates an enzyme, protein kinase A, that phosphorylates inactive phosphorylase-a to convert it into active phosphorylase-b. Phosphorylase-b starts the enzymatic conversion of glycogen to glucose.

Because muscle (but not the liver) lacks the enzyme glucose-6-phosphatase, lactic acid accumulates in it during exercise. Lactic acid is a local vasodilator. Its levels increase in the bloodstream, which conveys it to the liver. The liver converts lactic acid into glucose under the influence of E.

Epinephrine acting through β-adrenergic receptors and a lipase enzyme also releases FFA from stores of body fat, the heart, and the diaphragm. The FFAs are a rich source of energy for the organism. The action of E on fat stores is also regulated by the corticosteroids and CRF. Therefore, the function of E in the economy of the organism is to provide the necessary energy resources to carry out its actions under conditions of stressful experiences, exercise, and preparation for a fight or for flight. The action of the catecholamines is brief by virtue of their binding, diffusion, reuptake, enzymatic degradation in the liver by catechol-O-methyl transferase and MAO, and of their excretion. In humans, the effects of the catecholamines once secreted are counterregulated by the enkephalins and endorphins. Under basal, steady-state conditions the opioid peptides, or their antagonists, have no effect on BP, HR, or plasma catecholamine levels. As soon as this state changes, and even with mild to moderate challenge or activity, increases in plasma E and NE levels are potentiated by naloxone (Bouloux and Grossman 1989).

The enkephalins are localized with E in chromaffin granules in the adrenal medulla. Enkephalins and β-endorphin (Kosterlitz, Robson, and Peterson 1989) both act through μ-receptors, although the enkephalins also act through a δ-receptor. The μ-receptor is coupled to another (inhibitory) G-protein (Schramm and Selinger 1984), which is closely linked to the previously described G-protein for E. The inhibitory G-protein prevents the action of adenylate cyclase, and thus the synthesis of cAMP (Gilman 1987); in this manner, the opioid peptides counteract the action of E at the β-adrenergic receptor.

The catecholamines can also directly stimulate the release on ACTH from cultured cells of the anterior pituitary (Axelrod and Reisine 1984; Vale and Rivier 1977). They do so through a β_2-adrenergic receptor, which is cAMP- and calcium-dependent (Reisine et al. 1983). The stimulatory effects of E and NE on ACTH secretion also occur in vivo: Epinephrine and NE injected into the third ventricle of the brain of rats raise plasma ACTH levels. Their action seems to be mediated by β_2- and α_1-adrenergic receptors, respectively. But the release of ACTH is probably indirect, as the catecholamines (especially NE) first stimulate CRF secretion (Bouloux and Grossman 1989; Szafarczyk et al. 1987).

Epinephrine and ACTH form a part of a dual positive feedback mechanism, at the level of both the pituitary gland and the adrenal medulla. The former stimulates the release of the latter from the anterior pituitary gland, and ACTH induces PNMT in the adrenal medulla to hasten the conversion of NE into E (Axelrod 1971; Wurtman and Axelrod 1966). The validity of this last mechanism for our understanding of the role of the sympathetic and adrenomedullary system in stressful experience has been demonstrated by the study of novel or very acute stressful experiences and animals in preparation for activity that show anticipatory responsive patterns. Anticipation is associated with increases in systolic BP, HR, and catecholamine secretion— changes that are largely mediated neuronally. The mechanism underlying the increase in catecholamine secretion, especially NE, appears to depend on a sharp increase in the synthesis of NE from tyrosine (but not dopa), when sympathetic neurons are activated. However, no increase in TH activity occurs, so that either no new enzyme is formed, or formation is inhibited by its endproduct, NE. The absence of change in TH content of tissue during acute experiences stands in contrast to the change that is produced by sustained stressful experience or prolonged sympathetic nerve discharge. Drug-induced, reflex increases in sympathetic nerve activity over several days markedly stimulate TH activity in the adrenal medulla, in the superior cervical ganglion of the rat, and in the brain stem of the rabbit. The activity of PNMT is also increased in the adrenal gland. The changes in activity of these two enzymes in the adrenal gland and in the superior cervical ganglion are not only neuronally mediated, but also result from the formation of fresh enzyme protein. In other words, the increase in TH activity is transsynaptically induced (Mueller, Thoenen, and Axelrod 1969a, 1969b; Thoenen, Mueller, and Axelrod 1969). To a lesser degree, the two other biosynthetic enzymes, TH and DA-β-hydroxylase, in the biosynthetic pathway of the catecholamines are neuronally and hormonally controlled.

These results have been confirmed by the use of another—the restraint—technique: The biosyntheses of NE and E are dually controlled. Restraint-immobilization has potent effects on the content of biogenic amines in tissues, including the brain. The immobilization of rats for 90 minutes produces an increased urinary excretion of NE and E, associated with a decrease in adrenal E (but not NE) content that persists for 24 hours after the end of the procedure. After more prolonged immobilization, adrenal E content remains unaffected, but NE content increases (Kvetnansky and Mikulaj 1970). Apparently, the adrenal medulla enhances its ability to replace released E during repeated immobilization by increasing the production of its precursor. This adaptation appears to result in part from a neuronally dependent elevation of TH and PNMT in the gland. When immobilization is stopped, TH levels diminish with a half-life of about 3 days (Kvetnansky, Weise, and Kopin 1970). Following the end of one bout of immobilization a latent period of about 6 hours occurs before levels of TH and PNMT again increase in activity. Further elevations appear in the next 7 days, but after 6 more weeks of daily immobilization, the process has ceased. The long-term increase in catecholamine levels and secretion in the adrenal medulla produced by restraining rats is also under the control of ACTH. After hypophysectomy, E content is more rapidly depleted on restraint. Levels of TH and PNMT in the adrenal medulla also fall. On repeated immobilization TH, but not PNMT, levels rebound, but never to the point of equaling those of unoperated rats. The rise of TH levels in operated rats is mainly neuronally dependent; it can be demonstrated experimentally that the rise in PNMT levels depends almost entirely on ACTH. Restraint of 3 hours' duration also significantly accelerates the disappearance of radioactive NE from the heart and kidney.

Serum DA-β-hydroxylase is increased after one 30-minute period of restraining rats and continues to increase with daily restraint for 4 days. The source of this increase is not, however, the adrenal gland but sympathetic nerve endings.

The question of how immobilization is centrally translated into these neuronally and hormonally dependent peripheral changes is only partly answered (B. Welch and A. Welch 1968). Restraint is associated with greater elevations of brain NE and 5-HT turnover in mice that had previously spent 8–12 weeks in isolation, when their levels are compared to those of litter mates first housed in groups and then immobilized. This exaggerated response occurs despite the fact that the isolated mice have lower baseline turnover rates of these brain biogenic amines than do their social peers. The isolated mice are also behaviorally "hyperexcitable." But this observation does not mean that this form of behavior and the lower biogenic amine turnover rates are causally related. What it does indicate is that isolation leads to individual differences in brain biogenic amine responses as well as behavior.

Norepinephrine.

NE is stored in granules in sympathetic nerve endings that differ from those in the adrenal medulla. The nerve endings contain all the biosynthetic enzymes required for the production of NE. Once DA is synthesized from tyrosine, it is transported to the granules, stored in them, and converted by DA-β-hydroxylase into NE. The release of NE from granules and nerve endings following nerve stimulation depends on calcium ions and adenosine triphosphate (ATP). The release of NE into the bloodstream is a continuous process; very low levels of NE constantly circulate in the bloodstream (Axelrod 1971; Yuwiler 1976).

Norepinephrine acts predominantly, but not exclusively, via α-adrenergic receptors. In contrast to E, it raises the peripheral resistance, but it has little effect on HR and CO. It markedly raises systolic, mean, and diastolic BP, the SV of the heart, and the pulmonary artery pressure. It can increase coronary artery flow when BP levels are steady. It can incite cardiac arrhythmias (e.g., nodal rhythms, atrio-ventricular (A-V) dissociation, bigeminy, and ventricular tachycardia). The failure of HR to increase is due to vagal reflex activity stimulated by increased mechanoreceptor discharge.

The immune system (including the bone marrow, thymus, spleen, gut, and lymph nodes) is under neuronal control of the sympathetic nervous system. Postganglionic nonadrenergic fibers run between lymph nodules in gut lymphatic tissue, where they traverse the area that contains plasma, enterochromaffin, and T-cells. (In addition to NE, roles for 5-HT, acetylcholine, and aVP in the regulation of these immunocompetent cells in the gut have been found.)

Immunocompetent cells in the gut are mobile; they circulate in the body, and may enter the spleen. The spleen and splenic lymphocytes are innervated by sympathetic neurons (Aravich et al. 1986; Felten and Felten 1989). Lymphocytes and plasma cells in the gut and spleen may be locally regulated directly by the catecholamines and by peptide hormones, which also influence enterochromaffin cells that secrete chemicals (e.g., histamine and 5-HT) with direct influence on immunologically competent cells, and which produce inflammation.

Norepinephrine exerts its effects by means of three receptor systems—α_1, α_2, and β. The α_1 receptor is joined to a G-protein that activates the membrane-bound enzyme phospholipase C, whose action is to hydrolyse phosphatidylinositol-bisphosphate and to produce two second messengers, inositol triphosphate (IP_3) and diacylglycerol (Berridge and Irvine 1989). The former (IP_3) releases and activates intracellular (nonmitochondrial) stores of calcium ion via its own receptor. The released ion "feeds back" to block the receptor. Diacylglycerol activates the protein kinase C system—another messenger system—involved in phosphorylating many signal-transducing, receptor proteins, and a variety of enzyme systems. A protein kinase C inhibits IP_3 synthesis and also enhances its degradation. Finally, protein kinase C can phosphorylate itself to increase its sensitivity to rising calcium fluxes (Baraban, Worley, and Snyder 1989; Nishizuka 1986).

The protein kinase C system is involved in physiological functions of sustained duration, such as the contraction of muscle cells. The β-adrenergic system linked to the G-protein-adenylate cyclase-cAMP system had already been described for E. The α_2 receptor is tied to a second G-protein with a diametrically opposite action, inhibiting adenylate cyclase activity and thus cAMP synthesis.

The Glucocorticoids

The glucocorticosteroids, synthesized and secreted by cells of the adrenal cortex, are traditionally accorded status second only in importance to the sympathetic-adrenomedullary system in mediating stressful experiences. They were the central focus of Selye's work, because his various injurious procedures produced adrenal hyperplasia. In retrospect it is fairly certain that the excessive corticosteroid production was a consequence of the fact that his animals were severely injured and had no control over the experience.

Many years have been spent sorting out the various conditions under which corticosteroid secretion does, or does not, occur (Henry and Stephens 1977; Levine and Coe 1989) and determining their role in the economy of the organism. In actuality, they usually play an important modulatory and counter-regulatory, rather than a predominantly pathogenetic, one (Munck, Guyre, and Holbrook 1984).

The corticosteroids are secreted during very specific experiences, some of which may be life-threatening: when the animal is wounded or in pain, and when bleeding is acute, profuse, and rapid (Gann 1969); when it is infected; when it is faced with a novel experience for which, by definition, it is unprepared and has no behavioral response in hand; when experimental situations are set up in such a way that a warning signal is not predictably or invariably followed by a shock (Weinberg and Levine 1980); when unpredictable and uncontrollable electric shock is inescapable; when an animal has learned a behavioral response but is subsequently prevented from, or punished for, achieving it (Coe, Stanton, and Levine 1983). But the animal may also have experiences during which corticosteroid secretion is actually inhibited. Predictable events that end in a desired consummation—such as obtaining food or water—are associated in female rats with a fall in ACTH and corticosterone levels (Gray et al. 1978). Similar hormonal changes occur when an animal has been trained in an operant-conditioning procedure and receives its reinforcing reward (Goldman, Coover, and Levine 1973). And the reduction in glucocorticoid secretion can be taught to and learned by the animal (Levine and Coe 1989).

These observations make it possible to operationalize the meaning of control: It is the ability of the organism to make an active, preventive, or avoidant response (for which it may be rewarded) during or after a challenging, threatening, or painful experience.

The production and secretion of the corticosteroids is principally, but not exclusively, under the control of pituitary ACTH, acting through parallel receptor mechanisms consisting of two specific G-proteins, one of which is coupled to the adenylate cyclase-cAMP system, and the second of which is linked to the phospholipase C-IP_3-diacylglycerol, second messenger system. Cyclic AMP activates protein kinases involved in corticosteroid synthesis in the adrenal gland.

Cortisol in humans is synthesized by adrenal cortical cells in five steps from cholesterol and progesterone. Corticosterone in animals and humans, however, also derives from cholesterol and progesterone but utilizes a separate pathway consisting of a series of four different enzymes.

Dissociations between plasma ACTH and cortisol levels have, however, repeatedly been described (Dallman and Yates 1969; Fehm, Voigt, and Bron 1987). Cortisol secretion is also believed to be stimulated by a sympathetic innervation to the adrenal cortex (Kiss 1951; Unsicker 1971). In rats these sympathetic neurons use VIP as the neurotransmitter (Holzwarth 1984). The peptide is colocalized in neurons with acetylcholine and can also stimulate steroid production in adrenocortical tumor cells in tissue culture (Morera et al. 1979). A second stimulus to corticosteroid secretion may be ACTH produced by immunocompetent cells (Smith and Blalock 1981).

The corticosteroids exert negative feedback control on ACTH, β-endorphin, and aVP production and secretion (Munck, Guyre, and Holbrook 1984; Simantov 1979). They inhibit transcription of the proopiomelanocortin (POMC) gene (Eberwine and Roberts 1984). The regulation of ACTH production and secretion is under the influence of a number of other positive and negative feedback mechanisms (see chapter 9). The feedback effect of the corticosteroids on ACTH is both rate- and concentration-sensitive (Yuwiler 1976).

The secretion of the corticosteroids is rhythmic. The rhythm is a double one: The first is circadian; it is under the control of a pacemaker in the SCN (Moore-Ede, Sulzman, and Fuller 1982). Circadian variations in plasma corticosteroids are paralleled by similar rhythms in corticosteroid-binding receptors in the rat's hippocampus. Superimposed on this rhythm in humans are five to seven rhythmic bursts of cortisol secretion during any 24-hour period, which are in part generated by ten rhythmic increases in ACTH secretion (Krieger et al. 1971) that reflect the same numbers of CRF pulses (Mortola et al. 1987).

Only one-third of the cortisol secreted by the human adrenal gland circulates in a free form; the rest is inactive because it is bound to a carrier associated with albumen and a corticoid-binding globulin. The action of the free corticosteroids is wide-ranging. They pass through the cell membrane, possibly by endocytosis, and are bound by a specific cytosolic glucocorticoid receptor (Crabtree, Smith, and Munck 1981), which consists of a complex of three different proteins, 319 kilodaltons in size. When released by dissociation of the complex, one of these proteins, with the glucocorticoid it binds, attaches itself to a specific site on a 96-kilodalton transcribing protein to induce gene transcription (Schüle et al. 1988). A third protein of 132 kilodaltons containing the steroid binds to transfer RNA (Ali and Vedeckis 1987). These complexes regulate and induce the genes coding for at least twenty-six different enzymes in the brain, adrenal gland, liver, muscle, and adipose tissue (Yuwiler 1982). The enzymes are involved in the biosynthesis of the indolamines and the catecholamines (e.g., tryptophane-5-hydroxylase, TH, and PNMT) and in carbohydrate, fat (lipoprotein lipase), and liver aminoacid metabolism (e.g., tryptophane-5-hydroxylase, -oxygenase, and -aminotransferase).

Thus the metabolic effects of the corticosteroids are extensive and patterned. But during stressful experiences enzyme induction is not indiscriminate but discrete: Starving or shaking a rat raises corticosteroid levels and increases the liver's tryptophane oxygenase activity, but not that of tryptophane or tyrosine transaminase. Isolating animals elevates levels of the two transaminases but not that of the oxygenase (Yuwiler 1982).

The physiological actions of the corticosteroids are specific to each tissue. They have dual actions on the liver—inhibiting one system (e.g., protein synthesis) and enhancing another (e.g., urea formation). They act to counterregulate the action of insulin by inhibiting its production. In concert with E and glucagon, whose output they stimulate they increase glucose production by the liver. They also enhance glycogen formation from amino acids and lactic and pyruvic acid. They increase cholesterol levels and FFA production from fat stores in concert with E, and they decrease glucose utilization by the liver, muscle, fat, and lymphatic tissue. In the liver, they enhance RNA synthesis, while in the thymus and the spleen they diminish it. They affect ion transport and metabolism by inhibiting calcium absorption by the gut; and they reduce sodium and increase potassium excretion by the kidney. They enhance the synthesis of angiotensinogen and pepsinogen. They sensitize arterioles to the action of AT-II. They also potentiate the effects of E and NE at β-adrenergic receptors in the heart, and they increase capillary tone.

The corticosteroids have antiinflammatory properties, inhibiting prostaglandin production and the release of arachidonic acid (Hirata et al. 1980), bradykinin, 5-HT, histamine (from human basophils), and enzymes such as collagenase (Munck, Guyre, and Holbrook 1984). But they enhance platelet adhesion.

Glucocorticoid receptors are present on the pyramidal cells of the hippocampus, granule cells of the dentate gyrus, cell bodies of the PVN, and the pituitary gland. The actions of the glucocorticoids on the learning process, attack behavior, mood, thought, and other aspects of brain function are not fully established, except in disease states with excessive production, or when they are administered in very high doses. Their effects on enzyme systems in the brain are usually less apparent than on those in other organ systems. They are capable of inducing tryptophane and tyrosine hydroxylase in the brain, thereby respectively enhancing 5-HT and catecholamine synthesis. But they have deleterious effects in very young animals on brain size and DNA and RNA synthesis (Yuwiler 1976, 1982).

To summarize: The glucocorticosteroids have metabolic, antiinflammatory, and immunoregulatory effects. By their interaction with β-adrenergic receptors, they also enhance the cardiovascular effects of E (and NE). They increase blood glucose levels, but they also stimulate liver and brain glycogen production and animo acid uptake. They enhance ketone body and urea production and RNA and protein synthesis in the liver. They release FFA to be used for fuel in body heat production.

In the immune system they produce lymphocytopenia and monocytopenia. They act to redistribute lymphocytes in body compartments. They decrease nucleic acid synthesis of immunocompetent cells. They block the synthesis and secretion of IL-2 from T-lymphocytes (Smith 1988) and of γ-IF from macrophages, while enhancing its secretion by monocytes (Guyre et al. 1988).

The corticosteroids are also an agent in an important immunoregulatory feedback system (Uehara et al. 1987a, 1987b). Interleukin-1β produced by macrophages during the acute phase reaction acts—in addition to many other effects—to stimulate CRF, and thus ACTH release (Berkenbosch et al. 1987). Adrenocorticotropin enhances corticosteroid secretion, which inhibits IL-1 and IL-2 production. The function of IL-2 is to diminish its own secretion through a specific receptor, while producing the growth and activation of B- and NK-cells (Smith 1988). Corticosteroids are involved in regulating antibody production (Roess et al. 1982) and nonspecific cytotoxic activity. However, another lymphokine produced by macrophages—the transforming growth factor–β—acts upon adrenal cortical cells to reduce corticosteroid production and secretion (Bateman et al. 1989; Feige, Cochet, and Chambaz 1986).

It has been the purpose of this section to emphasize the involvement of the corticosteroids in complex regulatory functions and to correct the impression that they are pathogenetic of disease. In fact, the corticosteroids endow protection to animals when injured or infected with pathogenetic bacteria or viruses. In recent years their role in the economy of organisms has been completely reassessed. They actually have permissive actions under steady-state conditions; endow resistance to stressful experience by their metabolic effects; counterregulate and modulate the effects of insulin in lowering blood

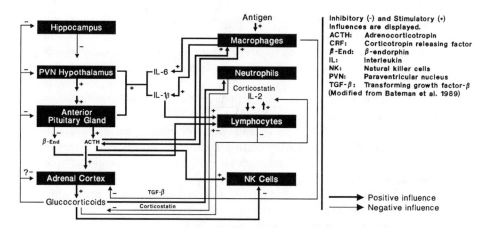

Figure 2. Regulatory Interactions Between the Hippocampal-Hypothalmic-Pituitary-Adrenal Cortical and the Immune System and Its Products

sugar, and of aVP when fluid loss or hemorrhage occurs; and modulate the immune and inflammatory responses to infection, allergy, and tissue damage. They counteract the effects of poisons. Thus their action is to regulate many bodily systems involved in providing the organism with the initial line of defense against threats to its survival (Munck, Guyre, and Holbrook 1984).

Once they have done so their actions are designed to stop. Persistent elevations of the corticosteroids may be associated with cortisol resistance due to inactivation of the cytosolic glucocorticoid receptor (Gormley et al. 1985) and with termination of their response to stressful experience brought about by feedback inhibition of the CRF-ACTH circuit via the hippocampus (Sapolsky, Krey, and McEwen 1984, 1986).

However, their chronic elevations are different in dominant than in subdominant male baboons (Sapolsky 1990). The more submissive animals continue to have elevated corticosteroid levels. Their system does not seem to shut off, possibly because their receptor in pituitary cells is resistant or inactivated.

Decalcification of bone, a redistribution of adipose tissue, muscle wasting, high BP, immunosuppression, impaired fertility, and altered moods and cognitive functioning in human beings can occur when high corticosteroid levels persist for prolonged periods of time (e.g., in Cushing's disease).

The Gonadal Steroids

Some of the bidirectional changes in gonadal steroids with stressful experience have already been discussed throughout this book and will briefly be recapitulated. Mason (1968) demonstrated that during a 72-hour session of training male rhesus monkeys in a conditioned-avoidance procedure, T and estrone levels are depressed. Once the trial is over the T levels rebound above control levels. Merely adapting animals to a restraining chair markedly lowers estrone levels for the first two weeks of the procedure; after that a biphasic rise is seen.

Of particular moment are the observations on the effects of stressful intra-uterine experience on male rats, which culminate in female mating behavior when they are sexually mature (Ward and Ward 1989); on raised levels of T in the dominant male squirrel monkey housed together, especially after a female is introduced into the group (Mendoza et al. 1979); and on the suppression of the reproductive cycle, LH levels, and progesterone in subordinate marmoset monkeys (Abbott 1987). Anovulation and amenorrhea in women occur after many different challenges—with disease, hemorrhage, and malnutrition, dur-ing wartime and pregnancy, and while nursing infants.

In some animals, such as lizards, fighting by two males in sight of a female changes her from being sexually receptive to not being so (Crews 1975; Crews and Moore 1986). Crowding rodents together reduces mating behavior and ovulation, but only in the subordinates. In men, diminished LH and T levels may occur in anticipation of surgery. The fall in T levels cannot be corrected by the administration of LHRH, suggesting that inhibition of secretion occurs at the levels of both the pituitary gland and of the testis (Levine and Coe 1989). Changes in blood flow in the testis occur. (The LH increases flow in this organ, and cortisol reduces it, thus regulating the secretion of T.)

Most studies, except of dominant male primates, have concerned them-selves with decreased LH and FSH gonadal steroid levels, or with altered or diminished mating behavior. But very subtle, species-specific enzymatic dif-ferences are associated with dominance: For example, the (reductase) enzyme that converts T to dihydrotestosterone is active only in the dominant gorilla, not in subordinate males.

Short-term increments in T levels occur in victorious male monkeys (Rose, Bernstein, and Gordon 1975). But the matter in men is by no means settled, and is controversial. Winners in competitive sports may show transient eleva-tions of T levels (Mazur and Lamb 1980). However, prolonged exercise, such as marathon running, may actually depress them (Nieschlag 1979). Danger-ous activities (e.g., parachute jumping) are associated with a fall in T levels in all men as they engage in the first jump. They continue to be low only in those men who fail the training course (Ursin, Baade, and Levine 1978).

To summarize: Sexual reproduction is the basis of variation. Yet ovulation and mating can only occur under optimal conditions that assure the offspring's survival; they are influenced by both the physical and social environment. In many animals, LH and FSH levels are affected by the environmental tempera-ture, sunlight, and the presence or absence of conspecifics of the same or the opposite sex. Generally speaking, and even in higher vertebrates, T levels are raised in male animals by the presence of a female and decreased by the presence of other males. Female mice housed together may become anestrus—a condition that is reversed when a male is introduced into this rodent "harem" (Rosenblatt 1978). Fighting, especially over females, raises T levels in the victor who either is or becomes the dominant male. In some vertebrate species the female actually seeks out the dominant male in order to mate with him— apparently for good evolutionary reasons.

Therefore, the hypothalamic-pituitary-gonadal (HPG) axis is not sui generis. It is influenced by environmental signals. It is not only regulated by LHRH, LH and FSH, GAP, and gonadal and androgenic steroids of the adrenal gland, and a negative and mixed feedback system consisting of T, E_2, and inhibin and other peptides. Prolactin inhibits the axis and is itself inhibited by GAP (Nikolicz et al. 1985). (The amenorrhea and anovulation occurring during lactation and nursing may in part be brought about by PRL.)

Of particular moment is the inhibitory effect of CRF on the HPG. In rats, intermittent shock raises corticosterone and depresses LH levels—an effect that is blocked by the specific antagonist of CRF, α-helical CRF (Rivier and Vale 1984; Rivier, Rivier, and Vale 1986). The inhibitory effect of CRF on LH secretion is indirect: Both in rats (Petraglia, Vale, and Rivier 1986) and in monkeys (Gindoff and Ferin 1987) it is mediated by opioid peptides, presumably β-endorphin. It is assumed that this endorphin, whose secretion by the pituitary gland is itself stimulated by CRF, feeds back to inhibit further CRF secretion at the level of the median eminence.

The dominant male squirrel monkey is an (unstable?) peer group manifests higher T but also higher cortisol levels, presumably as a result of the activation of the HPA axis (Mendoza et al. 1979). Somewhat different results have been obtained in wild olive baboons. The serum T levels in the dominant male of this species increase during acutely stressful experiences and for about an hour thereafter; in subordinate males they fall. However, both groups of animals show a fall in LH levels under these conditions, due to the inhibiting effects of β-endorphin. The rise in serum T levels in dominants is ascribed to an increase in blood flow through the testis, brought about by increased catecholamine and LH secretion and by the blocking of the counterregulatory influence of cortisol (which inhibits the secretion of T). The increase in blood flow speeds the delivery of LH to the testis.

As time goes on the resting plasma cortisol levels are lower in the dominant than in subordinate olive baboons, but they rise more rapidly whenever acutely threatening situations are experienced by him. In the dominant male the testis eventually becomes resistant to the action of cortisol and testicular flow increases due to the enhanced delivery of LH. No such resistance to cortisol is seen in the subordinate male. He eventually manifests low T levels. In subordinates, the inhibitory (negative feedback) action of cortisol and of dexamethasone on the HPA is reduced and excessive secretion of ACTH continues to sustain the high plasma cortisol levels. However, individual differences in behavior and physiology in dominant male olive baboons are observable: Some dominant males also have high resting plasma cortisol levels; they are the ones for whom every move on the part of their male conspecifics is threatening (Sapolsky 1990).

9

The Selection of the Signal and the Mediation of Stressful Experience by the Brain: The Generation of Patterns and the Integration of Behavior and Physiology

Throughout this book a comprehensive biological approach to the understanding of stressful experience has been emphasized. According to this view the whole organism, not one or the other of its subsystems, is the proper focus of study. Its behavior is as important as is its physiology; the one cannot be separated from, and does not "cause," the other. Behavior and physiology are two part functions of an integrated whole designed by nature for a special purpose—to allow an organism to overcome, avoid, or escape potentially damaging or fatal experiences, or to protect the organism from them. The organism attempts to survive by virtue of its behavior. The physiology during this endeavor is appropriate to the specific task confronting it. In the end, as Darwin knew, one cannot disengage physiology from behavior; they are inseparable.

The behavior is usually attuned and appropriate to the signal that elicits it (Tinbergen 1951). The organism selects the signal(s), and usually (depending on the context) the appropriate behavior follows. The process of signal selection will be discussed in this chapter, and the neural basis of patterned behaviors will be described.

The fact that a particular pattern of behavior may be elicited by more than one signal does not mean that either the signal or the behavior lacks specificity. Many different signals connote danger to the same organism, and the behavior has evolved to overcome, avert, avoid, or escape it. These statements should not be construed to mean that the relationship of the signal(s) and the behavior is fixed, reflexive, or invariant; far to the contrary.

The organism's behavior is in part determined by its status in the social hierarchy, or the context in which it finds itself: In rhesus monkey colonies, the appearance, direction, and expression of "attack" behavior that follows a painful, electrical shock to the skin or stimulation of the periaqueductal area of the midbrain depends on an animal's rank in the hierarchy. If the dominant male animal is stimulated in this manner it attacks the subordinate. A subdominant beast shows submissive behavior on stimulation in the presence of a dominant conspecific (Plotnick, Mir, and Delgado 1970). Such observations make it difficult to determine the neural substrates subserving behavioral response patterns observed during stressful (i.e., painful) experiences and the context in which they occur.

An additional, conceptual problem also arises: An increase in serum corticosterone levels in rats may follow uncontrollable electric shock. This change has been used as a criterion independent of behavior, such as squealing or cowering, for determining whether an animal is stressed. But no independent criterion (other than the behavior itself) exists when an investigator attempts to identify the neural circuitry or other brain mechanisms that underlie the behavior. A tautology is inherent in this endeavor.

Nonetheless, progress has been made in understanding the manner by which the organism selects a signal of danger, threat, or challenge so that it may carry out the appropriate behaviors. Some of the neural circuitry underlying defensive, submissive, and attacking behavior has been traced out. And genuine progress has been made in knowledge about the integration of the behavior and physiology of organisms.

Selection of the Signal in the Predator-Prey Relationship

Wild rodents in the presence of a natural predator such as a hawk become immobile (chapter 7). The particular signal for freezing is the hawk's moving shadow falling on or near its prey. Immobility has survival value, because the retinal cells of the hawk's eye respond predominantly to moving (not stationary) objects. Therefore, one may ask: How do the retina and brain of a hungry hawk respond selectively and rapidly to its potential victim's movement? The rodent must selectively transform its perception of moving shadows and their context into manageable and meaningful structures, or categories, that promote survival. The signals emitted by the actor are processed by its audience in a reciprocal manner.

The retina is a selective signal processor: A visual signal moving from left to right will excite only one of an array of retinal bipolar cells while inhibiting others in the network, due to the activation and intervention of an (inhibitory) GABAergic amacrine cell. But if the signal moves from right to left, the entire network of bipolar cells will be excited, as no inhibitory amacrine neurons intervene (Gottlieb 1988). In the former case, the signal is too weak to excite the ganglion cell, and no output to the brain occurs. Many excitatory inputs from the array of bipolar cells must converge for a ganglion cell to fire and relay the signal to the brain. The arrangement described exemplifies how some visual signals are processed in parallel, i.e., by the simultaneous excitation of both the bipolar and amacrine retinal cells.

The first stage in the treatment of raw visual information about the world is carried out by the retina. Through further analysis and refinement, the data are transformed in a series of steps to create a picture of the visual world (Altman

1987). These transformations proceed according to a program that has evolved over millions of years: It is not a fixed program because it is modifiable by experience (Hubel and Wiesel 1965; Wiesel and Hubel 1965).

The transformations are initially carried out by the retina, which transduces electromagnetic radiation into chemical signals that in turn give rise to electrical ones. The electrical response varies with the intensity of photons falling on an array of 10^8 different points (cones and rods) in two-dimensional space (Marr 1982). Immediately the incident light is segregated. The cones respond to the frequency (hence color) of the light waves, but the rods do not.

The retina also separates the input into ON and OFF channels. The input signal from the rods and cones is then channeled into 10^6 bipolar and ganglion cells. The neural activity pattern of the bipolar and ganglion cells constitutes an abstraction of visual space, additional to the analysis that is carried out by of the rods and cones. Because the bipolar and ganglion cells are organized into receptive fields, they respond to light and dark contrasts and to movement, but not to the intensity or frequency of the light. Each receptive field has an excitatory center, whose cells discharge more actively, and an inhibitory surround, whose cells discharge less vigorously. The contrast is created by the gradient between the center and the edges of these circular receptive fields in space (Marr 1982; Zeki 1984).

As the result of this arrangement information about light intensity is transformed into coarser receptive field information consisting of shapes and forms in space external to the viewer. But the retina can do even more: It can "compute" and hold constant the color of an object despite changes in the intensity of illumination and in incident wavelength. It does so by separating the illumination of the object from its inherent reflectance.

Further processing occurs in the lateral geniculate nucleus, where, as in the primary visual cortex (area V1), neurons exist that respond mainly to bars of finite lengths. The bars are greater in length than the diameter of the circular receptive fields of retinal ganglion cells; convergence has occurred. Some primary visual cortical cells also signal contrasts along moving straight lines of various orientations, while others—the "complex" cells—only respond to parallel sets of lines. Somewhat anterior (in area V4) to the primary visual cortex neurons in V1, neurons exist that respond to the color (wavelength) of the stimulus (Zeki 1984). Thus in these two visual areas, groups of cells, intermingled with each other, selectively respond to separate attributes of the stimulus—its color, its orientation, and/or its direction of movement.

But that is not all: Each parameter of the stimulus is processed in parallel and mapped several times in different parts of the cerebral cortex (Allman, Miezin, and McGuinness 1985). Variation occurs in how each of perhaps twelve visual receptive fields emphasizes or analyzes the different attributes of the stimulus (i.e., its size, shape, form, color, position in space, and direction of movement). Every one of these characteristics is in turn processed in parallel in different (albeit overlapping) streams and fields—parietal neurons process the position in space of the stimulus, and temporal neurons its form and color (Ungerleider and Mishkin 1982). Prefrontal neurons provide a delay circuit for the short-term maintenance of information, especially when it is novel (Fuster 1980). Premotor neurons are organized to initiate collective motor programs (actions) based on the integrated information about the signal.

The cortex makes a map of the world and the objects in it. This map covaries with the internal state of the organisms (e.g., "attention") (Llinás 1988). At lower levels of the nervous system that map is topographic; at higher levels more abstract attributes of stimulus objects are processed. The number and organization of the various fields vary from species to species; such variation reflects what is relevant for the members of each one (Altman 1987).

The retina is not only connected to the brain by the "classical" visual neuronal pathways. A parallel set of neurons pass from the retina to the SCN—the generator of several circadian rhythms. By virtue of this pathway light acts as an entrainer of such rhythms (chapter 7). The retinohypothalamic pathway diverges and passes from the retina via the inferior accessory optic tract and the medial forebrain bundle to the medulla and then to the superior cervical sympathetic ganglion and back into the brain to innervate the pineal gland and determine diurnal variations of melatonin synthesis (Moore et al. 1967).

The implications of these data are profound (Weiner 1972), because the experience of a signal (light) does not necessarily determine the physiological response. Light is processed by parallel pathways, which are temporally but are not necessarily causally correlated.

The Nature of the Signals for Fight, Defense, Flight, and Submission: Behaviors Are Patterned

The kinds of signals processed by animals are not only shadows or threatening postures. A rat that perceives the vibrations of the vibrissae of another (often familiar) rat assumes an upright posture, but it does not lunge at the other or bite its nose, as it does on different occasions. Therefore, the postural pattern is expressed while another behavioral sequence (lunging and biting) is inhibited in this particular social interaction (Kanki and Adams 1978).

Postures, gestures, the emission of vocal sounds, changes in pupillary size, snarling, the erection of hair on the back or the tail, and the excretion of urine, pheromones, or feces are directed at a threatening target or used to define territory by various species of mammals.

Examples of some of these specific behaviors have already been described while discussing the different endocrine changes that occur in the resident and in the intruding rat (chapter 7), but the details of such behaviors were not given. What actually happens is that the intruder stops at the first movement in its direction made by the resident. It may freeze, then flee, or it may freeze and roll on its back. It becomes analgesic. It squeals audibly while also uttering high-frequency sounds, which the human observer cannot hear. These ultrasonic vocalizations signal for the resident rat to cease and desist (Lehman and Adams 1977). Before doing so, however, the home-cage rat goes on the offensive by approaching the intruder sideways. Its hair stands up. It bites at and kicks the intruder.

Some of these behaviors are specific to this particular context; others are not. Away from the home cage, two rats may fight. The loser may freeze or flee. It may assume an upright posture while emitting squeals and other noises. But rarely does it roll over on its back. Occasionally it may lunge and bite at the attacking rat in self-defense, or as a last resort. Defensive behaviors are designed to avoid injury or detection by predators; they may consist of immobility or flight to the safety of a nest or burrow (Adams 1977).

Threats or challenges to the dominant status of an animal, to food supplies, or over mates are not the only signals that incite fighting. The urine of male rodents contains a pheromone that elicits fighting among males. Because it is absent in castrated males it is believed to be an androgen. Fighting can be restored by injections of T in castrated males. It also appears in androgenized female mice (Mugford and Navell 1970a, 1970b). Fighting does not take place when a male mouse's sense of smell is destroyed.

The resident rat attacks the intruder that submits. The dominant male rat or mouse maintains its status by biting the subordinate in the flank or the root of the tail. Having staked out its own territory by urinary pheromones, the dominant rat respects the territory of another dominant male animal on its side of the demarcation line. Rodents may fight among themselves and defend themselves by flight, submission, or biting. Other species, such as cats and dogs, may "choose," or not, to fight an opponent. They may also assume a threatening posture that induces their opponent to flee or slink away without a fight.

Each animal is able to attack, submit, or defend itself in different contexts. It can switch from one of these behavioral configurations to another. Therefore, it has been suggested that three different, or separate, neuronal system exist that subserve each of the patterns and their autonomic and hormonal correlates (Adams 1979).

Some of the cardiovascular and hormonal patterns associated with fighting, victory, and defeat, were described in chapter 7. To recapitulate: Patterned cardiovascular changes occur while a cat is preparing to fight another; they differ from those observed during the actual fight. In turn, the defeated animal's hormonal and cardiovascular patterns are not the same as the victor's. The specific and integrated physiological patterns are under the control of separate neural circuits in the brain, which subserve both them and the coordinated behavioral patterns. The neural circuitry underlying the "defense" reaction (Hess 1957) passes from the dorsomedial nucleus of the amygdala via the striae terminalis to the lateral (perifornical) hypothalamus in the cat, but in the rabbit the pathway ends in the VMN of the hypothalamus (Schneiderman 1983). From there, neurons travel to the central gray neuronal complex of the brain stem, and then to the intermediolateral nuclei of the medulla.

A second behavioral pattern observed in rabbits is associated with immobility and a fall in BP and HR. It is mediated by a pathway that runs from the nucleus centralis of the amygdala to the lateral hypothalamus, the lateral zona incerta of the diencephalon, the parabrachial nucleus, and finally to preganglionic vagal (cardioinhibitory) motorneurons. A third and somewhat different pattern in the rabbit manifests itself by complete immobility, except for orienting movements of the head, attended by pupillary dilatation, and by bradycardia in the face of an increase in BP. This behavioral pattern is reminiscent of the one seen when rabbits are startled and then become vigilant. It also occurs in response to unsignaled electrical shocks with restraint when the animal is prevented from coping (von Holst 1972), and in anticipation of the shock when the animal is first restrained and then shocked. It can be elicited by electrical stimulation of a broad band of neurons that runs from the anterior to the posterior hypothalamus (Schneiderman 1983).

Separate neural circuits have been described that each subserve exercise-induced or orthostatic cardiovascular responses (Doba and Reis 1974) and a conditioned emotional response (CER) (LeDoux 1989). By pairing a sound with an electric shock, marked increases in BP and "freezing"—the CER—are observed in monkeys. The auditory cortex is not necessary for the CER to occur, but the medial geniculate nucleus (MGN) is. The neural circuit subserving the response passes from the MGN to the caudate nucleus, the putamen, and the lateral nucleus of the amygdala, then to its central nucleus, the lateral hypothalamus, the central gray matter of the brain stem, and (presumably) the intermediolateral nuclei of the medulla.

Although the integrated behavior and cardiovascular responses that comprise the CER are usually one and indivisible, they can be dissociated experimentally (LeDoux 1989). A lesion of the hypothalamus eliminates the BP increase but leaves immobility unaffected. A different lesion placed in the central gray area of the brain stem produces the opposite effect. One may conclude that although the behavior and physiology (the CER) are usually integrated, they can also be dissociated.

Smith and his colleagues (1980) have also been able to separate out the motor behaviors (bar pressing) of baboons from the correlated cardiovascular responses (increases in HR, BP, and CO) during another kind of CER, induced by the threat of electric shocks. The cardiovascular changes, but not the bar pressing to avoid shock, are abolished after placing a lesion in the posterior hypothalamus. But the circulatory responses elicited by pressing bars, or by feeding the animal, are not.

The circulatory responses to exercise are known to pass from the motor cortex to the subthalamus, posterior hypothalamus, and ventral brain stem (Cohen 1981). By lesioning the fields (H2) of Forel the cardiovascular patterns of change in anticipation of, but not during, exercise are abolished. Another and separate neural circuit subserves the integrated cardiovascular responses elicited by orthostasis. It begins at the vestibular apparatus, then passes via the eighth nerve and the vestibulocerebellar pathways to the cerebellum and the paramedian reticular and vasomotor medullary neurons (C1), and down the spinal cord to sympathetic preganglionic nerves (Doba and Reis 1974).

These observations are particularly instructive for reconceptualizing the effects of stressful experience. The brain circuits that subserve the components of the CER are arranged in parallel. However, the activity of one component may precede the other. The observer is, therefore, prone to believe that such a temporal sequence either implies causality or not: If the BP response comes first the observer may infer that it is the "cause" of the behavior (or is "caused" by the signal); but if the behavior antecedes the BP response, it is causing it. None of the two responses after the signal are due to the fact that the parallel circuits subserving them contain different numbers of neurons and synapses. Therefore, the responses may not occur simultaneously. The discrepancy in the time of occurrence of the two responses cannot be construed as implying causality. Temporal relationships, or covariances, do not necessarily imply causality.

What can be learned from this new information? Although Darwin was correct that behavior and physiology form an indivisible whole, these analytic studies teach us that separate but parallel pathways in the brain subserve some behaviors and their associated cardiovascular responses. Even the responses of peripheral sympathetic nerves are highly discriminated and under separate central control. Sympathetic discharge to muscle, producing vasoconstriction, is regulated by changes in baroreceptor and phrenic nerve activity. But the sympathetic innervation to the skin, which is involved in the modulation of its blood flow, sweating, and thus body surface temperature, is regulated by and associated with fluctuations in ambient temperature, vibratory and tactile stimulation, and emotional expression (Jänig 1987; Wallin 1987).

Yet this topic is even more complex. Although local sympathetic cardiac reflexes attenuate baroreceptor reflexes—designed to lower BP and HR—they are in turn modified by intraindividual differences in behavior and during different behaviors and states of the organism. The sensitivity of the baroreceptor reflex in human beings is blunted with age and during exercise (Bristow et al. 1971) and mental arithmetic (Brooks et al. 1978). It is greatest during sleep, intermediate during eating, and least during mild exercise (Stephenson, Smith, and Scher 1981). As reflex sensitivity is lowered, BP and HR rise; as it increases, they fall.

The baroreceptor system is located in the large vessels of the heart, particularly in the carotid sinus. By means of the carotid sinus nerve (N. IX) the baroreceptors are linked to the NTS of the medulla oblongata, whose cells are involved in the tonic regulation of BP. (The neurotransmitter of the carotid sinus nerve is L-glutamate). From the NTS, GABAergic neurons pass to nucleus C1 of the medulla. A system of adrenergic neurons links C1 to cells lying in the intermediolateral column of the spinal cord. From there, cholinergic preganglionic sympathetic fibers pass to spinal ganglia, which give rise to postganglionic neurons innervating the heart and the arterial tree. Postganglionic sympathetic neurons release NE and NPY.

Electrical stimulation of C1 neurons raises the tonic BP level, and their destruction lowers it. They relay baroreceptor reflexes: An increase in pressure within the carotid sinus lowers the BP and HR, suggesting that reflex inhibition of C1 neurons occurs via the NTS (Reis and LeDoux 1987).

The Neuronal Basis of Attack and Defense

Chronically decerebrate cats are prone to respond to sensory input by poorly directed attacks on animate and inanimate objects. This behavior was first thought to depend upon the integrity of the hypothalamus and the midbrain (Bard and Rioch 1937). The function of the cerebral cortex is both to direct an accurate attack to the target and to modulate or suppress it (Bard and Mountcastle 1948). Later these conclusions were refined: Coordinated, but poorly directed, attacks are still observed in a rat after destruction of its hypothalamus (Olivier 1977); only the integrity of the midbrain is required for the behavior to be manifested.

Usually attack behavior in wild rodents is set off by pheromones. The smells are mediated by two parallel olfactory pathways, one to the main, and the other to the accessory, olfactory bulb. From the former, axons pass to the olfactory tubercle and anterior olfactory nucleus. From the accessory bulb, neurons course to the corticomedial portion of the amygdala (Gloor 1978). Both sets then converge on the preoptic region of the lateral hypothalamus, and from there they run to the central gray complex of the upper midbrain.

Competition and fighting for food and water requires the integrity of both the amygdala (Shipley and Kolb 1977) and fibers that traverse the striae terminalis and end in the lateral hypothalamus. The hypothalamic nuclei receive modulatory inputs from septal nuclei (Adams 1979) and the hippocampus. The motor patterns characteristic of attack behavior depend on pathways and circuits that lie downstream from the upper midbrain, but they have not as yet been clearly delineated.

Animals submit to conspecifics or to animals of other species, including human beings with whom they are familiar (Darwin 1872). Defensive stalking, hissing, and biting are elicited in domestic cats in the presence of unfamiliar animals, including members of their own species. These behaviors are more likely to occur in wild rats than in tame ones (Richter 1949); domesticated laboratory animals attack only when confronted by an unfamiliar animal or human being, or one who inflicts pain on them.

Submissive behavior and attack behavior, designed to defend the animal—attack being the best means of defense—are subserved by different and parallel circuits; "switching" from one to the other is readily accomplished (Adams 1977). The inhibitory circuits of defense behavior in domesticated rats appear to be activated by visual signals—e.g., the sight of another rat's vibrissae vibrating—and smells.

A series of regulatory circuits inhibits neurons of the perifornical region of the hypothalamus from which the "defense" reaction (Hess 1957) can be elicited in cats. They run from the septal nuclei, anterior hypothalamus, and VMN to the tegmentum of the midbrain. Additional inhibitory inputs emanate from the VMN to the central gray region of the midbrain. They are counteracted by excitatory inputs from the dorsomedial nucleus of the amygdala and the septal nuclei, which travel to the perifornical region of the hypothalamus and the VMH (Adams 1979).

Rostral brain circuits also seem to inhibit ongoing behavior to produce submission: Inhibition seems to rely upon neurons that pass from the dorsomedial nucleus of the thalamus to the frontoorbital area of the cortex (Roberts 1962), and also upon neurons that travel from the anterior nucleus of the thalamus to the cingulate cortex and then to the hippocampus (Adams 1979).

However, a full understanding of the role of these circuits has not been obtained. Many of the components that together constitute the totality of submissive behavior or defensive attacks can be elicited separately by electrical and chemical stimulation of the same regions. Or, stimulation by these two different means may have opposite effects: Chemical stimulation (by carbachol) of the perifornical region of cats may elicit a submissive posture, while electrical stimulation produces an attack (Baxter 1967). These conflicting results are not easily explained. However, in making such observations, the context in which the particular stimulus is applied should be taken into account.

To summarize: The brain circuits that underlie "defense" and submissive behaviors consist of a series of negative and positive feedback loops, activated by specific signals. The separate circuits for these behaviors seem to be able to "switch" from one to the other. Their output consists of identifiable integrated configurations of behavior, associated with autonomically mediated and hormonal secretory patterns that are exquisitely attuned to the signal and the context in which it appears (chapter 7). The main components of the behaviors are generated by the brain stem, cerebellum, and spinal cord. Their output patterns are inhibited, modulated, or "switched" by more rostral circuits organized in parallel. A signal, or a stressful experience, is necessary to elicit these behaviors, whose expression is also determined by the social context and whether the animal is, or is not, familiar with the source of the signal.

However, it is too early to generalize across species. Rats may fight for food, but other rodents hoard it, store fat in their bodies, or both. Assuring food supplies is essential for survival, in the same manner as survival is essential for reproduction.

The Biology of Mating and Reproduction

Each genus and species has a different way of harmonizing mating behavior with the production of gametes. Mating behavior in turn is coordinated with signals specific to each genus. But in some genera and species the signal is predominantly internal and hormonal.

Internal communication systems for reproduction exist, consisting of hormonal and neuronal signals. But the organism also receives mating signals (sounds, displays of courtship behavior, smells, and bites) that signify the conditions favorable for mating and the care of the offspring. Both sets of signals are species-specific. Behavior and physiology are inextricably bound together.

Mating and the care and survival of the young are under intense selective pressure. In the terminology of this book the activities are prone to stressful experiences brought on by predators, the need to assure adequate food supplies, and the availability of security and protection.

The physiological regulation of ovulation is a complex time-dependent mechanism. In mammals it involves the participation of ovarian hormones, LH and FSH, GnRH, and its associated peptide (GAP) (chapter 2). The two releasing hormones are located in neurons of the preoptic and arcuate nuclei of the hypothalamus, which terminate in the external, lateral layer of the median eminence (Nikolicz et al. 1985). Ovulation in the female rat and sheep, and in women, is brought about in a cyclic manner by an internal positive feedback mechanism leading to a massive signal of LH in midcycle. Estradiol levels progressively rise under the pulsatile influence of LH and FSH during the follicular phase. At the same time the pituitary gland is "primed" by E_2 and progesterone to become more responsive to LH. Finally, E_2 stimulates the release of a massive pulsatile signal from LHRH to LH. This pulse in turn is the product of the integration of adrenergic and noradrenergic neurons activating GnRH and GAP release and the removal of the tonic inhibitory influences of opioid peptidergic neurons.

However, the description of this complex signaling system fails to indicate the purpose of ovulation: It is to provide gametes for reproduction. Sexual reproduction creates variation. In evolutionary terms reproductive success is the gold standard of fitness (Huxley 1942).

Mating and ovulation must sooner or later be harmonized. Their coordination, carried out in many different ways by different species, does not, however, assure reproductive success. Breeding must also occur at times that favor or are optimal for the survival and care of offspring: Successful breeding requires environmental conditions that assure food supplies, housing (nesting) of offspring, the right temperature conditions, and a relative protection from predators (Crews and Moore 1986).

Many strategies have been devised by nature for coordinating ovulation and mating, and to assure the optimal conditions under which birth occurs and the young survive. In rat, sheep, and human females, ovulation is the product of a complex coordination of hormonal and neural signals that occur "spontaneously." In other species, ovulation is promoted at the time of mating. In the red deer, the bellowing of the rutting stag is the signal that triggers ovulation in the doe. In the sea otter, the male bites the nose of the female during copulation, causing her to ovulate. Ovulation in the rabbit, cat, vole, and treeshrew is brought about by vaginal stimulation during intercourse.

To make the matter even more interesting, LHRH, while promoting ovulation, releases the characteristic lordosis behavior of the sexually receptive female rat. In some birds (sparrows), however, male mating behavior is completely independent of hormonal state: Mounting is released in them by solicitation displays of the female. In other birds (finches), hormones play only a permissive role in mating behavior: Rainfall is the signal that sets off mating and nest-building. In still other animals, gonadal maturation and ovulation are completely uncoupled in time from mating behavior, gametes are stored for a subsequent mating season, or mature gonads and gametes are kept in a viable state for long periods until favorable environmental signals (temperature, climate, food or nesting) are received (Crews and Moore 1986).

In women, however, ovulation occurs independently of mating: Mating does not depend on ovulation; it occurs even when ovulation has ceased. Yet women seem to be more sexually receptive during the luteal phase of the reproductive cycle (Benedek and Rubenstein 1942).

The signals emanating from the environment and from an animal's glands may also signify unfavorable conditions for mating. A sexually receptive female lizard who has elevated gonadotropin levels becomes unreceptive, and the levels plummet when she perceives two males fighting. In some species of monkeys, progesterone and LH levels are undetectable, and no cycling occurs in the subordinate (but not in the dominant) female (Abbott 1987) (chapter 7). The complex ovarian cycle in women is also remarkably sensitive to disruption (Weiner 1989c): Anovulation, oligomenorrhea, and amenorrhea occur in (some) women with stressful experience, exercise, weight loss, obesity, malnutrition, chronic disease, migration, depressive mood states, and head injury. Presumably, the extreme sensitivity of this system of such conditions has evolved because they may be unfavorable to reproductive success.

The Role of the Peptide Hormones in the Integration and Pattern Generation of Behavior and Physiology

The discovery about twenty-five years ago of certain gastrointestinal hormones involved in the regulation of gastric secretion and motility opened a new chapter in biology. It has led to the description of an ever-growing number (now about eighty) of peptide molecules present virtually everywhere in the brain and body—in the pituitary gland, immune system, heart, pancreas, gut, and kidney. Some of these molecules are conserved throughout evolution. Their function is to act as communication signals, which participate in the regulation and modulation of every function (Brown and Fisher 1984). Their effects are broad and not confined to any one cell, organ, or system. They are present in synaptosomes in nerve terminals in the brain, to which they are transported from the cell body down the axon. They are colocalized with the classical neurotransmitter signal system in peripheral nerve terminals. Monoamines and neuropeptides coexist in neurons: (a) DA with NT, CCK, and enkephalin; (b) E with enkephalin, NT, and NPY; (c) NE with enkephalin, VIP, and NPY; (d) 5-HT with SP, TRH, and enkephalin; (e) acetylcholine with VIP, LHRH (in preganglionic sympathetic C fibers), and TRH. The actions of the neurotransmitters are brief, but those of the peptides are of longer duration.

Peptides can act as neurotransmitters, autocrine and paracrine signals, or, when released into the bloodstream, as hormones. When secreted into the lumen of the gut they act to regulate its many activities. They are also produced by activated cells of the immune system and regulate them. They have the ability to stimulate cell growth (Sporn and Roberts 1988).

Different combinations of receptors for these peptides are located on virtually every cell. Their effect depends on the predominant function of these cells or cell groups, the nature of the receptor on their surfaces and the second messenger systems to which they are linked, and the context in which they are released. A protein may transport the peptide signal from its site of synthesis (within, for example, a nerve cell) to its site of release at a distance. Different proteins may transport the peptide's metabolic products back to the site of synthesis.

The discovery of the peptide hormones has provided new insights into how certain specific interactions between animals produce analgesia—for example, in the intruding animal but not in the one resident in its home cage (Smelik 1985)—and how certain stressful experiences perturb the organism to activate specific behavior patterns and their coordinated configurations of changes in bodily function. The diverse transformations brought about by centrally administered CRF exemplify this assertion. In all likelihood, it mediates the effects of many stressful experiences—unavoidable shock, restraint, cold, etc. (Weiner 1982, 1989a). On the other hand, cardiovascular responses elicited by different stressful experiences also fall into different patterns and are specific to them. They are generated, as previously described, by different neural circuits whose messenger signals are still not fully elucidated (Reis and LeDoux 1987; Zanchetti, Baccelli, and Manci 1976).

The peptides have provided us with the empirical tools for understanding how behavior and physiology are coordinated. In the rat, CRF increases motor activity in a familiar environment and during the autonomically mediated changes characteristic of the "defense" reaction (Hess 1957). Thyrotropin releasing hormone is secreted when the ambient temperature falls (chapter 7) to stimulate the secretion of TSH and thus of T_4, which is converted to T_3. As a result energy metabolism for maintaining the body temperature is increased, which in turn generates the need for caloric fuel in the form of food. At the same time, TRH in the DMV promotes gastric acid secretion and motility (chapter 7). Therefore, this sequence can be conceptualized as follows: The cold organism is coordinating its increased energy requirements provided by food by preparing the stomach for receiving and digesting it.

Angiotensin II acts in the rat's hypothalamus to promote the drinking of water and the eating of salt; it also raises the BP. Partly by these behavioral means it counteracts a decrease in blood volume. Insulin, a main regulator of blood glucose levels, indirectly regulates glucose intake. Following a carbohydrate meal, insulin levels rise. Insulin promotes the preferential transport of the amino acid tryptophane through the blood-brain barrier. Tryptophane is the precursor of 5-HT, one of whose actions in the VMH is to suppress the eating of carbohydrates by rats (Fernstrom and Wurtman 1972).

Peptides also have both tonic and phasic signaling functions; e.g., NGF tonically maintains the integrity of sympathetic and sensory neurons. Its level phasically increase in mouse serum during fighting to enhance sympathetic activity and to increase the weight and size of, and induce TH in, the adrenal medulla. Nerve growth factor also promotes the secretion of renin (Aloe et al. 1986).

Hormones act at a distance from their sources. They form components of a wide-ranging communication system within the organism. The main glands producing hormones are centrally controlled by a system of hypothalamic releasing factors and hormones, some but not all of which are peptides. In turn, these signals stimulate the secretion of a series of pituitary (peptide) hormones involved in the regulation of functions as diverse as milk ejection, water and salt excretion, energy metabolism, responses to stressful experiences, ovulation, BP regulation, immune function, and behavior.

The secretion of releasing factors is also under the control of signals coming from within the body and from the environment. One of the main functions of these factors is to produce patterned rhythms of hormone secretion and of behavior. Each of these patterns has its own characteristic and relatively stable form, frequency, and amplitude. Each pattern oscillates during any 24-hour period in a characteristic manner. The mature pattern of many hormones also follows a developmental sequence.

CORTICOTROPIN RELEASING FACTOR (CFR). The regulation of hypothalamic CRF secretion—a peptide composed of 41 amino acids—is extraordinarily complex, being the result of the integration of many signals. It is localized in, and released from, cells in the parvocellular region of the PVN by a wide variety of neuronal signals coming from receptors for smell, light, sound, pain, and touch (Feldman 1985); by visceral afferent, neural signals from the heart, liver, and gut through the NTS; by peptides and steroid hormone message signals, which pass through the circumventricular and the subfornical organs and the blood-brain barrier. Some of these inputs are inhibitory, and some stimulatory, of CRF release. The principle of parallel processing is nowhere more apparent than in this system.

The PVN has direct and important direct neuronal connections to critical brain stem nuclei; of special note are the bidirectional ones between it and the LC and the NTS. Corticotropin releasing factor is found in the terminals of the former, where it is believed to modulate α-adrenergic receptors. The pathway to the NTS uses OT as its neurotransmitter; it is one arc of a circuit, while the other one consists of NTS neurons that end in the PVN. Thus the PVN regulates two important nuclei in the brain stem that play a critical role in controlling autonomically mediated functions.

Corticotropin releasing factor can also be found in many other regions of the brain—the cerebral cortex, hippocampus, brain stem, (Sawchenko 1989), and sympathetic neurons (Udelsman et al. 1986). Specific cortisosterone receptors are present in the hippocampus to inhibit CRF release and terminate the response to stressful experiences (Keller-Wood and Dallman 1984; Sapolsky, Krey, and McEwen 1984, 1986).

It was initially believed that the main function of CRF was to act as a signal for the secretion of ACTH from the anterior pituitary (Hökfelt et al. 1983; Taylor and Fishman 1988). Because ACTH is but a segment contained within the prohormone POMC, within which other hormones—β- and γ-lipotropin, α, β, and γ-MSH, β-endorphin, and the enkephalins—are contained, it is not the only hormone CRF regulates. In fact, ACTH, β-lipotropin, and β-endorphin secretion occur simultaneously, at least in some animals exposed to specific stressful experiences. Immunoreactivity for CRF is diminished in the PVN following exposure to them (Chappell et al. 1986).

Simple stimuli are mediated by specific neuronal circuits in the brain that stimulate CRF release. The CRF-containing neurons in the parvocellular

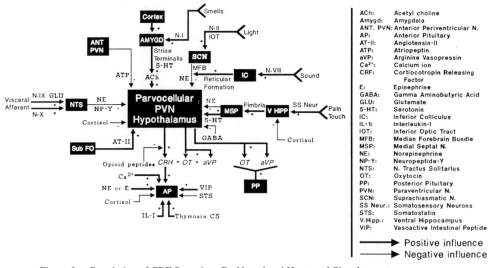

Figure 3.   Regulation of CRF Secretions By Neural and Hormonal Signals

region of the PVN are impinged upon by afferent neurons of the median forebrain (MFB) bundle. Photic stimuli pass via the inferior bundle of the accessory optic tract to its terminal nuclei, and from there via the mamillary peduncle to the MFB. Auditory stimuli travel via the reticular formation to the MFB. Olfactory stimuli are transmitted to the amygdala, and then via the striae terminalis to the PVN. Somatosensory (including painful) stimuli are mediated via the ventral hippocampus, fimbria, precommissural fornix, and medial septal nuclei to the PVN (Feldman 1985, 1989). Visceral afferent input to the PVN is relayed from the NTS, which collects fibers arising from noradrenergic (A1, A2, A6) and adrenergic (C1, C2) cell groups in the brain stem. The noradrenergic neurons also contain NPY and galanin. The NTS sends afferents to the central nucleus (CN) of the amygdala, which contain neurons staining for CRF, SP, and the enkephalins. Efferent projections from the CN of the amygdala travel to the pontine parabrachial nucleus, the central gray matter of the medulla, and the DMV, thereby completing another neural circuit involved in central autonomic control.

The release of CRF from PVN neurons is probably stimulated by 5-HT (via the 5-HT$_2$ receptor) (Feldman 1985) and inhibited by E and NE (Axelrod and Reisine 1984). Neurons from the PVN to the external layer of the median eminence system also contain enkephalins, NPY, and an intestinal porcine peptide (PHI-27) that is believed also to regulate PRL secretion. In fact, ACTH and PRL are secreted simultaneously in some animals during stressful experiences (Hökfelt et al. 1983).

Centrally administered CRF, by promoting ACTH secretion from the ante-

I. BEHAVIOR:
  Motor Activity ↑
  (Familiar Envt)

  Grooming ↑
  Food Intake ↓
  CHO Intake ↓

II. NEUROTRANSMITTERS:
  Epinephrine:
    Central   ?
    Peripheral ↑

  Norepinephrine:
    Central   ↑
    Peripheral ↑ +NPY

  Dopamine:
    Kidney ↑
    Fat   ↓

III. ENDOCRINE SYSTEM:
  ACTH↑   ⎫
  β-Endorphin↑ ⎪
  CLIP ↑   ⎬ Released
  MSH ↑   by
  GH ↓   Pituitary
  LH ↓   ⎪
  FSH ↓   ⎭

  Somatostatin ↑↓ Hypothal
  TRH   ↓ Medulla

  Insulin   ↓ ⎫
  Glucagon ↑ ⎬ Pancreas
  Blood Glucose↑

  Corticosteroids   ↑
  Androgenic steroids ↑

IV. CARDIOVASCULAR:
  Heart Rate   ↑
  Blood Pressure ↑
  Cardiac Output ↑
  Stroke Volume ↑
  Peripheral Resistance ↓

V. GASTROINTESTINAL:
  Gastric Acid Secretion ↓
  Pepsin Secretion   ↓
  Gastric Motility   ↓
  Gastric Erosions   ↓
  (Counteracts TRH 's
  effect on these)

VI. IMMUNE:
  NK cells ↓
  (Cytotoxicity)

Figure 4.   Effects of Intracerebroventricular Corticotropin Releasing Factor (CRF) on Behavioral and Physiological Patterns (Rat and Dog)

rior pituitary gland, regulates the secretion of cortico- and androgenic steroids but inhibits aldosterone secretion by the adrenal cortex (Aguilera, Fujita, and Catt 1981). Within the brain CRF increases STS activity, thereby reducing GH release from the pituitary gland (Rivier and Vale 1985). It inhibits LH and FSH secretion in male rats (Rivier, Rivier, and Vale 1986) and baboons, probably through the mediation of β-endorphin acting at the level of the median eminence (Rivier, Rivier, and Vale 1986; Sapolsky 1989). It promotes the secretion of E, NE, and NPY into the bloodstream, and of DA by and in the kidney. It increases oxygen consumption. It reduces fever. It depresses insulin secretion and raises blood glucagon and glucose levels (Brown and Fisher 1985, 1989).

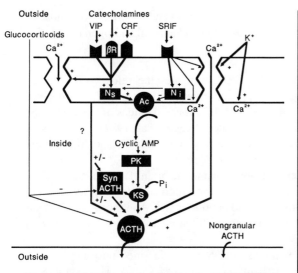

The release of ACTH can be stimulated (+) by various hormones such as CRF, catecholamines acting on β-adrenoreceptors (β R) or α,-adrenoreceptors (not shown), VIP, or vasopressin (not shown). Each agonist acts on separate and specific receptors. The hormone-induced secretion of ACTH involves a multitude of intracellular second messengers. Secretagogues can activate adenylate cyclase (Ac) to form cyclic AMP. A guanine nucleotide stimulatory protein (Ns) is required for hormone activation of Ac. Cyclic AMP activates protein kinase (PK), which catalyses the phosphorylation (Pi) of a protein substrate (KS). The phosphorylated KS may induce ACTH synthesis (Syn ACTH) or the release of granular ACTH (in the circle). The secretion of nongranular ACTH appears to be regulated differently from granular ACTH. Hormones and membrane depolarization, induced by extracellular potassium (K⁺), may stimulate calcium (Ca2⁺) influx or mobilization from intracellular compartments. Other intracellular events (?) induced by secretagogues may involve changes in phospholipid methylation, protein carboxymethylation, phosphatidylinositol turnover, protein kinase C, and glycosyltransferase activity. ACTH release can be inhibited (-) by at least two hormones. Glucocorticoids can inhibit ACTH synthesis or release. Somatostatin (SRIF) blocks the activation of Ac or Ca2+ mobilization. A guanine nucleotide inhibitory protein (Ni) mediates SRIF's inhibition of Ac. Coupling of Ni with SRIF receptors leads to either a direct blockage of the catalytic subunit of Ac or an inhibition of Ns activity (Modified from Axelrod & Reisine, 1984).

Figure 5.   Molecular Mechanisms Involved in ACTH Release

At least in animals, CRF raises HR but diminishes the peripheral resistance and thus BP, while raising the CO. Acting through β-adrenergic receptors it mobilizes brown fat, thereby increasing heat production. It inhibits gastric acid and pepsin secretion (Taché, Stephens, and Ishikawa 1989) and reduces gastric motility in the resting (Garrick et al. 1988) or the hypoglycemic rat (Stephens et al. 1989). It reduces (splenic) NK-cell cytotoxicity—an effect mediated by NE, and not by the corticosteroids (Irwin, Vale, and Britton 1987). It increases grooming behavior. It stimulates food, especially carbohydrate, intake (Morley and Levine 1982). It promotes attack behavior in two rats subjected to electric shocks (Tazi et al. 1987).

The changes brought about by CRF are patterned. Its broad actions exemplify the principle that peptides enhance (e.g., CRF, aVP, and VIP) or inhibit (CRF and TRH, CRF and LH) each other's activities, while coordinating an animal's behavior and physiology.

ADRENOCORTICOTROPIN (ACTH). The CRF regulates the release of pituitary ACTH via specific receptors. ACTH is also secreted from the gland under the direct influence of catecholamines acting through α_1- and β-adrenoreceptors, aVP, OT, bombesin, VIP, IL-1β, extracellular potassium, and calcium. Each agonist has its own receptor or channel on corticotrophs that are coupled to different intracellular second messenger systems and protein kinases (Axelrod and Reisine 1984). The antagonists of ACTH secretion are the glucocorticoids, STS, and an unidentified peptide inhibiting factor (CIF).

The bodily effects of ACTH are both similar to and different from those of CRF. ACTH mainly promotes corticosteroid and adrenal androgen production and secretion.

OPIOID PEPTIDES. The CRF stimulates the release of not only ACTH but also the opioid peptides, β-endorphin, and the enkephalins derived from the same precursor molecule, POMC. These peptides are released and their receptor sites in the brain are occupied (Seeger et al. 1984) in animals by stressful experiences, such as bodily injury, unavoidable and intermittent shocks, fear (Smelik 1985), and pain (Madden et al. 1977).

Since the enkephalins were first identified in the brain (Hughes et al. 1975), there has been a virtual explosion of information about them and the endorphins. Four families of these opioid peptides exist. And recently, MS itself has also been identified in the brain and adrenal gland of cattle (Goldstein et al. 1985).

The endogenous opioid peptides, and MS are classified into five groups, each with separate receptors (Chang and Cautrecasas 1979; Holaday 1985). (1) One group is composed of three endorphins. Beta-endorphin has a specific (ε-) receptor, but it also binds to the μ-receptor. (2) The five enkephalin derive from a common precursor, proenkephalin A. Leu-enkephalin binds to the δ-receptor, and met-enkephalin to the i-receptor. (3) The three dynorphins and two neo-endorphins are contained in prodynorphin. Dynorphin (1-17) binds to a κ-receptor. (4) MS, which is not a peptide but an alkaloid, has a specific receptor (μ). (5) The three morphins make up a group whose precursor and receptors are not known. (A sixth (σ) receptor has been identified, but its naturally occurring agonists are unknown.)

Under ambient or resting conditions, the opioid peptides are not secreted into the bloodstream in humans. But serum β-endorphin-like immunoreactivity shows a circadian rhythm in animals, which parallels that of ACTH and of cortisol. Nicotine, caffeine, painful stimuli, acupuncture, intermittent electrical shock (Lewis, Cannon, and Liebeskind 1980; Rossier et al. 1977), cold-water restraint, injury, a fall in blood glucose levels, strenuous exercise, infection, and danger (Smelik 1985) activate the opioid system at different bodily locations.

Life-threatening "shock" produced by bodily and spinal cord injury, pain, sepsis, hemorrhage, and anaphylaxis can be reversed by the antagonist naloxone. By the use of selective antagonists, and analysis can be carried out revealing which opioid receptors are activated during the various forms of "shock;" the δ- and κ-receptors mediate the effects of dire injury or life-threatening infection.

Cold-water immersion with or without restraint, or raising the ambient temperature to 36°C, increases blood levels of β-endorphin immunoreactivity in rats. When injected with an opioid antagonist, rats exposed to heat become progressively more hyperthermic, suggesting that opioids are involved in lowering increases in body temperature (Holaday 1985).

Beta-endorphin (31 amino acids) is given off from the anterior lobe of the pituitary in humans, and from its intermediate lobe in the rat. Its secretion from the anterior lobe is regulated by CRF; in human beings it is not always expressed at the same time as ACTH. It also has other sources than the pituitary gland, because it can be identified in the bloodstream, cerebrospinal fluid, and semen; in fact, it is present in cells in the placenta, pancreas, heart, gut, and spleen.

The (met-)enkephalins, however, are expressed by the adrenal medulla, along with E, chromogranin, NPY, dopamine β-hydroxylase, and ATP. Leu-enkephalin and the dynorphins are mainly of posterior pituitary origin in rats. Foot shock reduces the content of leu-enkephalin in the hypothalamus of rats (Rossier, Guillemin, and Bloom 1978).

Enkephalin neurons have short axons that are widely distributed throughout the brain. Of particular interest is their presence in the CN of the amygdala, the periaqueductal gray matter, the NTS, and the dorsal horn of the spinal cord. In the hypothalamus, they are to be found in the arcuate nucleus and the PVN, which contains the highest concentration of β-endorphin anywhere in the brain. The second highest content is found in NTS neurons. The axons of β-endorphin-containing neurons in the arcuate nucleus are long and are widely distributed to the CN of the amygdala, septal nucleli, periaqueductal gray matter, and the medullary nuclei involved in cardiorespiratory control.

Dynorphin-containing neurons are found in supraoptic and PVN neurons, colocalized with OT and aVP. They are also present in the arcuate nucleus, hippocampus, caudate nucleus, NTS, and spinal cord. Dopamine and enkephalins are found together in carotid body neurons. In the superior cervical ganglion, NE and enkephalins are colocalized. In the adrenal medulla β-endorphin inhibits the release, or action, of acetylcholine by either pre- or postsynaptic mechanisms. The actions of the opioid peptides and MS are counteracted by a number of other peptides such as ACTH, TRH, aVP, SP, CCK, and STS (Holaday 1985, 1989), some of which (ACTH and aVP) are in turn inhibited by them.

A likely central role played by the opioid peptides is in mediating stress analgesia. But β-endorphin also has wide-ranging modulatory activities on neurotransmission and hormone regulation within the brain. Beta-endorphin inhibits the release of acetylcholine, NE, DA, and GABA, and 5-HT locally in the hippocampus; however, it has the opposite effect on 5-HT in the hypothalamus and brain stem. Catecholamines are released into the circulation of rats after β-endorphin is administered centrally. But, as already mentioned, the rise in circulating catecholamines induced by exercise, the cold pressor test, or hypoglycemia in humans is opposed by the opioid peptides (Bouloux and Grossman 1989).

Beta-endorphin directly promotes the secretion of ACTH, GH, PRL, and aVP, but it counteracts the release of TSH, LH, and FSH in animals (Holaday 1985; Morley 1983). It may actually play a double role in inhibiting CRF expression and in indirectly lowering CRF-stimulated ACTH secretion. In human beings, ACTH, LH, and FSH secretion are tonically inhibited by β-endorphin, but opiate agonists do not influence TSH secretion.

Met-enkephalin increases GH and PRL and decreases LH, FSH, and TRH in animals. Morphine sulphate releases ACTH, GH, MSH, PRL, aVP, and OT but inhibits LH, FSH, and TRH secretion in rats (Holaday 1985). Opiate agonists raise insulin, glucagon, and blood glucose levels in humans.

The opiate peptides appear also to influence several aspects of the immune system. Opioid peptides suppress overall NK-cell cytotoxic activity in rats, and also reduce their specific (cytotoxic) action on tumor cells (Shavit et al. 1984, 1985). They cause CD8$^+$ cells to proliferate and suppress antibody responses. These in vivo experiments are, however, contradicted by the in vitro demonstration that β-endorphin, but not α- or γ-endorphin, enhances NK-cell cytotoxic activity. Beta-endorphin augments interferon production by large granular lymphocytes in the presence of mitogens (Mandler et al. 1986) and enhances IL-2 production (Morley, Kay, and Solomon 1989). Conversely, naloxone-binding by lymphocytes is counteracted by IL-2.

The proliferative response to mitogens of rat spleen cells is increased by β-endorphin. Beta-endorphin, dynorphin, and met-enkephalin stimulate monocyte and granulocyte chemotaxis. Beta-endorphin enhances antibody formation and modulates CD4$^+$ cell function. It binds to the C-9 terminal sequence of complement. It stimulates histamine release by mast cells. On the other hand, α-endorphins inhibit antibody formation by mouse spleen cells to sheep red blood cells (Heijnen, deFouw, and Ballieux 1986) or ovalbumen (Ballieux and Heijnen 1987). Therefore, α- and β-endorphin have opposite effects on antibody formation.

Opioid peptides (especially dynorphin) promote the eating of food, even in satiated animals (Morley 1983). Restraint inhibits, and the pinching of the tail of a rat (known to release β-endorphin) enhances, food intake—an effect that is reversed by naloxone. Opioid agonists seem to have both enhancing and suppressive actions on food ingestion depending on which receptor is being bound; e.g., stimulation of the μ-, δ- and κ-receptors suppresses and, of the ε-receptor increases, intake.

The current belief is that opioid peptides may have specific effects on the perception and intake of certain kinds of foodstuffs. Naloxone decreases feeding without altering the perception of hunger and the intake of palatable and fatty foods. Opioid peptides also appear to be involved in the recognition of edible foods; they therefore determine food preferences, rather than merely influencing the act of eating.

Enkephalins and dynorphins are present in the myenteric plexus of the gut, which innervates its smooth muscle. Met-enkephalin may increase gastric acid secretion, but other opioids may reduce gastric secretion and contractions. For many centuries it has been known that MS constipates by virtue of stimulating segmental contractions of the colon. In fact, naloxone may alleviate chronic constipation. The action of opioid peptides on the motility of the gut is by no means unique (Holaday 1985). An array of other peptides affects motility and/or secretion: Gastrin, CCK, and motilin increase motility, whereas glucagon, gastric inhibitory polypeptide, pancreatic polypeptide, and VIP decrease it (Taché 1988; Taché, Stephens, and Ishikawa 1989).

The opioid peptides depress respiration by diminishing the stimulatory effects of CO_2 on the medullary respiratory centers through the agency of μ- and δ-receptors. These peptides also have bidirectional effects on HR and BP, depending on which opioid is injected at what site in the brain. In general, stimulation of μ-receptors in the medulla produces bradycardia and hypotension, whereas stimulation of hypothalamic δ-receptors produces the opposite effects (Holaday 1985).

Injected into the lateral ventricles of a rat, β-endorphin and MS produce immobility and rigidity—a behavioral state that is reminiscent of the tonic immobility observed in many rodents when confronted with natural predators.

THE THYROTROPIN RELEASING HORMONE (TRH) AND THYROID-STIMULATING HORMONE (TSH). The effects of stressful experience on the hypothalmic-pituitary-thyroid axis has only recently been clarified. Before the isolation of TRH and the development of a radioimmunoassay for TSH, the activity of the axis could only be estimated by the measurement of iodinated (thyroid) compounds in blood plasma. In that era, their long-lasting changes were described during and after monkeys were subjected to 72 hours of conditioned-avoidance sessions, or prior to training while they were getting used to the novelty of a restraining chair (Mason 1968). In the next decade, increases in TSH and thyroid hormone levels were observed in rats placed in novel situations or exposed to a cold environment (Yuwiler 1976). Only recently has more definitive evidence been obtained that exposing rats to cold releases TRH into third ventricular fluid and markedly increases its content in the median eminence (Arancibia et al. 1983; Arancibia and Assenmacher 1987). Exposure to cold also stimulates the secretion of TSH from the anterior pituitary and increases T_3, more than T_4, levels in the bloodstream. The rise in free T_4 levels is mainly the result of its displacement from a binding globulin by FFAs, which are first released by the animal's exposure to cold (Yuwiler 1976). In addition to releasing TSH from the anterior pituitary gland, TRH promotes PRL secretion.

Multiple signals regulate TRH secretion from neurons in the preoptic nucleus of the hypothalamus: NE inhibits its release; NE and DA are in turn liberated from synaptosomes in the brain by TRH; 5-HT is a weak inciter, and β-adrenergic blocking agents, glucocorticoids, and STS are inhibitors of TRH secretion. At the level of the pituitary gland itself the secretion of TSH is promoted by DA and 5-HT. In the body, glucocorticoids block the peripheral conversion of T_4 to T_3, while T_3 regulates the number of β-adrenergic receptors particularly on cardiac cells.

Thyrotropin releasing hormone is widely distributed throughout the brain and spinal cord, in addition to being present in the dorsomedial nucleus of the hypothalamus (Hökfelt, Johansson, and Goldstein 1984). Approximately 12% of the total content of TRH in the brain is to be found in the brain stem, especially in the NTS, the DMV, the nucleus ambiguus, and the raphé nuclei (Kubek et al. 1983).

In rodents, TRH increases spontaneous motor activity and diminishes the amount of their sleep. It inhibits conditioned avoidance behaviors. It wakens hibernating animals. It opposes the hypnotic, hypothermic, and potentially lethal effects of barbiturates and counteracts the action of ethanol, diazepams, and other sedative and hypothermic agents (Guillemin 1978; Krieger and Liotta 1979; Vale, Brown, and Rivier 1977). In vertebrates, including the rat, it stimulates gastric motility, pepsin and acid secretion, and pancreatic secretion and increases duodenal, jejunal, ileal, and colonic propulsive contractions. When injected into the cisterna magna or the DMV of rats it enhances gastric emptying and mucosal blood flow. It produces gastric erosions that are prevented by cutting both the vagus nerves (Taché 1985, 1987, 1988; Taché, Vale, and Brown 1980; Taché et al. 1983, 1988; Stephens et al. 1988).

Thyrotropin releasing hormone raises catecholamine levels in the bloodstream, and raises the HR and BP, when injected into the cisterna magna. It inhibits baroreceptor reflexes, but it can also reverse the endotoxic shock of overwhelming bacterial infection (Holaday and Faden 1983). Therefore, the action of TRH introduced into that area of the brain stem is to enhance both vagal and sympathetic efferent activity.

SOMATOSTATIN (STS) AND GROWTH HORMONE (GH). The stimulation or inhibition of GH secretion has also been related to behavioral states and environmental contingencies. In the waking state, exercise and stressful experiences trigger its release (Martin et al. 1978). Conversely, the maternal deprivation syndrome in children is characterized by tonic inhibition of GH release.

In primates GH secretion is promoted by exercise, examinations, danger (chapter 4), and potentially life-threatening conditions such as hypoglycemia, infection, anemia, fractures, and other injuries. Noise and drugs such as ether, chlorpromazine, and E also promote it (Yuwiler 1976). In rats, however, GH release is inhibited by stressful experiences.

As its name suggests, GH has wide-ranging growth-promoting activities on bone, the mucosa of the stomach, and other tissues. It also elicits lactation in mammals. The actions of STS are of special interest because it is present in both the hypothalamus and the amygdala and in other brain regions, as well as in the gastrointestinal tract and pancreas.

Somatostatin inhibits the secretion of GH and TRH by the pituitary gland, but not of PRL, the gonadotropins, or ACTH. It counterregulates glucagon and insulin expression by pancreatic islet cells and the action of gastrin and secretin by the stomach and the duodenum (Guillemin and Gerich 1976). In addition to STS, GH release is inhibited by NPY and calcitonin-gene-related peptide.

The actions of GH are multifarious. For the particular subject under discussion, only a few of its interesting properties will be mentioned. Its episodic secretion from the pituitary gland of human beings during the first slow-wave sleep period is under multiple stimulatory and inhibitory control. Stimulation is thought to be brought about by a chemically unidentified releasing factor colocalized with DA, as well as by a number of peptides. In some circumstances TRH and LHRH release it; in others aVP, the α-MSH, glucagon, substance P, neurotensin, met-enkephalin, and β-endorphin are responsible. Morphine sulfate, insulin hypoglycemia, L-DOPA, and arginine are potent stimuli to GH secretion; they are counteracted in humans and animals by STS (Martin et al. 1978). The action of STS is under the control of afferent monoaminergic neurons to the hypothalamus. Norepinephrine, DA, and 5-HT inhibit STS. The catecholamines exert their effects primarily through α-adrenergic receptors in the hypothalamus, which also mediate GH release by insulin hypoglycemia, arginine, aVP, L-DOPA, exercise, and stressful experiences. Inhibition of GH secretion is, however, mediated by β-adrenergic and dopaminergic receptors (Meister and Hökfelt 1989).

PROLACTIN (PRL). The principal natural stimulus to PRL secretion in mammals is the nursing of an infant at its mother's breast. The pulsatile release of PRL occurs in connection with the intermittent sucking of the infant to produce milk ejection. Suckling also stimulates TRH, hGH, ACTH, and β-endorphin secretion. In human adults, PRL is secreted somewhat irregularly during the night, especially before morning awakening, and out of phase with GH secretion. In birds, however, PRL has growth-promoting properties. In many vertebrates it suppresses mating behavior. The administration of PRL in relatively high doses is followed by depression of LH and FSH and involution of the gonads. Progesterone secretion by the corpora lutea of rodents is at first stimulated by PRL. But progesterone also inhibits the spontaneous secretion of PRL by the pituitary gland (Giguere et al. 1982).

Many stressful experiences promote PRL secretion in vertebrates, and in women more than men. They include novel experiences, danger, restraint, exercise, surgery, and life-threatening ones such as bodily injury, hemorrhage, and exposure to cold. In the relatives of dying patients, serum PRL levels may

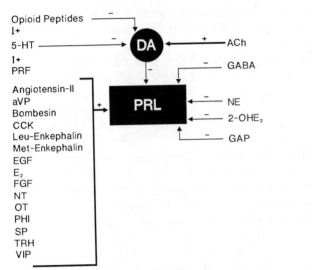

Opioid Peptides
|+
5-HT
|+
PRF
Angiotensin-II
aVP
Bombesin
CCK
Leu-Enkephalin
Met-Enkephalin
EGF
E_2
FGF
NT
OT
PHI
SP
TRH
VIP

ACh
GABA
NE
$2\text{-}OHE_2$
GAP

The principal inhibitor of secretion is dopamine (DA). Acetyl choline (ACh) acts indirectly through DA to increase inhibition. Serotonin (5-HT) has the opposite effect, and its action is furthered by the opioid peptides and the prolactin releasing factor (PRF). The net effect is to promote PRL secretion. Gamma aminobutyric acid (GABA), norepinehprine (NE), 2-hydroxyestradiol $(2\text{-}OHE_2)$ and the gonadotropin associated peptide (GAP) inhibit PRL secretion. The exact means by which angiotensin-II, arginine vasopressin (aVP), bombesin, cholecystokinin (CCK), the enkephalins, epidermal (EGF) and fibroblast growth (FGF) factors, estradiol (E_2), neurotensin (NT), oxytocin (OT), peptide histidine isoleucine (PHI), substance P (SP), thyrotropin releasing hormone (TRH), and vasoactive intestinal peptide (VIP) stimulate PRL release are unknown.

→ Positive influence
→ Negative influence

Figure 6.   Regulation of Prolactin (PRL) Secretion

be depressed for weeks, while serum cortisol levels are elevated (Theorell 1989).

Rats that have been hypophysectomized demonstrate a depression of antibody production and humoral and cell-mediated immune responses. These immune functions can be restored by injections of PRL (Grossman 1984, 1989), suggesting that it has a tonic effect on them.

Prolactin is contained in cell bodies in the AN. Prolactin secretion is under multiple control; fourteen known factors influence it. It is promoted by β-adrenergic stimulation (Smelik, Tilders, and Berkenbosch 1989), TRH, E_2, OT, VIP, aVP, and other peptides. The effect of TRH is mainly seen in higher vertebrates, but only under certain conditions. Dopaminergic fibers of the tuberoinfundibular tract, arising from the AN of the hypothalamus, exert tonic inhibitory control over PRL secretion, mediated by an unidentified inhibitory factor. Acetylcholine and GABA also play inhibitory roles. And in addition, DA and T_4 directly act on the anterior pituitary to prevent its release. The GAP, as we have seen, inhibits PRL secretion within the hypothalamus, thus counteracting the possibility of simultaneous PRL and gonadotropin secretion.

ARGININE VASOPRESSIN (aVP). Arginine vasopressin was the second hormone to be implicated in the response of the organism to stressful experiences, specifically painful ones. Later it was shown that it was also released during conditioned avoidance procedures, electric shocks, and hypoxia (produced by any reduction in blood volume and the osmotic pressure of blood), or by a fall in blood sugar levels induced by insulin (Plotsky, Bruhn, and Vale 1985). Its release is in part promoted by angiotensin II (Gibbs 1986;

Renaud 1978), and inhibited by GABA. But in contrast to its sister hormone, OT, it is not secreted in rats on immobilization or enforced swimming (Gibbs 1986).

Arginine vasopressin–containing neurons (some of which also store NE) are principally found in the magnocellular portion of the PVN and project to the posterior lobe of the pituitary gland. But aVP is additionally present in cells of the parvocellular part of the same nucleus in rats (colocalized with CRF), where their axons project to the median eminence. The expression of aVP from cells in the parvocellular portion of the PVN is tonically inhibited by corticosteroids (Kiss, Mezey, and Skuboll 1984; Sawchenko 1989; Sawchenko, Swanson, and Vale 1984). Although adrenalectomy enhances the expression of aVP in the parvocellular section of the PVN, it has no such effect on magnocellular cell bodies containing aVP or OT (Sawchenko 1989).

The colocalization of aVP and CRF makes "good sense," as the former modulates the stimulatory action of the latter on anterior pituitary cells to release ACTH via separate receptors. The question of the obligatory and simultaneous coupling of CRF and aVP release from parvocellular PVN neurons is not completely settled. During insulin hypoglycemia they seem to be secreted together, but IL-1β seems only to release CRF (Smelik, Tilders, and Berkenbosch 1989).

The main action of aVP is to promote water reabsorption by the distal convoluted tubules of the kidney: It thus plays a central role in the regulation of blood volume, BP, and the osmotic pressure of the extracellular fluid. But it may also play a role in elevating BP, acting through pathways that link the PVN to central autonomic nuclei in the brain stem.

Some Other Peptide Hormones Involved in the Integration of Behavior and Physiology with Stressful Experience

ANGIOTENSIN II (AT-II). Angiotensin II is produced in the body by the action of the renal enzyme, renin, on a circulating protein, angiotensinogen. Angiotensin II, by its action on adrenal cortical receptors, releases the potent mineralocorticoid aldosterone. Angiotensin acts directly on arterioles to produce vasoconstriction. It releases catecholamines from adrenergic nerve terminals. By its various coordinated actions, it is critically involved in BP and blood volume regulation and in salt and water metabolism.

The hypothalamus contains a complete renin-angiotensin system capable of synthesizing AT-II. The peptide, when injected into the brain, is an extremely powerful inducer of thirst, and therefore of drinking behavior, and is involved in the maintenance of BP levels (Ganten et al. 1971; Ganten, Schelling, and Ganten 1977; Phillips et al. 1977; Snyder 1978). The massive pressor effects of AT-II infused into the vertebral arteries of dogs (McCubbin 1967; Sweet and Brody 1971) probably are mediated by enhanced sympathetic efferent discharge from the brain stem, because they can be averted by pretreatment with reserpine (Ferrario et al. 1969; Gildenberg 1971). Increased sympathetic activity of this kind in turn stimulates the secretion of renin by the kidney (Bunag, Page, and McCubbin 1966). The intracerebroventricular infusion of AT-II has different cardiovascular effects than does CRF; they are not prevented by sympathetic ganglionic blockade.

Angiotensin II incites the secretion of aVP from the magnocellular portion of the PVN, and it also promotes ACTH secretion (Lind, Swanson, and Sawchenko 1985). Angiotensin II is present in the PVN. It may be synthesized there. It may also enter the brain via the subfornical organ or the area postrema (Joy and Lowe 1970). The release of aVP by AT-II is counteracted within the brain by another peptide, atriopeptin (Saper 1989).

ATRIOPEPTIN. The heart, in addition to its principal function, is also an endocrine organ. In response to an increase in pressure within the atrium,

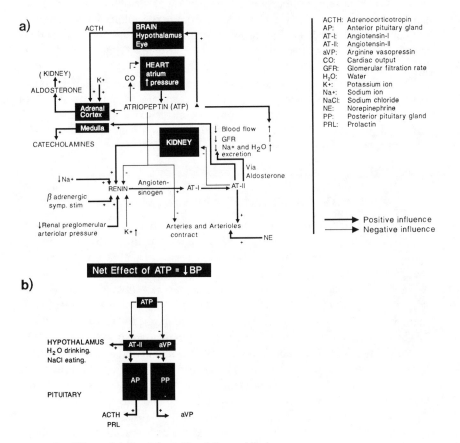

Figure 7.   Effects of Atriopeptin on Circulation and Brain

promoted by a rise in blood volume or BP, or by restraining a rat, a 28-amino-acid peptide—atriopeptin—is secreted to produce diuresis and natriuresis, a reduction of blood volume, BP, and vasodilatation. Atriopeptin, therefore, counterregulates all the physiological effects of the renin-angiotensin-aldosterone system. Atriopeptin also inhibits peripheral renin and catechola-mine secretion and inhibits central aVP secretion (Saper 1989). Receptors for atriopeptin are present in the adrenal medulla and in the glomeruli, Henle's loop, and collecting ducts of the kidney.

Atriopeptin is also present in the rat's brain, particularly in the N. peri-ventricularis of the thalamus, N. habenularis, PVN, preoptic nucleus, bed nu-clei, mammillary nuclei, N. anteroventralis periventricularis (AV3V), lateral dorsal tegmental, interpeduncular nuclei, and NTS—nuclei that are all known to be involved in the integration and regulation of autonomic and endocrine function.

Immunoreactive-like atriopeptin levels are reduced in the hypothalamus of rats on a high-salt diet. Atriopeptin is present particularly in the AV3V region of the hypothalamus, lesions of which produce hypodipsia and hypernatremia. In the PVN, it is colocalized with AT-II, aVP, OT, NPY, and CRF. From the PVN axons run to the LC, whose terminals also contain CRF, and to the medullary cardiovascular control centers (Sawchenko 1989).

Injection of atriopeptin-28 into the third ventricle of rats suppresses the drinking of water induced by increases in osmotic pressure or by AT-II in-jected in the PVN. Peripherally released atriopeptin can probably enter the brain via the organum vasculosum and the subfornical organ (Saper 1989; Standaert, Saper, and Needleman 1985). Receptors for the peptide have been identified on cells of the pituitary gland.

NEUROPEPTIDE-Y (NPY). This 36-amino-acid peptide is widely distributed throughout the brain in high concentrations, and in nerve plexuses around the cerebral and coronary blood vessels. It is colocalized with nor-adrenergic sympathetic neurons throughout the body. It is present in cell bodies in layers II–VI of the cerebral cortex (which also contain STS), whose terminals end in layers I and IV. It can be identified in nerve terminals in lim-bic structures, especially in the medial amygdala, N. accumbens, and hippo-campus.

Neuropeptide-Y cell bodies are also prominent in the arcuate nucleus and PVN. The peptide is thus colocalized with LHRH, GnRH, and DA neurons in the former, and CRF neurons in the latter. Neuropeptide-Y terminals reach the dorsomedial and preoptic (TRH-containing) nuclei, the anterior preoptic (TRH and LHRH) and periventricular (STS) nuclei, and the SCN. Neurons containing NPY are present throughout the brain stem; of particular interest is their presence in the parabrachial nucleus, the LC, the A1, A2, A4 (with NE), and the C1 and C3 (E) medullary cell groups. They are also present in the NTS (A2 and C2), ventrolateral medullary (A1 and C1), DMV, and MFB.

Neuropeptide-Y is found in the adrenal medulla where it is stored and released together with NE and met- and leu-enkephalin. It is present in sympathetic ganglia and terminals in the spleen, ovary, vas deferens, cardiac atria, and the submucosa and mucosa of the gut (Gray and Morley 1986).

Neuropeptide-Y has multiple physiological functions. It is released by any stressful experience that activates sympathetic neurons (chapter 8). It is cosecreted with NE, whose action it potentiates and prolongs. Calcium channel blockers prevent its actions, but α_2-antagonists do not. At the present time, it is believed that the physiological action of NPY in humans is particularly prominent on the smaller coronary arteries, where it produces prolonged vasoconstriction, which NE does not.

When given intravenously to rats, NPY increases BP, HR, and the strength of myocardial contractions (Gu et al. 1983). It constricts the cerebral and coronary arteries. It potentiates the secretion of T_4 when stimulated by either TSH, isoproteronol, or VIP. It counterregulates the release of insulin produced by raised glucose levels. And it inhibits the contraction of the uterine cervix and the vas deferens (Morley 1989).

Neuropeptide-Y also has behavioral effects when administered into the brain. It sedates. It increases carbohydrate intake when injected into the VMN and the PVN, possibly by promoting the action of NE and the opioid peptides in these nuclei. For reasons not fully understood, its stimulation of eating is not attenuated by vagotomy or adrenalectomy, procedures that eliminate the promotion of eating by NE.

It increases fluid intake and reduces the body temperature. When injected into the third ventricle, it lowers the BP, seemingly counterregulating the central effects of AT-II and the vasoconstriction and hypertensive effects of NE. It depresses the RR. It reduces grooming and lordosis behavior and the excessive secretion of LH in ovariectomized rats. But when such rats are first treated with E_2 and progesterone, NPY, like NE, raises LH levels in the blood. Normally NPY modulates the release of GnRH and thus LH and FSH. Gastric contractions are inhibited by NPY. Thus the peptide has opposite peripheral and central effects, especially on cardiovascular function. And it also shares some of the properties of CRF and other peptides (Morley 1989).

The Peptides of the Immune System and Their Interactions

Another class of peptides plays a crucial role in the self-regulation of the immune system, the activation and recruitment of fresh immunocompetent cells, and the division or differentiation of others, while also serving other functions not directly related to the immune system. They go by various descriptive names—growth factors, cytokines, or lymphokines.

The transforming growth factor-β, present in macrophages, promotes the controlled growth of fibroblasts and osteoblasts, while inhibiting T-cell expansion, Ig secretion, and the synthesis of adrenal corticosteroids. Neuro-leukin is found in the brain, denervated muscle, and salivary glands. It is secreted by T-cells. It induces B-cell maturation, Ig secretion, and the growth of sensory neurons and cells in the spinal cord (Sporn and Roberts 1988). The colony-stimulating factors promote the growth of various granulocytes and macrophages. Other similar (epidermal) factors inhibit the growth of hair follicle cells and the cells of a squamous cell carcinoma.

The interleukins act as stimulators (IL-1) of, or proliferative (IL-2) factors for, activated T- and B-cells. They play a permissive role in the multiplication of parent bone marrow cells (IL-3); they further the proliferation and differentiation of B-cells and resting T-cells, and enhance the activity of specialized cytolytic cells (IL-2 and IL-4); or they help suppress the expression of cell surface antigens and Ig secretion (IL-6).

The multifunctional nature of the interleukins may be understood by the fact that the cellular responses to them vary according to the nature of the target cell. This principle is illustrated by the actions of IL-1: In chondrocytes and fibroblasts it induces the synthesis of PGs and proteases; in lymphocytes it causes both the expression of the IL-2 receptor and IL-2 production; and in endothelial cells it promotes antifibrinolysis, adhesion, and coagulation. In order that some of these induced processes are not injurious to cells, IL-1 is tightly regulated by three related protein inhibitors that bind to its specific receptor without causing IL-1 expression (Hannum et al. 1990). Some of the interleukins also act as signals to the brain: For example, IL-1 induces fever and sleep (Moldofsky 1989). Interleukin-1 is released during slow-wave sleep. Both IL-1 and Il-6 stimulate the release of CRF from the PVN.

Another peptide—the tumor necrosis factor-α—is released by cytotoxic cells to kill tumor cells. But it also causes fibroblast and epithelial cells to proliferate. It has broad executive functions during inflammation. It induces fever and sleep but suppresses appetite. It enhances the breakdown of collagen and bone and inhibits the enzyme lipoprotein lipase (Sporn and Roberts 1988).

The interferons (α-, β-, γ-) are a fourth class of peptides. Some are involved in combating viruses. Others augment the activity of those cells (e.g., NK) that combat virally infected cells. And one of them, interferon-α, also has effects on the brain: It alters mood and causes fever (Dinarello and Mier 1987; McDonald, Mann, and Thomas 1987).

The four groups of peptides produced by cells of the immune system have a broad spectrum of signal functions. While they alter the functional state of immunocompetent cells and are involved in protecting the organism against infected and malignant cells, they also regulate cell and tissue repair and modulate each other's activities. They thus act as bidirectional communication signals informing the organism of infection (i.e., by fever) and the presence of neoplasia. Their activation and expression are independent of the specific nature of the antigen. Other (the B- and plasma) cells of the immune system, however, generate specific antibody responses (Nossal 1987).

A discussion of the peptides does not end here. The immune system, though diffuse compared to other systems (solid organs), can regulate itself following its activation by an antigen (Smith 1988). But it does not exist sui generis (Bateman et al. 1989). It is part of a larger communication system, consisting of afferent and efferent loops that also entail the sympathetic and neuroendocrine systems: CRF acting through a noradrenergic sympathetic pathway suppresses NK-cell cytotoxicity (Irwin, Vale, and Britton 1987). The CRF may act via the LC—a source of sympathetic neurons. In fact, lesions of the LC reduce cellular immune responses. The two peptides VIP (Rola-Pleszczynski, Bolduc, and St.-Pierre 1985) and β-endorphin (Matthews et al. 1983) enhance this form of cellular cytotoxicity. The pituitary peptides—ACTH, GH, β-endorphin, PRL—affect various other immune functions, including antibody production and mitogenesis (Bernton, Meltzer, and Holaday 1987). Some other peptides—SP, VIP, STS, the enkephalins—have wide-ranging effects on the immune system (Shanahan and Anton 1988), as do the gonadal steroids (Grossman 1989).

In view of the broad effects of some of these peptides and steroids, one would expect them to alter patterns of lymphocyte function, involving migration, secretion, antibody production, and cytotoxicity, while indirectly influencing phagocytosis. In fact, many of the peptides and neuropeptides (e.g., insulin growth factors, SP, aVP, β-endorphin, GH) also regulate cell proliferation.

Equally consequential is that all lymphatic tissue and the thymus are densely innervated by sympathetic nerve fibers (Felten et al. 1985). Many different cells of the immune system have surface receptors for catecholamines and peptides.

But to complicate the matter further, immunocompetent cells, in addition to their autocrine, paracrine, and growth-promoting activities, also have hormonal functions. Messenger RNAs for POMC gene products are present in the thymus and spleen. Monocytes and macrophages produce ACTH and β-endorphin, but leukocytes do not (Bateman et al. 1989; Lolait et al. 1986; Smith and Blalock 1981). (These hormones may, however, only be secreted when the organism is threatened by infection.)

Furthermore, so-called thymosins are composed of a number of hormones and transforming factors for B-cells. They are produced by the thymus. This family of hormones stimulates ACTH, and thus corticosteroid, secretion (Bateman et al. 1989). The thymus also contains receptors for gonadal sex steroids. A reduction of both T and E_2 is thought to promote the expression of thymosins, which in turn stimulate LH production by their action of hypothalamic gonadotropin synthesis (Grossman 1989).

These data are relevant to the topic of stressful experience. Isolated female rats have diminished responses to mitogens and low E_2 levels. Crowding has the opposite effects (Joasoo and McKenzie 1976). But in male rats both procedures reduce this particular immune response.

To summarize: To date, the four classes of peptides produced by cells of the immune system have a positive and negative feedback effect on each other, recruiting and stimulating other components of the system, and modulating each other's actions. They also act in parallel. Yet each cell or component of the immune system is also closely integrated into a communication system of many peptide hormones and neurotransmitters with multiple and bidirectional interactions between each other, and between each and the brain.

Summary

The history of recent research on stressful experience, the new concepts that it has generated, and an explosion of knowledge about the systems that subserve the behavior and physiology of the organism during these have led to several generalizations. The behavioral and physiological responses of the organism to a particular stressful experience, unless overwhelming, are very specific (not general). They are also patterned. The varied patterns of cardiovascular changes, for example, are generated by separate and discrete neuronal circuits in the brain. Hormones are also secreted in a patterned manner in response to specific experiences. Their secretion subserves the metabolic and behavioral requirements of the organism in its efforts to survive and overcome danger and challenge. The regulation of autonomically mediated hormonal and immune patterns is carried out by a variety of peptides, catecholamines, and steroids present both in the brain and elsewhere in the body, acting locally and at a distance.

In addition to producing patterned physiological changes in a number of organ systems, peptides also regulate each other and are responsive to social and physical changes in the environment. Most important they integrate the behavior and the physiology of the organism.

The discovery of the peptides during the past twenty years has been revolutionary. New ones are daily being discovered. It has been calculated that there may be 1,500 or more yet-to-be-discovered peptides present in the brain and the body! This eventual plethora of peptides will pose an enormous intellectual challenge to those trying to understand and conceptualize their role in normal functioning, under conditions of stressful experience, and in the inception of illness and disease. In part that challenge is already upon us, and many difficult questions remain unanswered.

In view of the fact that several peptides are colocalized in the same neuron, what brings about the selective release of only one of them in response to a specific stressful experience (Gibbs 1986; Smelik 1985)? Is this selectivity determined by one of the many regulators of their release, such as the releasing or steroid hormones, the biogenic amines, or by the interactions at receptors (Meister and Hökfelt 1989; Reisine 1989; Sawchenko 1989)?

How is it possible that an intruding rat secretes only the peptide products of the intermediate lobe of the pituitary gland, while the home-cage rat has an increase in ACTH secretion, given that all of these peptides derive from a common precursor molecule? What determines the appropriate cleavage point of the precursor, POMC? Under what specific conditions does this occur other than those already mentioned?

Do specific contingencies and stressful experiences only promote the release of the stored peptides via one second messenger system, and not another (Drugan et al. 1989; Reisine 1989)? The potentiating interaction of CRF and aVP is known to be brought about because each peptide has its own second messenger system within corticotrophs. Other peptides inhibit each other's activities (CRF and the endorphins; CRF and TRH; STS and TRH).

To expand this thought somewhat: It may be necessary to classify the facilitatory and inhibitory actions of the peptides into two different kinds, either phasic or tonic. The opioid peptides, for example, phasically inhibit the products of the sympathoadrenal and pituitary-adrenal axes in humans during conditions associated with heightened activity such as mental arithmetic and exercise, the cold pressor test, or hypoglycemia (Bouloux and Grossman 1989). However, the opioid peptides also inhibit pituitary-adrenal function in a tonic manner. They constitute a local counterregulatory system to the production of some hormones (CRF, LH, and ACTH).

On the other hand, GH and/or PRL seem tonically to maintain normal levels of NK-cell activity (Grossman 1989; Bernton, Meltzer, and Holaday 1987), based on the following lines of evidence: The intraventricular CRF administration suppresses NK-cell cytotoxic activity. The reduction in cytotoxicity is averted by a sympathetic ganglionic blocking agent. Following hypophysectomy, intraventricular CRF has no such effect, and baseline NK-cell levels are reduced (Irwin, Vale, and Britton 1987). But PRL and GH raise the levels to normal. Thus peptides may have a tonic inhibitory function on some systems, and a tonic facilitatory function on others. They maintain baseline levels upon which phasic responses and circadian variations in levels are imposed.

Some peptides may have both tonic and phasic actions. The nerve growth factor (NGF) regulates the growth of sympathetic and sensory neurons. But it also tonically maintains the integrity of sympathetic neurons. This particular growth factor is regulated by T_4 and T. In fact, the content of NGF in the salivary glands in the male mouse is six times greater than in the female (Levi-Montalcini 1987). Usually, NGF does not appear in detectable amounts in the bloodstream (Aloe et al. 1986). Injection of NGF causes an increase in the size of sympathetic neurons, the weight and size of the adrenal glands, the induction of TH in the adrenal medulla, and the release of renin.

Another major intellectual task confronting investigators of stressful experience is to understand how its perception leads to the release of brain peptides. An important beginning to answering this question is the mapping of the input circuitry to the PVN from sensory receptors on the surface of the body (Feldman 1989). These circuits are in turn mediated by different neurotransmitters. Hypothalamic noradrenergic neurons mediate photic, acoustic, and painful stimuli, whereas serotonergic neurons transmit information after sciatic and limbic stimulation. Both amines lead to the release of CRF from the PVN. The CRF neurons in the parvocellular portion of the PVN are in turn inhibited by corticosteroids—an effect partially mediated by the hippocampus. In some PVN neurons CRF and aVP are colocalized, and the release of aVP from the PVN is in part regulated by atriopeptin.

10 New Concepts about the Organism and Its Perturbation by Stressful Experience

In the course of reviewing the historical development of research on, and the concepts about, stressful experience, the generality and nonspecificity of Selye's formulations were emphasized. Regardless of the individual nature of the injury to his rats a virtually invariant triad of pathoanatomical lesions was produced, mediated by a general reaction (the GAS). Little or no attention was paid either to the fact that the agents of injury were unavoidable or to the behavior of his animals.

Much of the subsequent research on stressful experience concerned itself with measuring single behavioral and physiological variables—acute changes in levels of HR, systolic or mean BP, or a hormone, a catecholamine, or its metabolites; or changes in one or another immune variable (e.g., responses of lymphocytes to a mitogen, or the cytotoxic activity of NK cells) (chapter 4). Mason (1968) studied unfolding patterns of hormone secretion, or excretion, over time. Finally, as our knowledge has advanced, the focus of research has shifted to the study of the generation of behavioral and physiological patterns by the brain (chapter 4), which are the product of multiple regulatory processes.

The principle guiding this line of investigation was initially to isolate independent/dependent variables at one point in time, rather than to study the covariances of interacting systems over time. A principal purpose in writing this book is to explicate the nature of these interacting systems, which are tied together in communication systems, or networks, in the organism.

As soon as it was realized that stressful experiences need not only be equated with overwhelming injury and infection, it became apparent that disease was not their inevitable outcome (chapters 4, 5, 6). This conclusion was especially true when experiences could be anticipated, prevented, avoided, or mastered. Structural damage to the organism may be direct, or it occurs when experiences are novel, unexpected, unavoidable, and repetitive, or the avoidant responses to them are punished.

Stressful experiences are part and parcel of the daily lives of humans and animals. Most adult persons master challenge, change, threat, and danger; because all organisms differ from each other, some, however, do not cope with, or overcome, them (chapter 4). The most likely outcomes when the endeavor fails are ill health, changes in behavior, anxiety, and depression, but not necessarily disease (chapter 5). Chronic, unpleasant, uncontrollable, demanding experiences, upon which acute ones may or may not be superimposed, are especially likely to have adverse consequences, such as depression and IHD (chapter 6).

In most instances, stressful experiences are followed by coordinated and integrated response patterns designed to prevent injury and to promote survival; they have evolved over millions of years. They are presumably conserved because they have been successful. Animals solve problems—they build nests; attack, submit to, or flee enemies, competitors, and predators; and patrol and defend their territory and young. They anticipate nightfall and changes in the seasons. They respond with appropriate actions to very specific external and internal signals, depending on the context in which they are buried. The physiological patterns are designed to enhance the blood supply to muscles and the brain; provide immediately available sources of energy to organs according to need; mount an antibody and cellular response to the specific antigens of infectious agents or allergens; signal the organism of impending disease while promoting tissue repair; and clear the agent from the body. The immune patterns are specific to the nature of the (antigen) signal. Cardiovascular patterns also are. They differ in preparation for fighting a threatening antagonist, during actual combat, and after it. The behavior and the physiology of organisms to stressful experiences cannot be decomposed; they are inseparable.

As this more comprehensive perspective to behavior and physiology is taken, new questions arise about the generation of patterns and about the integration of behavior and physiology. Very specific tasks and the coordinated patterns they elicit are subserved by different neuronal circuits in the brain. The peptides, on the other hand, carry out the task of integrating behavior and physiology in very specific ways (chapter 9). Even E has broad metabolic effects, which are obscured by studying only its actions on the cardiovascular system. But in addition, E is part of a complex interactive network involving CRF, ACTH, the corticosteroids, glucagon, insulin, and several biosynthetic and hepatic enzymes. It acts at the cell surface by two (not only one) receptors and second messenger systems (chapter 8).

The study of patterned changes in levels of E obscures the complexity of the interactions of this communication signal. Epinephrine is in turn but part of a larger intra- and extracellular communication system. The regulation of the production of signals is remarkably complex; most of the peptide hormones released from the pituitary gland (e.g., CRF, GH, and PRL) are under multiple negative, positive, and mixed feedback control (chapter 9). Furthermore, every one of them is frequency-modulated—it functions in a rhythmic manner over time. Rhythms are lost sight of by measuring changes in levels of the variable of interest, or its peak value. Little attention is paid in such studies to deviations and variations about a baseline, or about a mean, value. The rhythmic nature of the variable—a hormone or neurotransmitter—is obscured by the manner in which it is sampled, analyzed, and reduced.

Many examples of changes in rhythms with stressful experiences have been given throughout this book (chapters 5, 6, 7, 8). These new insights about the behavior and physiology of organisms have necessitated a shift in concepts. The various rhythms of sleep, body temperature, potassium excretion, cortisol, hGH and PRL, etc., covary and interact. They are generated by interacting oscillators consisting of cell groups within the brain. Rhythms are also observed within many individual cells (Berridge and Irvine 1989). They characterize the behaviors of cells: Mitosis, for example, is a cyclic process.

Rhythms are additionally produced by negative, positive, and mixed feedback systems (chapters 2, 6, 8). The interactive nature of signals operating in a rhythmic manner makes their perturbation likely. The subsystems of the organism that generate the fluctuating signals are in constant communication with each other; together they compose the organism. Because the organism is also in continuous communication with the dynamic environment, the subsystems appropriately respond when conditions change.

These perturbations, to which Bernard (1865) had alluded, require new ways of measurement and new concepts. They may be represented and modeled in terms of changes in form, frequency, and amplitude of a variable acting in a rhythmic manner, and not only in terms of its altered levels (chapters 5, 6, 7). Transformed rhythms characterize many states of ill health and disease. They reflect altered function, and not only structure.

In the remainder of this chapter, these assertions will further be specified and documented.

The Nature of the Organism

Stressful experiences should be studied in an organismic manner. They cannot be understood from a single categorical perspective—behavioral, psychological, or physiological. To restrict oneself to one or other of these three disciplines is to neglect biology.

However, it is incumbent on anyone who holds to an integrated biological point of view to present some vision of what constitutes the organism: One may not merely hide behind vague holistic concepts. A notion, concept, or theory must be presented that defines the organism in its full panoply of functions. A consistent language must be spoken to describe it. Should this be possible, a different and unified way of conceptualizing and speaking about stressful experiences might be found.

The organism is a dynamic evolving system, and not merely an anatomical structure. It exists in an ever-changing environment. A dynamic system is one best described by a series of interrelated subsystems that also function in a rhythmic manner over time. To repeat, the interrelationship of the subsystems is brought about by a large variety of communication signals emitted in a regular, or irregular, rhythmic manner and arranged in a series of feedback loops (chapters 2, 9). Stressful experience perturbs these rhythms (chapters 5, 6) and may result in illness and disease. As rhythms are perturbed they undergo transitions to different modes over a period of time. Some of these transitions are also brought about by altered communication between cells, organs, or the organism and its environment. Dynamic biological systems and changes in them are best modeled by nonlinear mathematics (Garfinkel 1983; Glass and Mackey 1988; Rapp 1979).

Further progress in conceiving the organism in this way will depend on the design of studies of covariances of behavioral and physiological patterns carried out over various time scales, and not only in terms of covariates. More data is needed about these patterns and how they are affected by perturbing the organism or one of its subsystems. The transition in patterns to new rhythmic forms characterizes changes in function, which in turn lead to alterations in structure, or, conversely, and in some still poorly understood and incomplete manner, result from structural alterations (Glass and Mackey 1988).

The most important feature of the behavior of complex biological systems is not any single feature, or their material components per se, but the interrelationship and interconnections between their subsystems. According to this view the organism is seen as an intricate communication system of information exchange by means of signals, which regulates its own behavior and that of its components—genes, cells, and organs. Cells communicate with one another by many different kinds of coded messenger signals (chapters 8, 9). By these means cells influence their own and each other's activities locally and at a distance. The emissions of these signals are themselves carefully regulated.

These messenger signals reach other cells where they are transduced by membrane-bound structures—specialized receptors, coupling proteins, and permeable ion channels. At these membrane structures the signal is integrated with a variety of other modulating signals, external or internal to the cell. The signal is transformed into the digital language of ion channels, leading to changes in the electrical potential of the cell membrane. This transformation is carried forward in the interior of the cell by a series of interconnected second messenger systems, often acting in parallel. The second messenger system may activate a cascade of enzymes (Nishizuka 1986) or other biochemical reactions, and indirectly induce, or suppress, gene expression. However, some (steroid) messenger signals directly switch genes on or off. Genes encode protein products. The initiation and expression of genes, and the activity of enzymes and the messenger system, are also closely regulated.

The output signal (e.g., secretion of a hormone, contraction or change in the electrical properties of a muscle) from the cell matches the input signal; it is the computed product of a variety of regulatory processes. The signal may influence the cell that emitted it, as well as neighboring and distant cells. Organs regulate their own activities and each other's to carry out their specialized functions. Many specialized messenger signals (e.g., peptides) are produced by, or act upon, the brain through a variety of channels to regulate behavioral patterns, or to integrate them with the appropriate change in physiological patterns (chapter 9).

Every cell and organ is a subsystem of a larger, complex communication system. In these systems and at every level, parallel processing of signals occurs (chapters 7, 9). The ultimate test of the thesis is to determine whether the same principles apply to the brain and its functions. It is generally accepted that the brain, composed as it is of 10^{14} neurons, some of which have 10^4 synaptic connections, is the most complex communication system of all. One of the brain's essential features is the parallel processing of signals. An "intelligent" system of multiple translation, integration, and processing characterizes most of its activities.

The organism is integrated into a larger system of information exchange mediated by the brain. The brain receives signals from every part of the body and from the environment. Visual inputs and images (e.g., gestures and postures) are also transduced and digitized into the "language" of membrane potentials, as are smells, tastes, sounds, tactile sensations, changes in environmental temperature, the position of body parts, etc., and the multiple chemical and mechanical (e.g., pressure) signals that emanate from the interior of the body. By parallel processing, and by the integration of all of these subsystems, an intelligent, self-regulating organism is established. The brain and the rest of the organism are not qualitatively different in their ability to compute information, but show only quantitative differences in their purposiveness.

The organism's task is ultimately to survive and reproduce. These activities can be carried out in many different ways and by many different brains, which have evolved not only to respond selectively to external signals (chapter 9) but also to the context in which these are buried.

The received signals are coded digitally in afferent (sensory) nerves to spinal pathways whose transmitters are amino acids and peptides. Other signals emanate from every organ, solid or hollow (e.g., the gut), via sympathetic and vagal afferent inputs. The brain monitors the metabolic activity of the body. Some of the metabolic and hormonal signals have direct contact with the brain in those tiny areas (e.g., the area postrema and the subfornical organ) where no blood-brain barrier exists. Other signals are selectively passed through the barrier. The brain monitors the height of an antigen-antibody response occurring in the body. It integrates each of these signals. Many examples of these processing and integrative activities have already been presented earlier in this book during the discussion of reproduction (chapter 7): Ovulation is ultimately regulated in parallel in the preoptic and arcuate nuclei of the hypothalamus *and* the anterior pituitary gland. The secretion of GnRH, LH, and FSH generates a patterned output (in the rat) consisting of both ovulation and mating behavior. The brain thus integrates and coordinates the appropriate behavior with the relevant physiology.

The integrated behavioral-physiological response patterns are specific and appropriate to the external signal and the context in which it appears. A particular perturbing experience elicits a pattern of hormonal responses that differs depending on the nature of the challenge (Gibbs 1986). Much remains to be learned about the manner in which signals perturb or activate hormonal or behavioral pattern generators. Patterned behavioral and cardiovascular responses to signals and contingencies are subserved by separate neuronal circuits (chapter 8), but the (control) pattern generators of each of these circuits remain to be identified.

In lower vertebrates sequential motor patterns are released by very specific signals (Tinbergen 1951). They are closely regulated. They start and stop appropriately. In humans they may also be generated "at will." Motor patterns are the product of millions of neurons with huge numbers of degrees of freedom; yet the patterns take a coherent, organized, relatively simple (rhythmic) form (such as swimming) (McLennan and Grillner 1984).

Although the brain has usually been considered to control movement, its more interesting function is to generate actions—integrated, purposeful behavior patterns, subserving critical biological functions such as mating or attacking an enemy. In species other than the rat, behavioral and physiological mating patterns are also under the control of a variety of external signals. But such variations in detail do not vitiate the argument. Many other actions are acquired, and with practice become automatized; their purposiveness is nevertheless obvious.

One of the major advances in knowledge of recent years answers questions about the manner in which physiological patterns are generated by the brain. As mentioned, cardiovascular response patterns are under the control of separate and very specific neuronal circuits (chapter 9). And many of the behavioral and physiological patterns are also generated by the brain through the medium of peptide signals, which either promote, modify, or modulate each other's effects.

The mind-brain can also modify its own intrinsic physiological—not only the body's—activities. Persons can learn to increase their brain electrical rhythms and thus diminish their epileptic seizures (Sterman 1982). They can also learn to regularize tetanic contractions of their esophagus, abnormal breathing patterns, and some altered cardiac rhythms and can learn to correct a deficit in contraction of the anorectal sphincter (Whitehead and Schuster 1985).

The brain also generates its own signals, which inform it of its own state so that appropriate action is taken. It is capable of responding both selectively to one aspect of, or in toto to, external and internal signals depending on the context in which they occur. The response pattern is also regulated and appropriate to both the signal and its context. The organism can also control its own behavior in response to an internal signaling system (the emotions) informing it of its own state—i.e., whether it is in danger, angry, about to be discovered or injured, sexually receptive, hungry, or in need of sleep. It emits signals: These coded signals (though not necessarily chemical) are communicated from, and between, organisms by behavior (such as postures and gestures), sounds, smells, and by verbal and nonverbal means. Furthermore, behavior is not only self-regulated but is also regulated by others—especially when the organism is young (Hofer 1984)—institutions, and groups.

To summarize, the organism is a complex, self-regulating, communication system tied together by messenger signals of a number of categories. Their emission is variously regulated; and they are in turn involved in the self-regulation of cells, organs, and behaviors. The particular task (e.g., mating, submitting, fleeing) the organism must accomplish will determine the messenger signals that are emitted, and their duration. The speed with which it is accomplished is limited by the velocity of information exchange (e.g., neural transmission), the distance between organs, and the presence or absence of a veridical signal "protected" against background noise.

The principles that govern the communication between cells and the coordination of, and changes in, behavior and physiology are the result of altered, rhythmic patterns of messenger signals and changes in the state of the organism, not of any single signal. The second major principle characterizing organisms is their remarkable stability over time. (Yet at the same time they grow, change, and regenerate.) This stability may arise in a self-organized manner, without necessarily needing externally imposed commands (Eigen 1971).

In searching for a common language to describe these phenomena, the biological sciences have begun to borrow a mathematical language that describes the dynamics of nonlinear systems. These systems display self-organization, stability, and fluctuation (change). Neurobiologists have developed neuronal network theory and have also laid down the principles of parallel (distributed) information processing in the brain.

One of the most promising attempts to explain pattern generation in biological and behavioral systems—i.e., the behavior of cells, organs, or populations—is the mathematical concept of self-organization in nonlinear systems. Without going into detail, nonlinear characterization defines the conditions for stability, fluctuation, and phase transitions into other stable conditions, or those that favor the emergence of new properties of a system. Cooperative effects in nature, such as coordination and pattern generation, are typically independent of the particular molecular machinery or the material substrate that underlies them. Two examples illustrate this point. The first is locomotion, which is fundamentally a rhythmically coordinated pattern shared by most living animals. It is carried out by a wide variety of anatomical structures and neural mechanisms. Nonetheless, it is possible to understand and derive rhythmic locomotoric patterns by mathematical means once certain variables are computed with the help of nonlinear dynamics. The second is the phenomenon of complex cardiac arrhythmias such as atrioventricular block or fibrillation. They can be predicted and simulated using nonlinear mathematics. In contrast to the traditional approach that characterizes the regulation of various ion channels to explain cardiac electrical behavior, this mathematical approach achieves the same solution by conceptualizing the heart as a nonlinear system obeying complex dynamics. One need not necessarily know the details of the ionic mechanisms underlying the disturbance to understand the complex changes in rhythm that are generated by an excitable system (Winfree 1987). Nonlinear mathematics has also been applied to understanding a range of living and even nonliving systems—from the opening of plasma membrane ion channels, the firing patterns of neurons, the behavior of neuronal networks, and gastrointestinal motility rhythms, to complex human behaviors.

A second approach that has enlightened our understanding of signal transmission is the concept of the parallel processing of information by the brain (DeYoe and Van Essen 1988). Rather than drawing a homology between the brain and computers, computer scientists are now designing computers to mimic the brain's use of parallel (distributed) processing—a principle that evolved over millions of years. The great majority of conventional computers achieve their task by breaking it down into innumerable individual components, which are then processed sequentially in a linear decision-making manner. By using huge numbers of progressively more miniaturized computer elements both the size and the speed of today's computers have increased enormously. Despite the fact that the brain's individual neurons are apparently millions of times slower than electronic "neurons" (the microprocessors of the computer), nature has accomplished rapid computation by using the principle of parallel processing. This approach achieves its result by handling simultaneously all of the information in many parallel channels. Each channel also has direct access to a memory bank. Experimental work with prototypes of parallel processing computers demonstrates that different types of computations require their own pattern of connections, and that each processor must be able to communicate with another. Relevant also to the discussion is the fact that in some of these prototypes there are many equally efficient— apparently "redundant"—routes of communication between any pair of processors. If one route is already occupied in the transmission of a signal, the computer will "select" an alternate route by processing the information in a different sequence. Parallel processing not only increases computational speed by several orders of magnitude, but it displays other "biological" properties: complexity and flexibility!

Parallel processing of information enables a computational system to deal with the most complex problems in a flexible way—a characteristic of organisms. In addition, it increases the speed of the computation and reduces the size of the computational system. The ability to process information in parallel depends critically on the number of connections between individual processors, i.e., the amount of information exchange through communication channels. Furthermore, the behavior of such a machine does not obey the rules of linear decision-making, but it can be characterized in nonlinear mathematical terms.

The Mode of Operation of Communication Signals

Oscillations, Pacemakers, and Feedback Systems

Every cell, organ, and organism is under the control of multiple messenger signals, and each signal is the final product of an exactly computed process. These multiple signals and the information contained in them are processed in parallel. Therefore, parallel processing occurs in cells other than neurons, and in organs other than the brain. Redundancy is a characteristic of biological systems, such as circulation, but the meaning of this fact remains unclear. Although redundancy assures speed and flexibility, alternative explanations of its evolution have been put forward: It may express a "fail safe" system: Redundant signaling systems and circuits are only brought into play in unusual, extreme, or unexpected situations, or when one of several circuits fails, in order to assure the organism's survival (chapter 9). No consensus on this matter has been reached.

Communication Systems and Regulation

The principles of regulation, communication within and between genes, cells, and organs, and redundancy are everywhere present in nature. Information exchange between the organism and the social and physical environment is crucial for its survival and for reproduction. Yet the precise signals employed in the exchange are species-specific.

As the details of the communication systems within the organism have been elucidated, insights have been obtained about the integration of behavior and physiology within the organism. These principles will next be discussed.

Interaction of the Mediators of Stressful Experience with Self-Regulatory Functions of Cells and Organs

The communication systems within the brain and body consist of a multitude of signals of many different types (e.g., calcium ions, glucose, FFAs, steroid and peptide hormones, biogenic amines, and amino acids), which act as transmitters and modulators. The main communication systems are usually divided into four main classes—neural (both somatic and autonomic), neuroendocrine, endocrine, and immune. But as we have already seen, they cannot so neatly be compartmentalized (chapters 8, 9). They are actually in continuous interaction with each other. Many of these signals serve many different functions (chapters 8, 9). They are exquisitely responsive to, and coordinate and mediate the perturbations brought about by, stressful challenges, changes, tasks, and experience. They protect the organism against possibly life-threatening infection and injury. They promote the repair and regeneration of damaged tissue. They have wide-ranging, diverse, and rather specific behavioral effects—alerting the organism, promoting and subserving attack and defensive behavior or sleep, and influencing food intake and mating behaviors.

The organism is tied together by a complex communication system consisting of these signals. Left out in this account so far is that these signal-mediators of patterned responses are themselves regulated by positive, negative, and mixed feedback systems acting in parallel. These signals interact with other cells and cell groups, but they also regulate themselves in an autocrine manner. Some genes also have the function of regulating or suppressing the activities of other genes (Sager 1989). The induction of structural genes is also tightly regulated (Pardee 1989), as is their transcription to messenger RNA by at least five binding proteins (transcription factors) and by elongation factors external to them (Carcamo et al. 1989).

Self-Regulation of Genes, Cells, and Organs

Regulation of the Gene and Its Enzyme Product

The concepts of self-regulation and regulation are in part the result of an understanding of how gene activity is governed. The gene consists of the four constituent nucleotides (in groups of three) that code for amino acids. It is activated by substrates, steroid and peptide hormones and other signals. In the absence of substrate—the signal—the structural gene that codes for a protein is quiescent. Coding takes place in a discontinuous manner. In the presence of the signal the gene is induced, or repressed. Activation occurs indirectly through the medium of a protein "repressor" to which the substrate binds (somewhat as a neurotransmitter binds to its postsynaptic receptor). In the absence of the substrate-signal, the repressor is bound to a section of the chromosome known as the operator, which in turn inhibits gene expression. When substrate is present, the repressor undergoes a change in conformation and becomes detached from the operator, and the gene is said to be induced. The repressor is itself the product of a (regulator) gene (Jacob and Monod 1961). Other signals—e.g., sex steroids known to induce protein synthesis (ovalbumin in the oviduct, or pituitary hormones)—operate in a more complex manner by dissociating two receptor proteins, one of which then binds to "response" elements on the gene (Baulieu 1989).

The products of structural genes are proteins, including enzymes. The activity of an enzyme may also be regulated by the end-product of a sequence of enzymes; end-product)i.e. feedback) inhibition of the initial enzyme occurs8e.g., the enzyme th is inhibited by da or ne acting indirectly on th's cofactor.)th is also regulated by other means; whether it is phosphorylated or not, and whether it is free in the cytoplasm or bound to the inner aspect of the cell membrane.) in other instances, the synthesized end-product may activate the repressor, and enzyme synthesis itself ceases when the structural gene for the enzyme becomes inactive. in still others systems, both regulatory processes may occur; repression of enzyme synthesis mediated by messenger RNA at the level of the gene, and inhibition of the activity of the enzyme by the synthesized end-product (e.g., of the enzyme threonine deaminase by isoleucine). The site of inhibition of the enzyme's activity is separate from the catalytic site. Such enzymes and the repressor are called allosteric proteins, which are regulators of synthesis of amino acids, neurotransmitters, enzymes, and proteins (Monod, Changeux, and Jacob 1963).

The topic of gene regulation is actually much more complex. Genes regulate other genes. Furthermore, the whole concept of a gene has undergone revision since the discovery was made that several exons cooperate to produce one protein (e.g., an immunoglobulin or a receptor protein). Two genes can code for the same protein, which may exist in more than one conformation.

Genes, as is well known, code for enzymes that participate in the synthesis of several classes of messenger signals; for the prohormones of peptides, which play a prominent role in information exchange; and for proteins that are assembled to act as receptors for messenger signals.

Regulation and Self-Regulation at the Cellular Level

Communication signals exist within and between cells. Cells regulate their own (autocrine) and each other's (paracrine) activities. The information that reaches the cell from other cells and its own surroundings may first be translated at the cell membrane into a "digital" signal, a translation that is accomplished by either the opening or closing of ion channels and/or the depolarization of the cell membrane. The signal is also transduced into intracellular signals consisting of the second messenger systems (Berridge and Irvine 1989; Gilman 1987; Low and Saltiel 1987; Nishizuka 1986).

Some ion channels (e.g., sodium and calcium) are voltage-dependent, and some are not, being opened and closed by neurotransmitters and/or hormones. Some are both. The regulation of some ion channels is also multiple. Furthermore, ion channels exist in families; for instance, several potassium channels are known to exist (Dolly 1988). Ions such as sodium and potassium can indirectly change the permeability of the cell membrane: Extracellular potassium, for example, opens the voltage-dependent ion channel for calcium. A rise in intracellular calcium concentration can in some cases close an ion channel, or activate an enzyme that phosphorylates the channel protein to shut it. Some hormones will activate enzymes bound to the inner cell membrane,

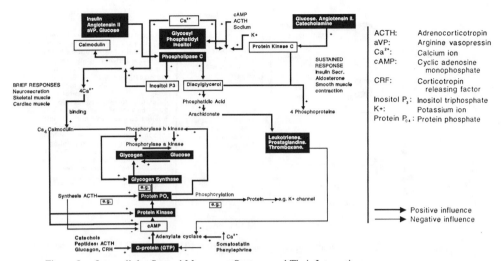

Figure 8. Intracellular Second Messenger Systems and Their Interactions

which in the presence of a specific ion (e.g., calcium) will mobilize one or more second messenger systems in parallel (Low and Saltiel 1987; Reisine 1989).

Ion channels consist of proteins bridging the cell membrane (Dolly 1988). They can be an integral part of the receptor structure, or they can be a separate membrane protein, which is connected to the receptor via intracellular or intramembranous coupling mechanisms.

Ion channels are selectively permeable to one ion, or several different ions, such as sodium, calcium, potassium, or chloride. The opening of such channels depends on changes in voltage on the surface membrane; others are regulated by ions such as intracellular calcium, changes in intracellular pH, or a variety of intracellular messengers (Rasmussen 1986). Ion currents through protein channels in cell membranes underlie nerve transmission (Hodgkin and Huxley 1952) and the activity of pacemaker cells in the heart, brain, and gut (Glass and Mackey 1988).

Other classes of receptors exist: Cholesterol is transported into the cell by clathrin-coated "pits." Steroid hormones somehow cross the cell membrane to bind to an intracellular, cytosolic receptor, which transports them to the cell nucleus (Baulieu 1989) where they promote or inhibit peptide or protein synthesis.

Still another class of receptors changes the metabolic machinery of the postsynaptic cell by releasing compounds (e.g., enzymes) bound to the cell membrane. These in turn stimulate the regulated synthesis of several second messenger systems—calmodulin, cAMP, cyclic guanosine 5'-monophosphate (cGMP), 1,2-diacylglycerol, IP_3, and multiple forms of protein kinase(s) C.

These second messengers (e.g., diacylglycerol–protein kinase C) relay the

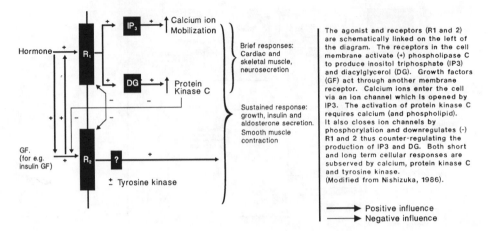

The agonist and receptors (R1 and 2) are schematically linked on the left of the diagram. The receptors in the cell membrane activate (+) phospholipase C to produce inositol triphosphate (IP3) and diacylglycerol (DG). Growth factors (GF) act through another membrane receptor. Calcium ions enter the cell via an ion channel which is opened by IP3. The activation of protein kinase C requires calcium (and phospholipid). It also closes ion channels by phosphorylation and downregulates (-) R1 and 2 thus counter-regulating the production of IP3 and DG. Both short and long term cellular responses are subserved by calcium, protein kinase C and tyrosine kinase.
(Modified from Nishizuka, 1986).

⟶ Positive influence
⟶ Negative influence

Figure 9.   Regulation and Counterregulation of Receptors and Three Second Messenger Systems

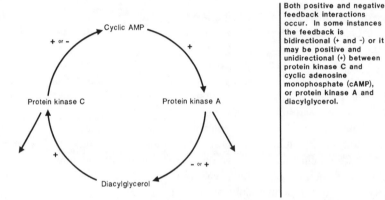

Both positive and negative feedback interactions occur. In some instances the feedback is bidirectional (+ and -) or it may be positive and unidirectional (+) between protein kinase C and cyclic adenosine monophosphate (cAMP), or protein kinase A and diacylglycerol.

Figure 10.   Feedback Regulation and the Interaction of Two Intracellular Second Messenger Systems

effects of catecholamines, glucose, and a variety of peptide hormones and growth factors, while at the same time they promote the secretion of enzymes (e.g., amylase), acetylcholine, catecholamines (e.g., DA, E, and NE), peptide hormones (e.g., ACTH, LH, PRL, GH, TSH, and insulin), steroid hormones (e.g., T, aldosterone); incite muscular contraction, gastric acid, and mucous secretion; release prostaglandins from platelets, histamine from mast cells; and activate lymphocytes (Nishizuka 1986).

The protein kinases C phosphorylate at least 45 different proteins and enzymes. Some of these are receptor proteins (e.g., the β-adrenergic, IL-2, and insulin receptors); others are membrane proteins (e.g., the sodium channel protein, and sodium/potassium ATPase), contractile proteins, enzymes (e.g., guanylate cyclase, TH, cytochrome P450), and proteins such as fibrinogen and the class of heat stress proteins. Protein kinases C are involved in the regulation of α_1-adrenergic, AT-II, and some growth-factor cell-surface receptors, and in the degradation of IP_3. And protein kinases C can both enhance and counterregulate the actions of cAMP, while the cAMP–protein kinases A system counteracts the diacylglycerol–protein kinases C cascade.

Of particular interest is that a hormone, such as ACTH, will activate a dual system: It strongly increases the generation of cAMP and weakly stimulates calcium influx. Potassium has the opposite effect. In the liver, cAMP (by inducing the production of the enzyme glycogen synthase) enhances glycogen storage and counteracts the calcium-calmodulin-regulated phosphorylase-a kinase enhancement of glucogenesis (chapter 8). Therefore, and in addition to counterregulatory intracellular processes, a parallel-processing system is present in cells. A system of this kind may be very subtle: It may be activated in series depending on the strength of the signal. When a neutrophil is exposed to a chemotactic peptide (f-Met-Leu-Phe) at low doses, the calmodulin system only is activated; at higher doses, the protein kinase C system is set in motion (Rasmussen 1986).

The principles of function enumerated here—signaling, regulation, modulation, and redundancy—apply at every level of organization.

Intracellular Regulation

In recent years, the central role of intracellular calcium in a wide variety of physiological processes, including muscle contraction and the secretion of steroid and peptide hormones, has been discovered. The cell is remarkably sensitive to fluctuations in the concentration of intracellular calcium. It main-

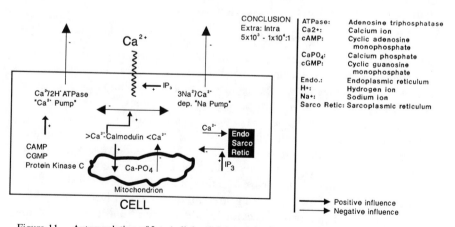

Figure 11.   Autoregulation of Intracellular Calcium (after Rasmussen 1986)

tains a very high concentration gradient between its external surroundings and its interior. Intracellular calcium concentration is carefully regulated. As its concentration rises within the cell, two enzyme transport systems are enhanced by three of the second messenger systems to expel the ion from the cell cytoplasm; more cytosolic calcium ions are taken up and inactivated within the mitochondrion and/or are bound to the endoplasmic and sarcoplasmic reticulum of (some) cells. When needed, however, the ion is liberated from its bonds by an IP_3 receptor–mediated mechanism as cytoplasmic calcium concentrations fall (Berridge and Irvine 1989; Rasmussen 1986).

Extracellular Self-Regulation of the Cell

The secretion of a neurotransmitter is a good example of the way a (nerve) cell regulates its own output signal. Once released in quanta from nerve terminals into the synaptic cleft, under the influence of calcium influx, the transmitter-signal binds to its special receptor, diffuses, and/or is degraded by a specific enzyme. But more important (for the self-regulatory principle), it is also taken up again by a receptor on the nerve terminal that released it. It is then stored for future use. The transport of choline (enzymatically cleaved from acetylcholine) back into the (presynaptic) nerve terminal is carried out by a voltage-dependent process in which calcium is bound by (membrane-bound) calmodulin, which in concert with a transporter returns choline to its storage vesicle. Other transmitter molecules have more specific high affinity receptors on the nerve terminal that passes them back into the neuron.

Other cells both secrete a specific chemical (e.g., a peptide) and synthesize and express the specific receptor for it on their surface: A T-lymphocyte activated by antigen expresses a receptor for the peptide IL-2. At the same time it secretes IL-2 to stimulate its own cell division and replication (Smith 1988). Interferon-α, another peptide produced by NK cells, enhances its own cytolytic activity via its own specific receptor (Dinarello and Mier 1987).

The Regulation of Cell Receptors

Three regulatory processes for receptors have been described: Ion channels undergo conformational changes so that they may either be in the open, closed, or desensitized state. An agonist, such as acetylcholine, will open an ion channel to allow the inward passage of sodium ions. The acetylcholine channel is closed when the agonist-signal is removed, or by phosphorylation. Closure may be more long-lasting (desensitization) due to raised intracellular calcium ion levels, the action of certain drugs or peptides (such as thymopoietin), or (in disease) an antibody against the channel protein. On the other hand, SP may counteract the desensitization of the nicotinic acetylcholine receptor in the adrenal medulla during stressful experience (Livett et al. 1989). The cytosolic glucocorticoid receptor is "mopped up" and translocated toward the nucleus, making the cell resistant to cortisol when high levels of the corticosteroid are present in serum (Lowy et al. 1988). The number of membrane receptors may be either increased or decreased. In the presence of high levels of an agonist the number or response of these receptors may diminish. When the quantum of the agonist is decreased, or is unavailable, the number of receptors may increase. However, receptor number or response sensitivity is not only under the control of its specific agonist-signal. As noted, T_3 increases the number of β-adrenergic receptors in the heart, and possibly in the brain (chapter 8). And E_2 increases the number of receptors for progesterone in the pituitary gland (chapter 2).

Receptor activity and function are also under the influence of a wide variety of other signals emanating from every level of organization, including environmental ones, and are modified by the behavioral state of the organism. The potassium and calcium ion channels are under multiple and antagonistic regulatory influences. A specific potassium channel on smooth muscle (M-current) is both transmitter-regulated and counterregulated, and voltage-sensitive. The calcium channel is both externally and internally regulated, through the medium of G-proteins, adenylate cyclase, and cAMP, by glycosyl phosphatidyl inositol, IP_3, arachidonic acid, and protein kinases C, as well as by intracellular calcium concentrations. It is opened by isoproterenol and cAMP but closed by the muscarinic action of acetylcholine, SP, bradykinin, and LHRH. These multiple influences on the channel, some of which emanate from afar (e.g., sympathetic nerves and the pituitary gland), interact to modulate each other's actions. The same statement is true for the GABA receptor and channel, which is bound to another protein, the benzodiazepine (BZD) receptor, to form a complex. Gamma-aminobutyric acid opens the ion channel to allow the influx of chloride ion into the cell, thereby heightening its negative intracellular electrical potential. The action of GABA is blocked by antagonists such as picrotoxin and bicuculline. The binding of BZDs to their own receptor alters the conformation of the chloride ion channel and augments the action of GABA. Barbiturates and alcohol seem to act directly upon the channel to promote chloride influx. Analgesic steroids (derived from both sex- and corticosteroids) apparently act through the BZD receptor to exert their effects. When rats are crowded together in cages BZD binding is increased. Conversely, shocking the feet of rats with electrical current diminishes binding in the hippocampus and cerebral cortex, and thus lowers the influx of chloride into the cell (Drugan et al. 1989).

Although we do not understand the signals that mediate the effects of group-housing or foot shock on the BZD receptor, these observations alert us to the fact that very specific experiences to which animals are subjected influence receptors. Such experiences may be naturally occurring ones: The binding of 5-HT to rat brain membranes exhibits circadian variation, being highest at midnight and lowest at noon. Serum concentrations of 5-HT show an inverse pattern. Sleep deprivation affects 5-HT binding, reducing it markedly at

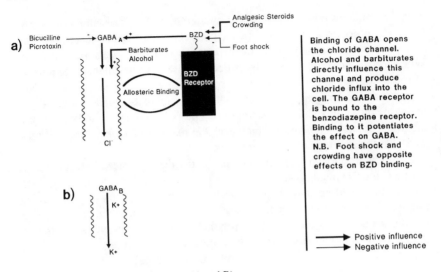

Figure 12.   The Two GABA Receptors (A and B)

about the halfway point (0700 hours) between the peak and the trough of its binding activity (Weseman et al. 1983).

In another system, the pineal gland of the rat, melatonin synthesis is also highest at night. Melatonin is a product of 5-HT. The activity of its biosynthetic enzyme, hydroxy-indole-O-methyl transferase, is greatest in the dark and inhibited by light. The biosynthesis of melatonin is also regulated by sympathetic activity: Norepinephrine promotes it; the activity of NE is greatest at night.

We have seen then that cells regulate their own activity by a series of internal messengers, which in turn are under the control of signal transducers: the receptors. These in turn are regulated and modulated in an exquisite and complex manner by many influences, including the behavior of the organism and environmental changes.

Cells Regulate Each Other

The focus of discussion has so far been on autocrine processes. A number of paracrine processes have been mentioned in passing—the effect of one nerve cell upon (a) another via synaptic signaling mechanisms, (b) smooth and striated muscle cells, (c) endocrine cells, and (d) splenic lymphocytes via sympathetic neurons.

However, adjacent cells also influence each other in a number of other ways. Their outer cell membranes are contiguous. They communicate with, and influence each other through gap junctions, which relay electrical and multiple chemical signals. Adjacent cells on contact inhibit each other's further growth, presumably by junctional communication, which appears to be regulated by a specific membrane-bound enzyme, tyrosine kinase. When the level of this enzyme is enhanced by a potential oncogenic virus, cell-to-cell communication diminishes (Azarnia et al. 1988). The importance of a diminished cell communication system may thus be critical in deregulating orderly cell growth.

The immune system is particularly instructive for the study of growth influences of its (component) cells upon each other: Each of the peptide colony stimulating factors, interleukins, or interferons secreted by some cells is either a growth factor or induces differentiation or the expression of cell components (e.g. surface antigens, or antibody) in a remarkably complex manner (Sporn and Roberts 1988) (chapter 9).

A characteristic paracrine signal operates between adjacent cells in the stomach: A STS-secreting cell inhibits an adjacent gastrin-secreting one through a gap junction, thereby maintaining inhibitory control on acid secretion. The STS-secreting cell is in turn inhibited by a vagal (cholinergic) signal. At the same time, a parallel vagal signal stimulates the gastrin-secreting cell via the gastrin-releasing peptide (Bunnett and Walsh 1988).

Cell-to-cell influences can occur via hormonal messengers, either in a paracrine manner or by communication at a considerable remove from each other. Adjacent islet cells in the pancreas secrete insulin, glucagon, and STS. Glucagon stimulates insulin and STS secretion in neighboring cells. And STS exerts negative feedback influence on both insulin and glucagon secretion, while insulin has the same effect only on the latter. The two cell groups respectively responsible for glucagon and insulin production are, at the same time, regulated by a variety of extraneous neural, hormonal, and metabolic signals, such as FFAs, E, NE, acetylcholine, electrolytes, and glucose, designed to maintain and alter glucose levels according to the need of the organ-

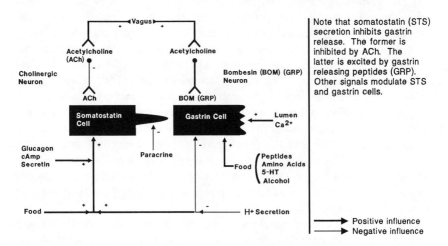

Figure 13.   Neurohumoral Control of Gastrin Secretion in the Stomach

ism (Unger, Orci, and Dobbs 1978). The diet, sleep, exercise, and the act of eating alter insulin secretion.

The amount of insulin and glucagon released is precisely proportional to the blood sugar concentration (Cryer and Gerich 1985). The mutual influences of insulin, glucagon, and STS secretion by the cells of the pancreatic islets are both facilitatory and inhibitory. Other examples have already been given (chapter 9) in discussing the mutual reinforcing influences of CRF, aVP, and OT in releasing ACTH (Gibbs 1986).

Some cells that produce two peptide hormonal signals combine to reinforce each other's stimulatory action on another cell. But only one of the two peptide signals inhibits a second cell group secreting another hormone: the GnRH and its associated peptide (GAP) cooperate to stimulate LH secretion from pituitary gonadotrophs (chapter 2). But only GAP inhibits PRL (Nikolicz et al. 1985).

To recapitulate, the cell regulates its own activity and internal milieu by an elaborate series of communication signals. Cells are also coupled, regulated, and perturbed by their surroundings through the agency of various receptors and ion channels, and internally by releasing (second) messenger signals initially bound to the cell membrane. The cell membrane is the medium that contains the messengers that activate a series of phosphorylating enzymes that sets its metabolic machinery into motion. Multiple influences play on receptor mechanisms and alter the context of the signal—that is, modulate them. By intimate contact with each other, cells influence one another's activities, as well as others' at a distance, through an elaborate communication system of nerve impulses, metabolites, hormones, biogenic amines, and peptides. They are also influenced by the behavioral activities and state of the organism.

The descriptions provided so far do not do justice to the exquisite manner in which multiple signals are integrated to provide a precisely "computed" output signal. The β-cell of the pancreas is regulated by a number of hormones, neural signals, and changing blood sugar, fatty acid, and electrolyte levels. The blood sugar levels are first transduced across the β-cell membrane into second messengers to activate ion channels, which alter the electrical potential of the cell membrane. Other ion (calcium) channels open, "translate" the blood sugar levels into increased intracellular calcium levels, and activate protein kinase systems to induce the genes coding for insulin to synthesize it. The cell secretes just the amount of insulin proportional to the increase in blood sugar concentration. But the β-cell is also coupled electrotonically to its neighbor and influenced by the electrical fields of hundreds of other cells: In essence, it is affected by their "computations." It is also densely innervated by autonomic nerves releasing neurotransmitters, which potentially mediate the brain's effects.

The blood sugar level is a complex oscillating signal integrated from such variables as the carbohydrate content and composition of the meal; the absorption of carbohydrate by the stomach and gut; the amount being stored in, or

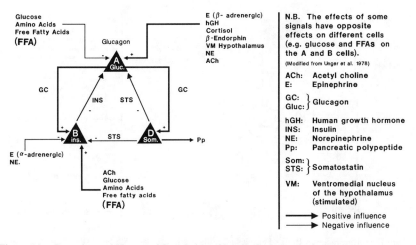

Figure 14.   Paracrine and Hormonal Regulation of Insulin Secretion in the Pancreas

released by, the liver and used by muscle; the secretion of counterregulatory hormones (i.e., those that raise blood glucose levels when they are too low) (chapter 8); blood electrolyte levels; the metabolic rate, body weight, and temperature of the person; and the functional state of the kidney and its threshold for glucose excretion. Oscillating glucose patterns are species-specific; they are perturbed by changes in diet to become chaotic.

The complexity and elegance of this subsystem in computing the appropriate rate of insulin secretion and blood glucose changes is astonishing. The system clearly "takes" innumerable variables "into account." A multiplicity of information is processed and transduced in parallel, integrated into a self-regulated, purposive subsystem—one of a number that compose the organism—and then further integrated with other systems.

Communication and Regulation at the Organ Level

Fluctuation is a characteristic of organ function, not only of cellular function. In the heart, the signals are mechanical (controlling pressure), ionic and electrical (controlling rates and rhythms), and neural and hormonal (controlling rates and pressure). The heart has its own pacemakers, perturbed by many local and distal influences. Imposed on pacemaker activity are circadian rhythms of HR and BP. Mechanoreceptors are present within both the heart and aorta; they have a positive feedback effect by β-adrenergic sympathetic signals on HR, BP, and myocardial contractility (Malliani, Pagani, and Berganaschi 1979), which are counteracted by negative feedback carotid sinus mechanoreceptors acting reflexly through the medulla by a chain of neurons whose messenger signals include L-glutamate, acetylcholine, GABA, NE, and NPY (Reis and LeDoux 1987). Baroreceptor reflex "sensitivity" in turn is perturbed by age, exercise, and mental arithmetic, which lower BP, and by sleep

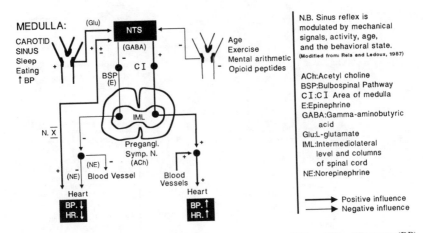

Figure 15.   Baroreceptor Reflex Pathways Regulating Heart Rate (HR) and Blood Pressure (BP)

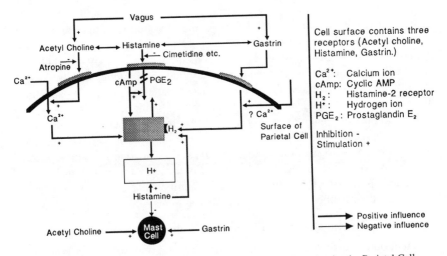

Figure 16.   The Parallel Signals for, and Regulation of, Acid Secretion by the Parietal Cell

and the postprandial state, which raise BP. The regulation of BP and blood volume is also carried out by the heart through the agency of atriopeptin, a 28-amino-acid peptide secreted by cells in the right atrium when pressure in it rises (chapter 9).

In the stomach hydrochloric acid secretion is triply controlled by gastrin, acetylcholine, and histamine. Local perturbations (distension of, or the presence of food, calicum, or alcohol in, its lumen) induce acid secretion. Rhythmic gastric contractions are under dual pacemaker control and are altered by the sight, smell, taste, and intake of food.

Acid secretion is also self-regulated by the stomach: Increases in luminal acid concentration diminish gastrin secretion. At least in the rat's stomach, 5-HT is cosecreted with, and counterregulates, acid output (Stephens et al. 1989). The secretion of acid is also under the control of an array of neural, pancreatic, and other hormonal signals. The neural signals emanate from the brain stem and hypothalamus, mediated by the vagus nerves. These nerves transmit the perturbations produced by stressful experiences and by everyday activities such as sleep and the reception and digestion of food.

Thus the stomach, like the heart, has an intrinsic control system that is influenced (and can be perturbed) by a variety of signals (visual, acoustic, thermal, etc.) emanating from the environment and processed by the brain. The

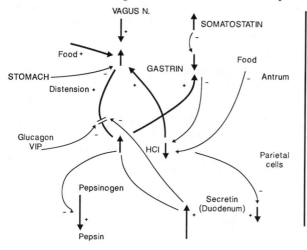

Gastrin is released (↑) by increased vagal discharge (+), food (especially protein), gastric distension, and a diminished gastric acidity (↓). Increased gastrin levels stimulate the secretion of hydrochloric acid by the gastric parietal cells (↑). In this acid medium, pepsinogen is converted into pepsin. Food in the stomach neutralizes hydrochloric acid (↓). Increased acidification of the gastric antrum inhibits gastrin secretion (↓). As the duodenal contents become acid, secretin is released, inhibiting the stimulating effect of gastrin on the parietal cells (=). Glucagon and the vasoactive intestinal peptide (VIP) act like secretin.

Figure 17. The Gastrin-Hydrochloric Acid Negative Feedback System That Normally Controls Gastric Acid Secretion

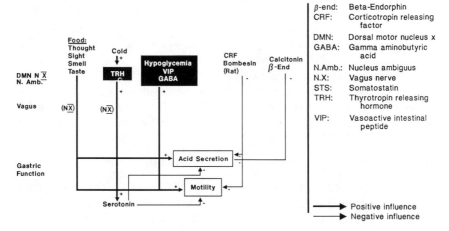

β-end: Beta-Endorphin
CRF: Corticotropin releasing factor
DMN: Dorsal motor nucleus x
GABA: Gamma aminobutyric acid
N.Amb.: Nucleus ambiguus
N.X: Vagus nerve
STS: Somatostatin
TRH: Thyrotropin releasing hormone
VIP: Vasoactive intestinal peptide

Figure 18. The Regulation and Counterregulation of Gastric Secretion and Motility by Signals via the Vagus Nerve and by Signals from Higher Brain Levels

ultimate signal transmitted to the stomach by the vagus nerve is the end-product of a variety of excitatory and inhibitory peptides and biogenic amines (Soll 1981; Taché, Stephens, and Ishikawa 1989).

The stomach is, therefore, a subsystem of another communication network. Signals are sent to it by the senses via the brain, from the duodenum and pancreas by a complex network. Acid secretion and its associated function—motility—are products of an elegant network, in which behavior (eating) and its anticipation, changes in ambient temperature, and a fall in blood sugar (to promote eating) are integrated with innumerable local and distant signals from the brain and the environment to generate an appropriate, regulated response.

To summarize: All cells and organs (limited examples of which have been discussed) regulate their activities by a complex and parallel system of information exchange and transfer. These regulatory processes may occur within the confines of the cell. Electrical and chemical signals are exchanged between cells; they are transduced by ion channels and cell surface receptors, which are then activated or shut off. The receptor is itself not a fixed structure: Receptor number is regulated by the signal. Receptors may remain closed for some time to remain desensitized. Many additional signals modulate receptor function, and thus signal transmission and transduction. Among the most important signals acting at a distance are hormones, whose synthesis and secretion by cells are promoted in a complex manner, and which act through specialized receptors. Hormones are chemically diverse signals (e.g., peptides, proteins, phenathrene-ring-derived sex- and corticosteroids). They perform both specific and diverse functions. Because they are ultimately controlled by the brain, they are also responsive to signals and contingencies that derive from the environment. The regulation and the patterned secretion of hormones have a developmental history. Their circhoral, ultradian, or circadian secretory rhythms may be intrinsic or "programmed" by the brain.

Support for the thesis that the organism consists of an intricate communication network has been put forward. It consists of subsystems that regulate themselves and each other by an exchange of signals integrated into a larger system—the organism—and coordinated by the brain. The brain in turn is responsive to, and interacts mutually with, its ever-changing environment.

Left out in this account is the form that signals take. A recognition and description of their formal properties and how these may be perturbed by stressful experience is the subject matter of the remainder of this chapter.

The Coordination of Physiology and Behavior

One of the functions of the organism is to coordinate and regulate appropriate behavior and physiological patterns in response to stressful experiences encountered in the dynamic biotic, climatic, and edaphic environments. Their integration has been a major topic of this book. It was exemplified in detail by discussing the coordination of ovulation and mating (chapters 2, 9) and the circulatory responses to various phases of a fight between animals (chapter 9). These processes are respectively carried out by peptide hormones with both behavioral and physiological functions, which act on, and by, neural circuits within the brain.

However, the coordination of ovulation by neuronal and hormonal signals differs in different species. They must be integrated with the sight, sounds, smells, bites, and courtship and receptive displays of partners (chapter 6). The behaviors and the physiology of reproduction are also exquisitely sensitive to perturbation by the presence of predators or a dominant male, or the absence of sunlight, rain, or adequate food supplies. Exercise, malnutrition, migration, lactation, a recent pregnancy, injury and disease, and a depressed mood adversely affect the process of ovulation, mating, and the care of offspring.

The Nature and Generation of Rhythms

The principles that govern the communication between cells, and the coordination of behavior and physiology, are the product of changes in both patterns of messenger signals and the state of the organism. The preferred mode of the transmitted signal is rhythmic (i.e., oscillatory), stable, and patterned. Each can be described by its own waveform, frequency, and amplitude. To switch to a different metaphor, frequency modulation is more accurate (Rapp, Mees, and Sparrow 1981) and assures that habituation in communication systems does not occur. If amplitude modulation were the preferred mode, no such assurances could be provided. The organism is composed of many different interacting functions, each of which oscillates according to its own pattern with a different phase, frequency, amplitude, and waveform and over different time frames (e.g., BP oscillates from systolic to diastolic levels approximately 70 times a minute, but it also shows a diurnal rhythm). At the same time oscillations in BP are influenced by other rhythms—respiratory ones (e.g., to produce sinus arrhythmia), food intake, exercise, sleep, and age, mediated in part by changes in baroreceptor sensitivity.

Virtually every conceivable natural phenomenon is periodic: Annual population cycles occur; epidemics of infectious diseases are periodic; the seasons come and go; and night follows day. Even biolumenescence in an *Alga* is periodic; the cycle is 24 hours long, and the phenomenon depends on the periodic expression of an enzyme, luciferase (Johnson and Hastings 1986). The cell oscillates between mitosis and interphase (Murray and Kirschner 1989).

In vertebrates, the circadian pacemaker—the SCN—has its own intrinsic rhythms of neuronal and metabolic activity, which are both more active in daylight than at night (Green and Gillette 1982; Schwartz et al. 1983). Interestingly enough, the fluctuations in neuronal activity are not seen in the neighboring hypothalamic arcuate nucleus. Endogenous rhythms, both circadian and seasonal, of α- and β-adrenergic receptors have been described in forebrain and hypothalamic membrane preparations; they are independent of light and time cues (Kafka, Wirz-Justice, and Naber 1981). Serotonin receptors in the brain show diurnal variation (Wesemann et al. 1983).

Locomotion, chewing, eating, sleep and wakefulness, core body and skin temperature, menstruation, ovulation, breathing, HR, and BP all have their own particular rhythms. Perodicities in mood and feeling states are particularly evident in the major affective and anxiety disorders. Regular variations in attention and states of consciousness have been described.

Repetitive neuronal discharge is oscillatory—at times regular, at other times not. It varies with the behavioral state of the animal. Within cells, calcium levels fluctuate with many different rhythmic patterns. At times a rather constant but still fluctuating baseline level of the ion is observed, which is interrupted by large transients with periods of 5 to 60 seconds; they are presumed to be due to the release of free calcium. The form and frequency of these oscillations in calcium levels differ from cell to cell but are relatively constant for any single cell. They depend in part on the presence of an extracellular ligand, and the activation of the IP_3 cascade, which is in turn regulated by negative feedback (Berridge and Irvine 1989).

The electroencephalogram and the electrocardiogram record rhythmic electrical processes. Hormones and neurotransmitters are secreted in a cyclic manner over two or more time scales (Garfinkel 1983; Rapp 1979). The pituitary gland shows circadian variations in its ACTH response to CRF (DeCherney et al. 1985). The adrenal gland differentially secretes cortisol when stimulated by ACTH at different times of the day and night (Kaneko et al. 1981).

Diurnal variations in glucose tolerance and insulin response to glucose in humans (Carroll and Nestel 1973), and in the expression of the enzymes maltase and sucrase in the small intestine of rats, have been recorded (Saito, Murakami, and Suda 1976). Levels of these enzymes are low at night, increase one hour before feeding, and are high during the day. Starvation eliminates the expression of the enzymes, but it, in turn, can experimentally be synchronized with food intake (Stevenson and Firestein 1976).

Lymphocyte numbers in humans show circadian variations. The total number of T-, CD4$^+$, CD8$^+$, and B-cells, but not of NK cells, is high during the day and low at night. The diurnal variation in number is exactly the inverse of serum cortisol levels (Ritchie et al. 1983).

The responsiveness to, and toxicity of, drugs or a bacterial toxin, depends on the time of day (Halberg 1960; Moore-Ede 1973; Reinberg 1967). The sensitivity to drugs depends on the diurnal fluctuations of receptor numbers and rates of absorption, hepatic conjugation, and renal excretion. Even the amount of electrolyte excretion by the kidney shows circadian variations (Moore-Ede, Sulzman, and Fuller 1982). Conversely, many drugs—lithium, MAO inhibitors, and imipramine—alter circadian rhythms (Wirz-Justice and Wehr 1983).

To digress for a moment: The periodicities just enumerated depend minimally on two interacting (not single) variables (Garfinkel 1983; Holden 1988). Oscillations are everywhere to be found in nature (Pittendrigh 1962; Reinberg 1967), but they have until recently been neglected in biology and medicine. The preferred manner of thought for the past century has been to look for steady states that are the product of reducing oscillations to mean rates or levels, or to study single variables and their covariates, which in time will approach either their means or their steady states (Garfinkel 1983). But the behavior of a single variable—the signal (e.g., a hormone)—is actually the product of several (oscillating) processes (e.g., the secretion of a pituitary hormone). Thus physiological (including behavioral) functions are nonlinear, dynamic, periodic and time-related.

Oscillations endow the organism with the capability of synchronizing and entraining pacemakers whose many functional subunits beating in phase give them "phase" coherence. Collective organization of these units multiplies their effects, of which they would not individually be capable. It also endows them with an additional property: stability.

Several pacemakers are known to exist: e.g., two main ones in the heart and in the stomach, and (at least) six in the mammalian brain. Their rhythmic outputs are stable: They persist in form and function unless perturbed. Locomotion is a coordinated rhythm. Sleep, cortisol, and temperature rhythms unfold daily. How is this possible, if pacemakers are composed of populations of subunits (e.g., neurons)? The pacemaker has many degrees of freedom by virtue of this composition. These separate units are organized into a collective whole with a "low-dimensional" form that endows it with a stable formal and functional mode (Garfinkel 1983).

Implicit in this idea is that pacemakers produce patterned oscillations. Patterns of this kind are obscured by the study of single variables at one point in time. Two coupled pacemakers have been identified in the SCN of the mammalian hypothalamus: One controls the diurnal patterns of REM sleep, plasma cortisol concentrations, and core body temperature; the other drives diurnal patterns of rest and activity, skin temperature, and slow-wave sleep. Both pacemakers, each oscillating in a distinctive manner, are entrained, or impinged upon, by external cues such as light, the ambient temperature, social cues, alterations of clock-time, and shift work (Moore-Ede, Sulzman, and Fuller 1982). Another set of pacemakers for sleep is the product of the interactions of LC and brain-stem reticular neurons in negative feedback interaction with each other (McCarley and Hobson 1975).

The actual physiological basis of the genesis of oscillations in signals in any one system is both controversial and not fully understood (Glass and Mackey 1988). In a general sense, the phase, frequency, and amplitude of an oscillator are under the control of inputs to it—e.g., another cell electrically coupled to it, a chemical messenger signal, or a signal deriving from the environment.

However, the membrane voltage of isolated cells also oscillates due to changing ion (calcium and potassium) conductances across them. In the case of single axons, this fluctuation may or may not reach threshold; when it does, periodic, regular depolarization occurs (Hodgkin and Huxley 1952). In other nerve cells bursts of electrical activity are irregular and aperiodic.

Central neurons vary widely in their electrophysiological properties—in their voltage- and agonist-dependent ionic conductances—which endow some of them with their own individual pacemaker properties. By virtue of their coupling to, and resonance with, other neurons they are believed to participate in network oscillations. Oscillation and resonance in brain-stem (inferior olive), cerebellar, thalamic, and motor neurons are components of motor coordination, which is, in part, made possible by the fact that inferior olivary neurons innervate cerebellar Purkinje cells in a parallel and distributed manner. The hippocampus (Traub, Miles, and Wong 1989), thalamus, and cerebral cortex also have their own intrinsic rhythms. These are perturbed by, and provide the context and frame of reference for, incoming signals. Oscillators in the brain stem (additional to those in the SCN) are partly responsible for states of sleep and wakefulness and respiratory rhythms (Llinás 1988).

The intrinsic properties (oscillations) of individual pacemaker neurons are thought to cooperate and generate rhythms in populations of nerve cells. But another possible explanation is that both the time courses and the strength of synaptic currents are responsible for them. A synthesis of these alternative possibilities is that, at least in the hippocampus, a few cells fire synchronously, but most of the other neurons depend on synchronous excitatory and inhibitory inputs to generate rhythms (Traub, Miles, and Wong 1989).

The origin of individual patterns of motor activity, or of specific hormone secretion, is also not fully understood. Motor rhythms (such as swimming) do not necessarily require any sensory input; they can be experimentally generated by stimulation with a central electrical pulse (McLennan and Grillner 1984). Central pattern generators are believed to underlie such complex motor patterns. These generators are composed of either neural networks or pacemaker cells, or both: No decision has been made as to the correct alternative explanation (Glass and Mackey 1988). Currently, the favored view is that some oscillations are a product of the interactions (resonances) of cells within the network. In order for rhythmic oscillation to occur, the interaction between cells within a group should be excitatory, but it is inhibitory between groups of cells.

This scenario is the simplest possible. However, in some systems the matter is more complex. In the case of the oscillations in corticosteroid levels, CRF-secreting neurons in the PVN stimulate pituitary corticotrophs rhythmically. Fluctuating pulses of ACTH in turn stimulate adrenal cortical cells to secrete corticosteroids, which feed back to inhibit the release of CRF and ACTH. Furthermore, a circadian rhythm that is entrained by light is imposed on short-term hypothalamic-pituitary-adrenal oscillations (chapter 9).

The concept that guides the system just described, and that of central pattern generators, is of positive, negative, and mixed feedback carried out by a variety of chemically heterogeneous messenger signals, previously enumerated (chapter 9). Negative feedback in part produces oscillations by virtue of time delays that are built into some systems (Iberal 1975): The velocity of the transmission of nerve impulses is variable but finite, synaptic delays occur, genes do not express their peptide products instantaneously (some are further processed from prohormones), hormones have to be secreted by the cell and circulate in the bloodstream to glands at some distance from their origin (Garfinkel 1983; Mackey and Milton 1987). A single-loop feedback communication system is in principle capable of producing an oscillatory output provided that the negative (inhibitory) influence (e.g., of corticosteroid on CRF secretion) is sufficiently steep. But the matter is actually more complex: Multiple negative or mixed (negative-positive) feedback influences determine the oscillatory secretion of CRF, ACTH, and the corticosteroids (Reisine 1989) and many other systems (chapter 9). In fact, the number of known possible interactions impinging on the PVN is of the order of 350!

Despite the complexity of such concepts it seems relatively clear that they attempt to account for the temporal organization, functioning, and relative stability of interacting, rhythmic systems, known to occur within cells and organisms. The recognition of oscillations as phenomena to be considered in their own right, and not only the product of chance or "noise" (Glass and Mackey 1988; Halberg 1960; Pittendrigh 1962), has led to a radical revision of our concepts of the biology of the organism. In the classical tradition of biology and medicine, stability was previously ascribed to structure, or to the hallowed concepts of the constancy of the internal milieu and homeostasis; these ideas have been guided by Bernard's and Cannon's principles. The recognition that oscillations are a fact of life may force a revision of our concepts.

Two main reasons for doing so immediately come to mind. If oscillations are the preferred mode of the organism guiding its communication systems, how do they account for the transition from health to illness and disease? And, granting that oscillations account for stability, regulation, and information transfer, how are they affected by small, or large, perturbations, which the organism encounters daily? How do stressful experiences, for example, alter them? What happens when the usual *Zeitgebers*—entrainers— of some rhythms are withdrawn?

Bifurcations

Such questions call for answers if this line of thought has any validity. Consider the transition from normal sinus rhythm to the irregular, either fast or slow, oscillations of ventricular fibrillation, or that from the normal cyclic breathing patterns to Cheyne-Stokes respirations or hyperventilation (Glass and Mackey 1988; Mackey and Milton 1987). Why do rapid alternations of mood occur in some forms of major affective disorders? How does sequential, rhythmic esophageal contraction develop oscillatory instability, i.e., become tetanic? How do stressful experiences alter the usual temporal pattern of contractions of the stomach in animals to slow or irregular ones, or extinguish the migratory motor complex of the small intestine (chapter 5)?

In disease, or when stressful experiences occur, oscillations undergo a transition from their usual, regular mode to an irregular one, or from irregular to regular behaviors. New frequencies, amplitudes, or rhythms may appear. Old ones may reappear, or they may disappear. In the mathematical language of this new physiology these transitions are called bifurcations.

Further to understand bifurcations requires knowledge about the manner in which each system customarily oscillates: The electrical rhythm of the waking brain—its alpha rhythm—is continuous and irregular whereas it is periodic and regular in the heart. In psychomotor epilepsy, for example, it becomes slower, regular, and periodic. In ventricular tachycardia it speeds up, and in fibrillation it becomes fast or slow; and in both cases, it becomes aperiodic and irregular (Mackey and Milton 1987). As already mentioned, each bodily system and each signal has its own oscillatory mode with its own quantitative parameters (i.e., amplitude, frequency, phase, waveform, etc.).

In humans, sleep goes through regular cycles of one REM and three non-REM periods. In the adult, hGH is secreted in one single, peaked pulse at the time of the first slow-wave sleep period. Prolactin, on the other hand, has an irregular rhythm during the night, with a relatively large peak toward the early morning hours (chapter 9). Body temperature falls on going to sleep during the night, and it rises in anticipation of awakening and arising in the morning. Cortisol levels are virtually undetectable in the late evening hours, and increase thereafter in three or four pulses, superimposed on a rising base line, which achieves its apex at about 0600 hours. Renal potassium excretion is highest during the day, but it begins to fall at 2000 hours, and it reaches a low point at midnight, which persists until about 0600 hours only to rise once again (Moore-Ede, Sulzman, and Fuller 1982). These few examples demonstrate the individual nature of each of these rhythms, each with its own waveform, phase, frequency, amplitude, and regularity.

Bifurcations can be modeled mathematically by nonlinear differential equations that describe the evolution of a system over time, while also modeling the transitions in parameters occurring in the same system that terminates in bifurcations and in "chaos" (Garfinkel 1983; Glass and Mackey 1988).

The nonlinear concept of bifurcation entails a qualitative change from a stable oscillatory mode to another. An example of such a transition is the mid-cycle LH pulse that ends with ovulation—an intermittent process that cannot be accounted for by any single-loop, oscillatory system (chapter 2). To complicate the matter even further, a single variable may oscillate within two separate time frames: Five to six oscillations (with a mean duration of 28 min.) in plasma cortisol occur in humans during any 24-hour period. They are in turn superimposed on a circadian oscillation (also about 24 hours in length) whose nadir occurs in the first hours of the night. Of equal importance is that ACTH shows a similar circadian oscillation. Yet, and despite its close link to episodic corticosteroid secretion, ACTH oscillations are present ten times in a 24-hour period, with each oscillation lasting about 140 minutes (chapter 9). In addition, oscillatory systems may appear to be closely coupled—e.g., sleep and the circadian oscillation of cortisol secretion. We know, however, that these systems may be uncoupled (e.g., by sleep reversal).

The point at which bifurcations in a system occur—when the number or stability of cycles (i.e., oscillations) changes—is defined by the value of any one of its parameters. Perturbing the system is one antecedent of bifurcations. The consequences of that perturbation may, however, be quite unpredictable: When a cardiac cell is electrically stimulated its regular rhythm may stop temporarily, only to be reestablished at its original cycle, or it may permanently be annihilated (Glass and Mackey 1988). In other systems stimulation or external changes induce progressively irregular aperiodic—chaotic—rhythms.

In some physiological systems (e.g., the heart), and for some parameter values and starting conditions, aperiodic dynamics are almost inevitable. In patients with coronary atherosclerosis, everyday perturbations, tasks, and challenges (e.g., mental arithmetic, exercise, reading a book, or public speaking) may produce silent myocardial ischemia (chapter 6), characterized by perfusion deficits, or motion irregularities of the wall of the ventricles, and S-T segment changes in the EKG, which reflect rhythmic coronary vasospasm.

The heart is particularly vulnerable to the loss of its periodicity by perturbations that correspond in time with its partial depolarization (return of S-T segment to baseline). If a coronary artery is experimentally occluded in dogs, both α- and β-adrenergic excitation, falling during that period, are at first followed by repetitive (aperiodic) extrasystoles, and then by irregularly recurring ("chaotic") ventricular fibrillations (VF). At other times in the cycle, sympathetic stimulation fails to produce VF (Verrier 1989). Therefore, the timing of the perturbation is critical to its outcome.

The evolution of chaos in some systems depends also on its initial and deterministic conditions despite the fact that they may be very similar. But from two slightly different starting points the dynamics of the system unfold over time quite independently and unpredictably (indeterministically). Because the initial conditions of a physiological system also vary by virtue of the many other influences playing upon it, it is impossible to predict their evolution at two separate points in time (Garfinkel 1983). Chaotic dynamics can occur in almost every bodily system and in a variety of disease states (Glass and Mackey 1988; Mackey and Milton 1987).

The reasons for the perturbations of a system are many because all physiological subsystems of the organism interact, and/or vary, with several other subsystems and also with the environment. Oscillations in physiological systems are perturbed by virtue of interacting systems, or when the control parameters of the system are altered. The latter may come about by a variety of ways: Parameter changes occur as the state of the organism is altered with stressful experiences, sleep, activity, food intake, sexual intercourse, or aging. Changes in the quality (parameters) of rhythms, as mentioned, can be modeled mathematically by nonlinear dynamics. However, it is still not certain—except in some instances—which mathematical model is the best to apply to every and all physiological rhythms, because their parameters are so varied and complex and their genesis is still not fully understood.

New Insights into the Role of Stressful Experiences in Ill Health and Disease

During the past decade, a major reconceptualization of the nature of ill health and disease has also occurred (Garfinkel 1983; Glass and Mackey 1979, 1988; Mackey and Milton 1987; Melnechuk 1978; Moore-Ede, Sulzman, and Fuller 1982; Rubenstein 1980; Weiner 1977, 1989b; Weiner and Mayer 1990). The basis of this shift in thinking is that changes in the dynamic functions of the organism, and not only in its structure, underlie the transition from health to illness and disease. The first advantage of this line of thought is that disease need no longer be divided into two categories: "organic" (disease) and "functional" (ill health). Therefore, it now becomes possible to conceive of ill health and disease in a uniform manner. Altered rhythmic functions occur with or without structural changes in behavior (e.g., in sleep disorders, periodic psychoses, and major affective disorders), the brain (e.g., in epilepsy, athetosis, chorea, tremor), muscle function (e.g., with myoclonus, fibrillation, tetanus), the respiratory system (e.g., in apnea, Cheyne-Stokes respirations, hyperventilation), the esophagus, stomach, and colon (e.g., with "tetanus"), the heart (e.g., with bigeminy, fibrillation), bone marrow (in cyclic neutropenia, etc.), the eye (with hippus) and its movements (with nystagmus) (Garfinkel 1983; Glass and Mackey 1979, 1988). Some of these transitions from one characteristic rhythmic mode to another may come about by slight (not excessive, unusual, damaging, or overwhelming) perturbations of the organism, and are associated with stressful experiences induced by its interaction with the environment. In each species and in each individual belonging to it, the initial conditions of its subsystems differ. The consequences of any particular perturbation are unpredictable and individual—an insight that may provide the basis of variation (individual differences) in behavioral and physiological responses.

The changes in function—qualitative parametric changes in the dynamics of a communication system based on an exchange of signals—may take several different forms (Garfinkel 1983; Glass and Mackey 1988; Mackey and Milton 1987): (1) New periodicities and/or parametric characteristics may appear in an ongoing rhythmic process; (2) rhythmic processes may disappear (e.g., apnea, absence of MMCs in the gut); or (3) regular oscillations in a system not usually thus characterized may appear (e.g., hippus, muscle fibrillations). These three classes of change in periodic function characterize a new dynamical concept of disease (Garfinkel 1983; Glass and Mackey 1979, 1988) and ill-health.

Some of the major categories of functional disorders are characterized by transitions to new periodic rhythms. In the functional bowel disorders several such bifurcations have already been described (chapter 5), one of which consists of repetitive nonperistaltic, oscillatory instability (tetanus) in the form of high-amplitude contractions of the esophagus rather than the usual, sequential ones. Esophageal tetanus can be provoked experimentally. The regular, pacesetter potential in the gastric antrum may become arrhythmic and speed up, or it may become intermittent and faster in some forms of nonulcer dyspepsia. Tetanic contractions on inflation of the colon with air have been described in some patients with irritable colon syndrome. In other such patients, a lower frequency of myoelectric rhythms in the colon is observable at rest and after eating. The migratory motor complex of the gut is extinguished by meals and stressful experience (chapter 5).

In some forms of fibromyositis, new (α-) rhythms are interspersed with existing, slow-wave ones. In normal sleeping persons, this transition can be brought about by noise. It may occur spontaneously or be induced by pain and fear (chapter 5).

None of these changes in function is associated with anatomical changes. They illustrate that bifurcations from one rhythmic mode to another are brought about by perturbing the organism, or a subsystem.

Cheyne-Stokes respirations can result from a lengthened circulation time that delays the delivery of CO_2 to brain stem chemoreceptors and the respiratory oscillator. This form of irregular but periodic breathing is also seen in obese individuals and with diseases of medullary-pontine chemoreceptors. One may also conceptualize the oscillating movement (tremor) observed in demyelinating disease as a result of delay in nerve conduction in a complex feedback circuit. (The analogous phenomenon can be modeled in a simple system, such as a thermostat, built on feedback principles; a delay in the conducting circuit causes it to fluctuate widely.) On the other hand, in the chronic hyperventilation syndrome (associated with anxiety, grief, pain, excitement, etc.), the "sensitivity" of these chemoreceptors to small changes in $PaCO_2$ is increased, resulting in more rapid ventilation interspersed with irregularly occurring, high-amplitude inspirations.

Some forms of dynamical diseases come about by changes in physiological systems that operate on negative, positive, or mixed feedback principles (Garfinkel 1983; Glass and Mackey 1988): At any one point in the system upon which rhythms depend, perturbations alter rhythmic function. Changes in behavior and feelings, pain, and sensory stimuli may be associated with changes in various normal rhythms.

The concept of dynamical diseases is so far limited to those in which the "qualitative dynamics of physiological control systems" change despite the fact that the systems themselves remain structurally intact; characteristically, they are sensitive to slight differences in initial conditions and/or small changes in their control parameters. Because many of them consist of multiple feedback loops regulating the output of a single variable, such small changes occur frequently: A slight increase in amplitude of a single signal, or a delay in its arrival at its receptor, may eventuate in large oscillations (Glass and Mackey 1979, 1988).

Another set of new and related ideas about health and disease derives from viewing the organism as a complex communication network tied together by frequency-modulated signals. According to this view, illness and disease are impairment or disorder in communication networks (Melnechuk 1978; Rubenstein 1980), characterized by disturbances in their regulation (Weiner 1975, 1977) that may or may not lead to bifurcations. Most of the communication systems studied to date operate on the principle of negative and positive, or mixed, feedback (chapter 9). However, this point of view is more inclusive than the concept of dynamical diseases, because it incorporates the fact that the physiological control system may not necessarily remain intact. A synthesis of these two sets of concepts remains for the future; it will depend on studying transitions in specific rhythmic functions when communication networks, upon which they depend, are disordered (e.g., by changes in the structure of the signal or its receptor).

A variety of different disordered communication systems have already been described; some of these can provisionally be classified as follows.

1. A closed-loop system may become an open-loop one; it escapes feedback regulation. Such a change may occur when a toxin modifies a membrane-bound second messenger system: For example, the cholera toxin, acting upon the membrane of small intestinal cells, continuously activates the G-protein and thus adenylate cyclase by ribosylation with adenosine diphosphate. As a consequence, cAMP is continually formed. Activation of the cyclase enzyme and cAMP generates the uncontrolled excretion of water, chloride, and HCO_3^- ions into the lumen of the gut, resulting in dehydration and acidosis.

In other instances, the closed feedback system is preempted by an auto-antibody to create an unregulated open-loop system. Such is the case when a stimulating autoantibody binds to the TSH receptor in Graves disease, thereby taking over the function of TSH. Unregulated production and secretion of cAMP-dependent T_4 results.

When peptides are produced at an organ site where no local regulatory sub-system exists, or when they are secreted in excess, analogous regulatory disturbances occur: Tumors of the lung may produce ACTH or aVP; pancreatic tumors may secrete gastrin that escapes the usual, exquisite regulation of this peptide in the stomach.

Unregulated signals may also be amplified: Peptide growth factors (GFs) (e.g., platelet-derived and insulin-like) are now believed to play a significant role in the formation of a number of malignancies (Farber 1984). The GFs are products of oncogenes. They are unregulated, in part, because they differ in just a few amino acid sequences from normal GFs, which are themselves products of proto-oncogenes. (The latter are involved in normal, healthy cell growth and division.) Proto-oncogenes are usually under the regulatory control of growth suppressor genes; the absence of one of these regulators of growth antecedes the development of several tumors (e.g., retinoblastoma).

A cell producing GFs also expresses its own specific receptors, thus establishing a positive feedback system that amplifies its own peptide signals. Some classes of oncogenes promote the expression of cell surface receptors for GFs that are linked to a protein kinase C, second messenger system (Nishizuka 1986). However, these particular receptors are devoid of the binding site for GFs. They remain in an unregulated state, continually phosphorylating intracellular proteins to produce GFs (Farber 1984).

2. The blockade of a receptor that receives an excitatory, or an inhibitory, signal impairs function. In myasthenia gravis an autoantibody binds to the postsynaptic acetylcholine receptor, blocking neuromuscular signal transmission. Additionally, receptor number is reduced, as is the amplitude of the aperiodic, miniature end-plate potential (Newsom-Davis 1988). However, this molecular explanation cannot be the only one: Some neuromuscular junctions are (or only one is) preferentially affected, and the disease has an unpredictable, fluctuating course. In Huntington disease (HD), the access of a GABA-inhibitory signal to its receptor in the corpus striatum is impeded in a manner not fully understood. Whether this block alone explains the recurring (choreic) movements—cited as one example of irregular dynamics in disease (Mackey and Milton 1987)—also remains unclear. (Furthermore, cholinergic intrastriatal neurons are also affected in HD.)

Nonetheless, models exist that throw some light on the manner in which receptor blockade in the brain may perturb the dynamics of a rhythmic system that depends on recurrent, mixed feedback inhibition. When the GABA receptor on hippocampus pyramidal cells is blocked by penicillin, disinhibition takes place. As a result, regular bursting neuronal activity with different periodicities is replaced by sustained, irregular "firing" patterns (Mackey and Milton 1987).

3. Communication networks may be altered or fail because of several different kinds of altered receptor function. Receptors may be entirely absent, or defective, because their genes fail to express them at all, or do so incorrectly. This situation obtains, for example, in familial hypercholesterolemia, in which no surface receptors for LDL are present. As a result, LDLs accumulate in the

bloodstream. In homozygotes with this disorder, early onset of atherosclerosis occurs. In other forms the receptors (clathrin-coated "pits") are structurally defective, although their density and/or number on cell membranes is normal, and serum LDL levels rise (Brown and Goldstein 1986). Receptor number and/or density may be reduced: Obese individuals develop type II diabetes mellitus because insulin receptor number and concentration are diminished. Glucose "intolerance," hyperglycemia, and, frequently, hyperinsulinemia then develop. To conceptualize this process in another way, dysregulation of glucose and insulin secretion—a periodic process (Molnar, Taylor, and Langworthy 1972)—occurs. But as the patient loses weight, the number of insulin receptors increases, and the regulation and counterregulation of the glucose signal is restored.

Binding of a ligand signal to a receptor may be impaired: One form of diabetes mellitus, leading to the dysregulation of glucose patterns, comes about because the amino acid sequence of an insulin molecule is altered by virtue of a genetic mutation. The binding capacity of this mutant insulin molecule is less than the normal one. On the other hand, the binding capacity of the receptor for the insulin ligand may be diminished by (a poorly understood) receptor defect that occurs in ataxia telangiectasia. An ion channel may be structurally defective, as in the case of the chloride ion channel in cystic fibrosis.

Receptors may be present in excessive numbers or densities, and/or they may have an increased binding capacity for a signal: One or another of these possible alterations characterizes the postsynaptic muscarinic acetylcholine reception on bronchial smooth muscle in some forms of bronchial asthma. The consequence of this initial condition (bronchial hyperreactivity) is that a multiplicity of perturbing influences, mediated directly or reflexively by the vagus nerve, produce rhythmic bronchial spasm and the asthmatic attack, which is characterized by a transition from the usual regular respiratory rhythms to altered amplitudes, frequencies, and regularities of breathing. Perturbations leading to asthmatic attacks are incited by pulmonary infections, antigens of many different kinds, exercise, excitement, odors, and changes in personal relationships (for review, Weiner 1977). Bouts of asthma may be seasonal, or they occur regularly or irregularly. Yet they would not take place without the participation of bronchial hyperreactivity.

4. Messenger signals may be absent or diminished. As a result, the regulation of an entire subsystem, or the maintenance of rhythmic changes within certain parameters, is altered. In type I diabetes mellitus, the β-cells of pancreatic islets are destroyed by an autoimmune process. Insulin secretion diminishes or ceases. Hyperglycemia and wide fluctuations in blood glucose levels occur, incited by perturbations such as exercise and food (especially carbohydrate) intake.

An analogous example is the reduction of the lymphokines IL-I and γ-IF, and of the number of receptors for IL-2 on CD4$^+$ lymphocytes, in the course of HIV infection (Murray et al. 1984; Prince, Kermani-Arab, and Fahey 1984; Rook et al. 1983; Smith et al. 1984). The interaction of an infected cell with the (depressed) state of the organism is also different than a noninfected cell's (Kemeny et al. 1990).

Many kinds (e.g., neurological, endocrine, genetic) of diseases exist in which cells, for diverse reasons, do not produce messenger signals (Melnechuk 1978); the result of the failure to do so has not been conceptualized in terms of alterations in communication systems. Yet examples illustrating these new concepts do exist: In paralysis agitans, regular rhythmic movements (tremor) of a definite frequency appear in the resting steady state. During willed movements, or in sleep, the tremor disappears. It is assumed that as the state of the organism is altered, the control parameters change. The tremor is ascribed to a reduction in the DA signal in the nigro-striatal system (N-S). This oversimplified explanation fails to take into account that the N-S contains a positive-negative feedback system of neurons signaled by DA, GABA, and acetylcholine. Not even this more complex set of facts truly explains the appearance of rhythmic tremors where none had previously occurred.

Other examples exist that help us to understand how the absence of a signal alters a communication system otherwise characterized by mixed feedback. In Turner syndrome (TS) the E_2 signal is not produced. Nonetheless, the rhythmic secretion of LH goes through the same maturational sequence as in normal girls, but at a much higher initial level (Boyar et al. 1977) because of the absence of the negative feedback signal (E_2). Thus the central pattern generator for LH is intact, but the system is unregulated. The altered feedback system in TS is readily perturbed: As patients with TS develop AN, the initial high LH levels fall and the oscillations of LH become aperiodic and of low amplitude—a characteristic mode of the prepubertal stage of LH secretion.

The maturational sequence of normal LH rhythms is of some interest. During puberty, LH (and to a lesser extent FSH) levels become chaotic—the frequency, regularity, and amplitude of the oscillations markedly increase, and the waveform becomes complex. Imposed on these oscillations is a circadian rhythm. In later adolescence and adulthood the base levels of LH are higher than before puberty; its oscillations are slower, irregular, and of lower amplitude, and no circadian variation is observable. In AN a reversion of adult LH patterns occurs to the chaotic pubertal, or to irregular, low-dimensional, prepubertal, oscillations (Boyar et al. 1974). Many factors perturb LH patterns and the regulatory system in which it participates, including a variety of stressful experiences and weight loss (Garfinkel and Garner 1982; Weiner 1989).

To date, no deeper understanding of these observations exists. They suggest that transitions to chaos may not be unusual; in fact, in some subsystems like the one just described, they may occur during maturation, and are age-appropriate. However, the same chaotic phenomenon may be associated with disease when it occurs at another age, i.e., when it is age-inappropriate.

5. Circadian rhythms can assume low-dimensional forms or can undergo phase shifts in illness and disease. Phase shifts in rhythms occur in a variety of conditions, including stressful ones (Moore-Ede, Sulzman, and Fuller 1982). A dramatic example of this phenomenon is the polycystic ovary syndrome in adult women in which the pubertal crest of LH oscillations, usually seen during the night, occurs during the day (Zumoff et al. 1983). A triple transition is present—phase shifting, diurnal variation, and an age-inappropriate cyclic pattern of LH.

In some forms of major affective disorders the putative hypothalamic (SCN)-coupled pacemakers may be uncoupled (Ehlers, Frank, and Kupfer 1988). In patients whose moods swing widely, period-doubling bifurcations in sleep onset have been observed under the impact of imipramine (Wehr and Goodwin 1983). Body temperature or TSH circadian rhythms may be reduced in amplitude in some depressed states (Souetre et al. 1988); they assume a low-dimensional form. In some instances rhythms of GH in major depressive disorders (Mendlewicz et al. 1985) may return to previous patterns seen in adolescence, characterized by an increased frequency and a shift to daytime secretion. Phase shifting of some chronobiological rhythms is also believed to occur in at least some patients with the major depressive disorders (Wehr and Goodwin 1983). Transitions to period doubling of cycles of motor activity have also been described (Glass and Mackey 1988).

6. A negative feedback communication system may become a positive one in disease. This change has been described in Cushing disease (CD) (Fehm et al. 1979). Infused cortisol immediately inhibits ACTH secretion in normal persons. In CD, cortisol at first promotes ACTH production and secretion, and only later in time inhibits it. This unusual effect is also associated with (but not necessarily causally related to) a transition in cortisol rhythms in CD, which are characterized by high initial levels, the absence of circadian variation, and a transition from irregular to large-amplitude, regular fluctuations in cortisol values.

7. Altered mixed feedback systems have also been described: Several varieties of this phenomenon may exist in the same subsystem. In some forms of human DU disease, negative feedback is defective, exemplified by the fact that acidification of the gastric antrum fails to reduce the secretion of gastrin; thus, more rather than less hydrochloric acid secretion is promoted. In other forms of DU, histamine, peptides, or the taste of food has excessive positive (stimulatory) effects on gastric acid secretion (Grossman 1978). The initial (baseline) conditions of pepsin and acid secretion also differ in a proportion of patients with DU.

Concluding Remarks

After several centuries of studying ever smaller constituents of matter and of the material body, physicists (Prigogine 1980; Weinberg 1987), physiologists

(Garfinkel 1983; Glass and Mackey 1988; Winfree 1987), and physicians (Mackey and Milton 1987) have now turned their attention to phenomena that require integrative concepts that may begin to allow us to understand complex phenomena and whole systems such as the organism. Two somewhat different but related sets of ideas have been presented: nonlinear dynamics, and information exchange within the organism and between it and the environment by signals. Both of these concepts speak a language that expresses the basic characteristics of the dynamics of whole living organisms and other complex systems: function in its various forms; qualitative (parametric) changes in function; rhythmic and usually stable modes of functioning; and individual variations in function.

Integrative concepts have been needed in the field of stress research and theory in order to describe and capture the nature of functioning organisms in their daily, ever-changing mutual interactions with other organisms and the physical world: An integrated portrayal of the organism in its world was sought. Until recently no common language seemed to exist that described the functions of living organisms in all their components and interactions at one period of, and over, time. They seemed to be composed of many disparate-seeming functions carried out by minds, brains, and other bodily subsystems in the task of survival and reproduction. A long-sought-for language seems now to be evolving that may accomplish this unifying purpose.

Function is such a unifying and dynamic concept. In living organisms every function changes constantly. These rhythms have a recognizable form and pattern, which are usually stable. The organism also functions in an integrated, patterned manner. The patterns of physiology and behavior are inextricable. Patterns are rhythmic. Rhythms have qualitative properties by which they can be described and distinguished. The genesis of rhythmic patterns of biological and behavioral systems—i.e. the function and behaviors of cells, organs, or whole populations of organisms—can be described by the mathematical concept of self-organization in nonlinear systems. Nonlinear characterization of a system also defines the conditions for stability, fluctuation, and phase transitions of functions into other stable conditions, or those that favor the evolution and emergence of new properties of a system over time.

Nonlinear mathematical models are approximate descriptions of the dynamic functions of biological systems (Glass and Mackey 1988). It is acknowledged that a more realistic account of physiological rhythms is needed. Feedback, that in part accounts for them, is provided by information exchange within the organism and between organisms by signals of a large variety of kinds. In this way, the organism is kept informed about its own internal state and the condition of the external environment, in order to carry out the appropriate behaviors and their coordinated alterations in the subsystems that compose it. The information is contained in an elaborate system of signals that are frequency-modulated and the emitted product of complex modulations. According to this view, the organism is conceived to consist of a number of communication subsystems integrated by the brain into a larger system of information transfer and exchange with the environment in terms of coded signals of many different categories (from ions to words). The information transfer and exchange occurs within and between cells and organs, between them and the brain, and between the brain and the environment. The principles underlying these exchanges are everywhere the same. The separation between the brain (and its mind) and the body fall away when the organism is seen in such a totally integrated system of information exchange and processing. These signals allow it to regulate its own activities and those of others. The organism consists of an intelligent, integrated, self-regulated system designed by evolution for very specific tasks. Yet different species carry out the same tasks in very different ways.

Any perturbation of one component of the feedback loop may radically alter the quality of the signal. The concept of perturbation leading to a change in function is central to, and the basis of, stress theory (Weiner 1989, 1991b). It is a concept that allows us to understand how the human organism with its unique genetic and experiential history responds to perturbing experiences that allow it to remain intact, or to make the voyage from health to illness and/or disease, characterized by transitions in the parameters of rhythmic functions.

The change in rhythmic function over time of any system depends in part on its initial conditions, small variations in which may have quite different, individual, and unpredictable outcomes—a phenomenon well known to anyone investigating individual organisms. These individual differences according to this new line of thinking are to be studied in their own right; they need no longer be considered a nuisance, or be submerged by averaging them. Rhythmic functions manifest stability but, being dynamic, are capable of change. They are part of the ever-varying rhythmic activities and tasks of the organism (e.g., eating, sleeping, exercising, mating, working, and meeting threats and challenges), and they do not exist in isolation, but interact with each other. They are perturbable—some more than others. And some rhythms are under conscious control. As a result of these interactions rhythmic functions change into new modes. In some cases they may become chaotic and characterize the functioning of a subsystem in ill health and disease.

References

Abbott, D. H. 1987. Behaviourally mediated suppression of reproduction in female primates. J. Zool. (London) 213:1–16.

Abraham, R. 1983. Dynamical models for physiology. Am. J. Physiol. 245 (Regul. Integ. Comp. Physiol. 14):R467–72.

Abrahams, V. C., S. M. Hilton, and A. Zbrozña. 1964. The role of active muscle vasodilatation in the alerting stage of the defense reaction. J. Physiol. (London) 171:189–95.

Ackerman, S. H. 1981. Premature weaning, thermoregulation and the occurrence of gastric pathology. In Brain, behavior, and bodily disease, ed. H. Weiner, M. A. Hofer, and A. J. Stunkard, 67–86. New York: Raven Press.

———. 1989. Disease consequences of early maternal separation. In Neuronal control of bodily function: Frontiers of stress research, ed. H. Weiner, D. Hellhammer, I. Florin, and R. Murison, 85–93. Toronto: Hans Huber.

Ackerman, S. H., M. A. Hofer, and H. Weiner. 1975. Age at maternal separation and gastric erosion susceptibility in the rat. Psychosom. Med. 37:180–84.

———. 1978. Early maternal separation increases gastric ulcer risk in rats by producing latent thermoregulatory disturbance. Science 201:373–76.

———. 1979. Sleep and temperature regulation during restraint stress in rats is affected by prior maternal separation. Psychosom. Med. 41:311–19.

Ackerman, S. H., S. E. Keller, S. J. Schleifer, M. A. Schindledecker, M. S. Camerino, M. A. Hofer, H. Weiner, and M. Stein. 1988. Premature maternal separation and immune function. Brain Beh. Immun. 2:161–65.

Ackerman, S. H., and H. Weiner. 1976. Peptic ulcer disease: Some considerations for psychosomatic research. In Modern trends in psychosomatic medicine 3, ed. O. W. Hill, 363–81. London: Butterworths.

Adams, D. B. 1977. The conspecific defense modulator. Abstract. Am. Zoolog. 17:927.

———. 1979. Brain mechanisms for offense, defense, and submission. Behav. Brain Sci. 2:201–41.

Ader, R. 1963a. Plasma pepsinogen level in rat and man. Psychosom. Med. 25:218–20.

———. 1963b. Plasma pepsinogen level as a predictor of susceptibility to gastric erosions in the rat. Psychosom. Med. 25:221–32.

————. 1964. Gastric erosions in the rat: Effects of immobilization at different points in the activity cycle. Science 145:406–7.

————. 1967. Behavioral and physiological rhythms and the development of gastric erosions in rats. Psychosom. Med. 29:345–53.

————. 1980. Psychosomatic and psychoimmunologic research. Psychosom. Med. 42:307–21.

————, ed. 1981. Psychoneuroimmunology. New York: Academic Press.

Ader, R., C. C. Beels, and R. Tatum. 1960. Blood pepsinogen and gastric erosions in the rat. Psychosom. Med. 22:1–12.

Aguilera, G., K. Fujita, and K. J. Catt. 1981. Mechanisms of inhibition of aldosterone secretion by adrenocorticotropin. Endocrinol. 108:522–28.

Akil, H., J. Madden, R. L. Patrick, and J. D. Barchas. 1976. Stress-induced increase in endogenous opiate peptides: Concurrent analgesia and its partial reversal by naloxone. In Opiates and endogenous opioid peptides, vol. 1, ed. H. W. Kosterlitz, 63–70. Amsterdam: Elsevier.

Akil, H., D. J. Mayer, and J. C. Liebeskind. 1976. Antagonism of stimulation-produced analgesia by naloxone, a narcotic antagonist. Science 191:961–62.

Akil, H., E. Young, J. M. Walker, and S. J. Watson. 1986. The many possible roles of opioids and related peptides in stress-induced analgesia. Ann. N.Y. Acad. Sci. 467:140–53.

Ali, M., and M. V. Vedeckis. 1987. The glucocorticoid receptor protein binds to transfer RNA. Science 235:467–70.

Allen, A., and A. Garner. 1980. Mucous and bicarbonate secretion in the stomach and their possible role in mucosal protection. Gut 21:249–62.

Allman, J., F. Miezin, and E. McGuinness. 1985. Stimulus specific responses from beyond the classical receptive field. Ann. Rev. Neurosci. 8:407–30.

Almy, T. P. 1983. Clinical features and diagnosis of functional GI disorders. In Functional disorders of the digestive tract, ed. W. Y. Chey, 7–11. New York: Raven Press.

Almy, T. P., F. K. Abbot, and L. E. Hinkle. 1950. Alterations in colonic function in man under stress: Hypomotility of the sigmoid colon and its relationship to the mechanism of functional diarrhea. Gastroenterol. 15:95–103.

Almy, T. P., L. E. Hinkle, B. Berle, and F. Kern. 1949. Alterations in colonic function in man under stress: Experimental production of sigmoid spasm in patients with spastic constipation. Gastroenterol. 12:437–49.

Almy, T. P., F. Kern, and M. Tulin. 1949. Alterations in colonic function in man under stress: Experimental production of sigmoid spasm in healthy persons. Gastroenterol. 12:425–36.

Almy, T. P., and M. Tulin. 1947. Alterations in colonic function in man under stress: Experimental production of changes simulating the "irritable colon." Gastroenterol. 8:616–26.

Aloe, L., E. Alleva, A. Bohm, and R. Levi-Montalcini. 1986. Aggressive behavior induces release of nerve growth factor from mouse salivary gland into the bloodstream. Neurobiol. 83:6184–87.

Alpers, D. H. 1981. Irritable bowel syndrome—still more questions than answers. Gastroenterol. 80:1068.

————. 1983. Functional gastrointestinal disorders. Hosp. Pract. 18:139–53.

Altman, J. 1987. Cerebral cortex: A quiet revolution in thinking. Nature (London) 328:572–73.

Amir, S., and Z. Amit. 1979. The pituitary gland mediates acute and chronic pain responsiveness in stressed and non-stressed rats. Life Sci. 24:439–48.

Amkraut, A., G. F. Solomon, and H. C. Kraemer. 1971. Stress, early experience, and adjuvant-induced arthritis in the rat. Psychosom. Med. 33:203–14.

Anderson, D. E. 1982. Behavioral conditioning and experimental hypertension. In 1981 joint USA-USSR symposium, Hypertension: Biobehavioral and epidemiological aspects, 105. Bethesda, MD: U.S. Department of Health and Human Services.

Aneshensel, C. S., R. R. Frerichs, and G. J. Huba. 1984. Depression and physical illness: Multiwave, non-recursive causal model. J. Hlth. Soc. Behav. 25:350–71.

Anisman, H., A. Pizzino, and L. S. Sklar. 1980. Coping with stress, norepinephrine and escape performance. Brain Res. 191:583–88.

Anisman, H., A. Pizzino, and L. S. Sklar. 1980. Coping with stress, norepinephrine and escape performance. Brain Res. 191:583–88.

Anisman, H., G. Remington, and L. S. Sklar. 1979. Effect of inescapable shock on subsequent escape performance: Catecholaminergic and cholinergic mediation of response initiation and maintenance. Psychopharmacol. 61:107–24.

Antonovsky, A. 1979. Health, stress, and coping. San Francisco: Jossey-Bass.

Appley, M. H., and R. Trumbull. 1967. On the concept of psychological stress. In Psychological stress, ed. M. H. Appley and R. Trumbull, 1–13. New York: Meredith Publishing Co.

Arancibia, S., and I. Assenmacher. 1987. Sécrétion de TRH dans le troisième ventricule cérébral lors de l'exposition aigüe au froid chez le rat non-anesthésié. Effet des drogues alpha-adrénergiques. C. R. Soc. Biol. (Paris) 181:323–37.

Arancibia, S., L. Tapia-Arancibia, I. Assenmacher, and H. Astier. 1983. Direct evidence of short-term cold-induced TRH release in the median eminence of unanesthetized rats. Neuroendocrinol. 37:225–28.

Aravich, P. F., B. J. Davis, C. D. Sladek, S. Y. Felten, and D. L. Felten. 1987. Innervation of the gut: Implications for interaction between the nervous and immune systems. In Neuronal control of bodily function: Neurobiological approaches to human disease, ed. D. Hellhammer, I. Florin, and H. Weiner, 63–85. Toronto: Hans Huber.

Arnetz, B. B., T. Theorell, L. Levi, A. Kallner, and P. Eneroth. 1983. An experimental study of social isolation of elderly people: Psychoendocrine and metabolic effects. Psychosom. Med. 45:395–406.

Arrigo-Reina, R., and S. Ferri. 1980. Evidence of an involvement of the opioid peptidergic system in the reaction to stressful conditions. Eur. J. Pharmacol. 64:85–88.

Arthur, R. J. 1982. Life stress and disease: An appraisal of the concept. In Critical issues in behavioral medicine, ed. L. J. West and M. Stein, 3–17. Philadelphia: J. B. Lippincott.

Askevold, F. 1983. Personal communication.

Ax, A. F. 1953. The physiological differentiation between fear and anger in humans. Psychosom. Med. 15:433–42.

Axelrod, J. 1971. Noradrenaline: Fate and control of its biosynthesis. Science 173:598–606.

Axelrod, J., R. A. Mueller, J. P. Henry, and P. M. Stephens. 1970. Changes in enzymes involved in the biosynthesis and metabolism of noradrenaline and adrenaline after psychosocial stimulation. Nature (London) 225:1059–60.

Axelrod, J., and T. D. Reisine. 1984. Stress hormones. Science 224:452–59.

Azarnia, R., S. Reddy, T. E. Kmiecik, D. Shalloway, and W. R. Loewenstein. 1988. The cellular *src* gene product regulates cell-to-cell communication. Science 239:398–401.

Bahnson, C. B. 1969. Psychophysiological complementarity in malignancies: Past work and future vistas. Ann. N.Y. Acad. Sci. 164:319–34.

Baker, G. H. B. 1982. Life events before the onset of rheumatoid arthritis. Psychotherap. Psychosom. 38:173–77.

Ballieux, R. E., J. F. Fielding, and A. L'Abbate, eds. 1984. Breakdown in human adaptation to stress: Towards a multidisciplinary approach. Vol. 2. Boston: Martinus Nijhoff.

Ballieux, R. E., and C. J. Heijnen. 1987. Stress and the immune system. In Neuronal control of bodily function: Neurobiological approaches to human disease, ed. D. Hellhammer, I. Florin, and H. Weiner, 301–6. Toronto: Hans Huber.

Baraban, J. M., P. F. Worley, and S. H. Snyder. 1989. Second messenger systems and psychoactive drug action: Focus on the phosphoinositide system and lithium. Am. J. Psychiat. 146:1251–60.

Baran, A., L. Shuster, B. E. Elefteriou, and D. W. Bailey. 1975. Opiate receptors in mice: Genetic differences. Life Sci. 17:633–40.

Barchas, J. D., R. D. Ciarenello, J. A. Dominic, T. Deguchi, E. O. Orenberg, J. Renson, and S. Kessler. 1974. Genetic aspects of monoamine mechanisms. Adv. Biochem. Psychopharmacol. 12:195–204.

Barchas, J. D., and D. X. Freedman. 1963. Brain amines: Response to physiological stress. Biochem. Pharmacol. 12:1232–35.

Bard, P., and V. B. Mountcastle. 1948. Some forebrain mechanisms involved in expression of rage with special reference to suppression of angry behavior. In The frontal lobes. Res. Publ. Assoc. Nerv. Ment. Dis. 27:362–404.

Bard, P., and D. McK. Rioch. 1937. A study of four cats deprived of neocortex and additional portions of the forebrain. Bull. Johns Hopkins Hosp. 60:73–147.

Baroldi, G. 1975. Different morphologic types of myocardial cell death in man. In Pathophysiology and morphology of myocardial cell alteration, ed. A. Fleckenstein and G. Rona, 383–97. Baltimore: University Park Press.

Baroldi, G., G. Falzi, and F. Mariani. 1979. Sudden coronary death: A postmortem study in 208 selected cases compared to 97 "control" subjects. Am. Heart J. 98:20–31.

Barry, J., A. P. Selwyn, E. G. Nabel, M. B. Rocco, K. Mead, S. Campbell, and G. Rebecca. 1988. Frequency of ST-segment depression produced by mental stress in stable angina pectoris from coronary artery disease. Am. J. Cardiol. 61:989–93.

Bartrop, R. W., E. Luckhurst, L. Lazarus, L. G. Kiloh, and R. Perry. 1977. Depressed lymphocyte function after bereavement. Lancet 1:834–36.

Bassett, J. R., and J. D. Cairncross. 1975. Time course for plasma 11-hydroxycorticosteroid elevation in rats during stress. Pharmacol. Biochem. Behav. 3:139–42.

Bateman, A., A. Singh, T. Kral, and S. Solomon. 1989. The immune-hypothalamic-pituitary-adrenal axis. Endocr. Rev. 10:92–112.

Baulieu, E.-E. 1989. Contragestion and other applications of RU 486, an anti-progesterone at the receptor. Science 245:1351–57.

Baum, A. 1987. Toxins, technology, and natural disasters. In Cataclysms, crises, and catastrophes: Psychology in action, ed. G. R. Van den Bos and B. K. Bryant, 9–53. Washington, DC: American Psychological Association.

Baum, A., R. Fleming, and L. M. Davidson. 1983. Natural disasters and technological catastrophe. Envt. Behav. 15:333–54.

Baum, A., V. Lundberg, N. Gruenberg, J. Singer, and R. Gatchell. 1985. Urinary catecholamines in behavioral research in stress. In The catecholamines in psychiatric and neurologic disorders, ed. C. R. Lake and M. G. Ziegler, 55–72. London: Butterworths.

Baxter, B. L. 1967. Comparison of the behavioral effects of electrical or chemical stimulation applied at the same brain loci. Exp. Neurol. 19:412–32.

Bayon, A., W. J. Shoemaker, F. E. Bloom, A. Mauss, and R. Guillemin. 1979. Perinatal development of the endorphin and enkephalin-containing systems in the rat brain. Brain Res. 179:93–101.

Beach, F. A. 1950. Discussion. Res. Publ. Assoc. Nerv. Ment. Dis. 29:674–75.

Beacham, W., and E. R. Perl. 1964. Characteristics of a spinal sympathetic reflex. J. Physiol. (London) 173:431–48.

Beale, N., and S. Nethercott. 1986. Job-loss and health—the influence of age and previous morbidity. J. R. Coll. Gen. Pract. 36:261–64.

Bebbington, P. E., T. Brugha, B. MacCarthy, J. Potter, E. Sturt, T. Wykes, R. Katz, and P. McGuffin. 1988. The Camberwell collaborative depression study I. Depressed probands: Adversity and the form of depression. Br. J. Psychiat. 152:754–56.

Beebe, G. W. 1975. Follow-up studies of World War II and Korean war prisoners. Am. J. Epidemiol. 101:400–22.

Belle, D. 1982. Social ties and social support. In Lives in stress: Women and depression, ed. D. Belle, 133–144. Beverly Hills, CA: Sage.

———. 1987. Gender differences in the social moderators of stress. In Gender and stress, ed. R. C. Barnett, L. Biener, and G. K. Baruch, 257–77. New York: Free Press.

Benedek, T., and B. B. Rubenstein. 1942. The sexual cycle in women. Psychosom. Med. Monographs, vol. 3, nos. 1 and 2. Washington, DC: National Research Council.

Ben-Eliyahu, S., R. Yirmiya, Y. Shavit, and J. C. Liebeskind. 1990. Stress-induced suppression of natural killer cell cytotoxicity: A naltrexone-insensitive paradigm. Behav. Neurosci. 104:235–38.

Benjamin, S. B., D. C. Gerhardt, and D. O. Castell. 1977. High amplitude peristaltic esophageal contractions associated with chest pain and/or dysphagia. Gastroenterol. 77:478–83.

Benner, P., E. Roskies, and R. S. Lazarus. 1980. Stress and coping under extreme conditions. In Survivors, victims, and perpetrators: Essays on the Nazi Holocaust, ed. J. E. Dimsdale, 219–58. Washington, DC: Hemisphere Press.

Bennett, J. R., and M. Atkinson. 1966. The differentiation between oesophageal and cardiac pain. Lancet 2:1123–27.

Berkenbosch, F., J. van Oers, A. del Rey, F. Tilders, and H. Besedovsky. 1987. Corticotropin-releasing factor–producing neurons in the rat activated by interleukin-1. Science 238:524–26.

Berkman, L. F. 1980. Physical health and the social environment: A social epidemiological perspective. In The relevance of social science for medicine, ed. L. Eisenberg and A. Kleinman, 51–75. Boston: D. Reidel Publishing Company.

Berkman, L. F., and S. L. Syme. 1979. Social networks, host resistance, and mortality: A nine-year follow-up study of Alameda County residents. Am. J. Epidemiol. 109:186–204.

Bermudez, F., M. I. Surks, and J. H. Oppenheimer. 1975. High incidence of decreased triiodothyronine concentration in patients with nonthyroidal disease. J. Clin. Endocrinol. Metab. 41:27–40.

Bernard, C. 1865. Introduction à l'étude de la médecine expérimentale. Paris: Baillière et Fils.

Bernton, E. W., M. S. Meltzer, and J. W. Holaday. 1987. Permissive effects of prolactin on cellular immunity in vivo: Implications relating behavioral stress and host defenses. In Neuronal control of bodily function: Neurobiological approaches to human disease, ed. D. Hellhammer, I. Florin, and H. Weiner, 290–300. Toronto: Hans Huber.

Berridge, M. J., and R. F. Irvine. 1989. Inositol phosphates and cell signaling. Nature (London) 341:197–205.

Besterman, H. S., D. L. Sarson, J. C. Rambaud, J. S. Stewart, S. Guerkin, and S. R. Bloom. 1981. Gut hormone responses in the irritable bowel syndrome. Digestion 21:219–24.

Bettelheim, B., and M. Janowitz. 1964. Social change and prejudice. New York: Free Press.

Beutler, E. 1991. Glucose-6-phosphate dehydrogenase deficiency. New Engl. J. Med. 324:169–74.

Bianchi, G., U. Fox, G. F. DiFrancisco, U. Bardi, and M. Radice. 1973. The hypertensive role of the kidney in spontaneously hypertensive rats. Clin. Sci. Mol. Med. 45 (Suppl.):135s–39s.

Bibring, G. L., and R. J. Kahana. 1968. Lectures in medical psychology. New York: International Universities Press.

Binger, C. A. L. 1945. The doctor's job. New York: Norton.

Bixler, E. O., A. Kales, C. R. Soldatos, J. P. Kales, and S. Healey. 1979. Prevalence of sleep disorders in the Los Angeles metropolitan area. Am. J. Psychiat. 136:1257–62.

Blanchard, E. B., L. C. Kolb, T. P. Pallmeyer, and R. J. Gerardi. 1982. A psychophysiological study of post-traumatic stress disorder in Vietnam veterans. Psychiat. Q. 54:220–29.

Blazer, D. G. 1982. Social support and mortality in an elderly community population. Am. J. Epidemiol. 115:684–94.

Bliss, E. L., and J. Zwaniger. 1966. Brain amines and emotional stress. J. Psychiatr. Res. 4:189–98.

Bloch, S., and C. Brackenridge. 1972. Psychological performance and biochemical factors in medical students under examination stress. J. Psychosom. Res. 16:25–33.

Block, J. 1971. Lives through time. Berkeley: Bancroft.

Bloom, A. A., P. LoPresti, and J. T. Farrar. 1968. Motility of intact human colon. Gastroenterol. 54:232–40.

Blumberg, B. S. 1977. Australia antigen and the biology of hepatitis B. Science 197:17–25.

Bodnar, R. J., M. Glusman, M. Brutus, A. Spiaggia, and D. D. Kelly. 1979. Analgesia induced by cold-water stress: Attentuation following hypophysectomy. Physiol. Behav. 23:53–62.

Bogdonoff, M. D., E. H. Estes, W. R. Harlan, D. L. Trout, and R. Kirsher. 1960. Metabolic and cardiovascular changes during a state of acute central nervous system arousal. J. Clin. Endocrinol. Metab. 20:1333–40.

Bornstein, P. E., P. J. Clayton, J. A. Halikas, W. L. Maurice, and E. Robins. 1973. The depression of widowhood after 13 months. Br. J. Psychiat. 122:561–66.

Bosisio, E., M. Sergi, R. Sega, and A. Libretti. 1979. Respiratory response to carbon dioxide after propranolol in normal subjects. Respiration 37:197–200.

Bouloux, P.-M. G., and A. Grossman. 1989. Opioid involvement in the neuroendocrine responses to stress in humans. In Neuronal control of bodily function: Frontiers of stress research, ed. H. Weiner, D. Hellhammer, I. Florin, and R. Murison, 209–22. Toronto: Hans Huber.

Bourgault, P. C., A. G. Karczmar, and C. L. Scudder. 1963. Contrasting behavioral, pharmacological, neurophysiological, and biochemical profiles of C57BL/6 and SC-1 strains of mice. Life Sci. 8:533–53.

Bourne, P. G., R. M. Rose, and J. W. Mason. 1967. Urinary 17-OHCS levels: Data on seven helicopter ambulance medics in combat. Arch. Gen. Psychiat. 17:104–10.

———. 1968. 17-OHCS levels in combat: Special forces A team under threat of attack. Arch. Gen. Psychiat. 19:135–40.

Bowlby, J. 1963. Pathological mourning and childhood mourning. J. Am. Psychoanal. Assoc. 11:500–541.

Bowling, A., and J. Charlton. 1987. Risk factors for mortality after bereavement: A logistic regression analysis. J. R. Coll. Gen. Pract. 37:551–54.

Boyar, R. M., and H. L. Bradlow. 1977. Studies of testosterone metabolism in anorexia nervosa. In Anorexia nervosa, ed. R. Vigersky, 271–76. New York: Raven Press.

Boyar, R. M., L. D. Hellman, H. P. Roffwarg, J. L. Katz, B. Zumoff, J O'Connor, H. L. Bradlow, and D. K. Fukushima. 1977. Cortisol secretion and metabolism in anorexia nervosa. New Engl. J. Med. 296:190–93.

Boyar, R. M., J. L. Katz, J. W. Finkelstein, S. Kapen, H. Weiner, E. D. Weitzman, and L. Hellman. 1974. Anorexia nervosa: Immaturity of the 24-hour luteinizing hormone secretory pattern. New Engl. J. Med. 291:861–65.

Brackett, C. D., and L. H. Powell. 1988. Psychosocial and physiological predictors of sudden cardiac death after healing of acute myocardial infarction. Am. J. Cardiol. 61:979–83.

Bram, I. 1927. Psychic trauma in the pathogenesis of exophthalmic goiter. Endocrinol. 11:106–21.

Brand, D. L., D. Martin, and C. E. Pope II. 1977. Esophageal manometrics in patients with angina-like chest pain. Dig. Dis. Sci. 22:300–304.

Brautbar, N., H. Leibovici, P. Finlander, V. Campese, C. Penia, and S. G. Massry.

1980. Mechanisms of hypophosphatemia during acute hyperventilation. Clin. Res. 28:387A.

Breier, A., J. P. Kelsoe, Jr., P. D. Kirwin, S. A. Beller, O. M. Wolkowitz, and D. Pickar. 1988. Early parental loss and development of psychopathology. Arch. Gen. Psychiat. 45:987–93.

Brende, J. O. 1982. Electrodermal responses in post-traumatic syndromes. J. Nerv. Ment. Dis. 70:352–61.

Brenner, M. H. 1973. Mental illness and the economy. Cambridge, MA: Harvard University Press.

———. 1985. Economic change and the suicide rate: A population model including loss, separation, illness, and alcohol consumption. In Stress in health and disease, ed. M. R. Zales, 160–85. New York: Brunner/Mazel.

Breznitz, S., and O. Zinder, eds. 1989. Molecular biology of stress. New York: Alan R. Liss.

Bristow, J. D., E. B. Brown, Jr., D. J. C. Cunningham, M. G. Howson, E. S. Petersen, T. G. Pickering, and P. Sleight. 1971. Effect of bicycling on the baroreflex regulation of pulse interval. Circ. Res. 28:582–87.

Brod, J. 1960. Essential hypertension—hemodynamic observations with bearing on its pathogenesis. Lancet 2:773–76.

———. 1970. Hemodynamics and emotional stress. Biblioteca Psychiatrica 144: 13–33.

Brodie, D. A., and H. M. Hanson. 1960. A study of the factors involved in the production of gastric ulcers by the restraint technique. Gastroenterol. 38:353–60.

Bromet, E. 1980. Three Mile Island: Mental health findings. Washington, DC: NIMH contract no. 278–79, 0048 (SM).

Brooks, D., P. Fox, R. Lopez, and P. Sleight. 1978. The effect of mental arithmetic blood pressure variability and baroreflex sensitivity in man. J. Physiol. (London) 280:75P.

Brown, G. W., and T. Harris. 1978. Social origins of depression. London: Tavistock Press.

———. 1986. Establishing causal links: The Bedford College studies of depression. In Life events and psychiatric disorders: Controversial issues, ed. H. Katsching, 107–87. Cambridge, Eng.: Cambridge University Press.

Brown, J. J., R. Fraser, A. F. Lever, J. J. Morton, J. I. S. Rubinson, and M. A. D. H. Schalekamp. 1977. Mechanisms in hypertension: A personal view. In Hypertension, ed. J. Genest, E. Koiw, and O. Kuchel, 529–48. New York: McGraw-Hill.

Brown, J. T., and G. A. Stoudemire. 1983. Normal and pathological grief. JAMA 250:378–82.

Brown, M., and L. Fisher. 1984. Brain peptides as intercellular messengers. JAMA 251:1310–15.

———. 1985. Corticotropin-releasing factor: Effects on the autonomic nervous system and visceral systems. Fed. Proc. FASEB 44:243–48.

———. 1989. Corticotropin-releasing factor: Regulation of the autonomic nervous system. In Neuronal control of bodily function: Frontiers of stress research, ed. H. Weiner, D. Hellhammer, I. Florin, and R. Murison, 233–39. Toronto: Hans Huber.

Brown, M. R., L. A. Fisher, V. Webb, W. W. Vale, and J. E. Rivier. 1985. Corticotropin-releasing factor: A physiological regulator of adrenal epinephrine secretion. Brain Res. 328:355–57.

Brown, M. S., and J. L. Goldstein. 1986. A receptor mediated pathway for cholesterol homeostasis. Science 232:34–47.

Brown, W. A., and G. Heninger. 1975. Cortisol, growth hormone, free fatty acids, and experimentally evoked affective arousal. Am. J. Psychiat. 132:1172–76.

Brown, W. A., and G. Heninger. 1976. Stress-induced growth hormone release: Psychologic and physiologic correlates. Psychosom. Med. 38:145–47.

Bruhn, J. G. 1987. The novelty of stress. South. Med. J. 80:1398–1406.

Bruhn, J. G., B. Chandler, M. C. Miller, S. Wolf, and T. N. Lynn. 1966. Social aspects of coronary heart disease in two adjacent, ethnically different communities. Am. J. Publ. Hlth. 56:1493–1506.

Buchwald, D., J. L. Sullivan, and A. L. Komaroff. 1987. Frequency of chronic active Epstein-Barr virus infection in a general medical practice. JAMA 257:2303–7.

Bueno, L., J. Fioramonti, Y. Rukebusch, J. Frexinos, and P. Coulomb. 1980. Evaluation of colonic myoelectrical activity in health and functional disorders. Gut 21:480–85.

Bukhave, K., and J. Rask-Madsen. 1980. An approach to evaluation of local intestinal PG production and clinical assessment of its inhibition by indomethacin in chronic diarrhea. Adv. Prostaglandin Thromboxane Res. 8:1627–31.

Bunag, R. D., I. H. Page, and J. W. McCubbin. 1966. Neural stimulation of release of renin. Circ. Res. 19:851–58.

Bunnett, N. W., and J. W. Walsh. 1988. Regulation of gastric secretion: Humoral mechanisms. In Perspectives in behavioral medicine: Eating regulation and discontrol, ed. H. Weiner and A. Baum, 33–48. Hillsdale, NJ: Lawrence Erlbaum.

Butler, S. R., M. R. Suskind, and S. M. Schanberg. 1978. Maternal behavior as a regulator of polyamine biosynthesis in brain and heart of developing rat pups. Science 199:445–47.

Caffrey, C. B. 1966. Behavior patterns and personality characteristics as related to prevalence rates of coronary heart disease in Trappist and Benedictine monks. Doctoral dissertation, Catholic University of America, Washington, DC. University Microfilms, no. 67-1830, 45–48.

Campbell, S. M., S. Clark, E. A. Tindall, M. E. Forehand, and R. M. Bennett. 1983. Clinical characteristics of fibrositis, 1: A "blinded" controlled study of symptoms and tender points. Arthri. Rheumat. 26:817–24.

Cannon, W. B. 1914. The interrelations of emotions as suggested by recent physiological researchers. Am. J. Psychol. 25:256–82.

———. 1928. The mechanisms of emotional disturbance of bodily functions. New Engl. J. Med. 198:877–84.

———. 1929. Bodily changes in pain, hunger, fear, and rage. 2d ed. New York: D. Appleton.

———. 1935. The stresses and strains of homeostasis. Am. J. Med. Sci. 189:1–14.

———. 1939. The wisdom of the body. Philadelphia: W. W. Norton.

Cannon, J. T., G. J. Prieto, A. Lee, and J. C. Liebeskind. 1982. Evidence for opioid and non-opioid forms of stimulation produced analgesia in the rat. Brain Res. 243:315–21.

Cannon, J. T., G. W. Terman, J. W. Lewis, and J. C. Liebeskind. 1984. Body region shocked need not critically define the neurochemical basis of stress analgesia. Brain Res. 323:316–19.

Cantin, M., and J. Genest. 1986. The heart as an endocrine organ. Scient. Am. 254:76–81.

Carcamo, J., S. Lobos, A. Merino, L. Buckbinder, R. Weinmann, V. Natarajan, and D. Reinberg. 1989. Factors involved in specific transcription by mammalian RNA polymerase II—role of factors IID and MLTF in transcription from the adenovirus major late and IVa2 promoters. J. Biol. Chem. 264:7704–14.

Carette, S., G. A. McCain, D. A. Bell, and A. G. Fam. 1986. Evaluation of amitriptyline in primary fibrositis. Arthri. Rheumat. 29:655–59.

Carroll, K. F., and P. J. Nestel. 1973. Diurnal variation in glucose tolerance and in insulin secretion in man. Diabetes 22:333–48.

Carter, J. N., C. J. Eastman, J. M. Corcoran, and L. Lazarus. 1974. Effect of severe chronic illness on thyroid function. Lancet 2:971–74.

Cassel, J. 1976. The contribution of the social environment to host resistance. Am. J. Epidemiol. 104:107–23.

Castell, D. O. 1976. Achalasia and diffuse esophageal spasm. Arch. Int. Med. 136:571–79.

Chalmers, J. P. 1975. Brain amines and models of experimental hypertension. Circ. Res. 36:469–80.

Champion, P. 1973. Some cases of the irritable bowel syndrome studied by intraluminal pressure recordings. Digestion 9:21–29.

Chandra, V., M. Szklo, R. Goldberg, and J. Tonascia. 1983. The impact of marital status on survival after an acute myocardial infarction: A population-based study. Am. J. Epidemiol. 117:320–25.

Chang, K. J., and P. Cautrecasas. 1979. Multiple opiate receptors: Enkephalins and morphine bind to receptors of different specificity. J. Biol. Chem. 254:2610–18.

Chantler, J. A., A. J. Tingle, and R. E. Petty. 1988. Persistent rubella virus infection associated with chronic arthritis in children. New Engl. J. Med. 313:1117–23.

Chappell, P. B., M. A. Smith, C. D. Kilts, G. Bissette, J. Ritchie, C. Anderson, and C. B. Nemeroff. 1986. Alterations in corticotropin-releasing factor–like immunoreactivity in discrete rat brain regions after acute and chronic stress. J. Neurosci. 6:2908–14.

Chaudhary, N. A., and S. C. Truelove. 1961. Human colonic motility: A comparative study of normal subjects, patients with ulcerative colitis, and patients with irritable colon syndrome. Gastroenterol. 40:1–17.

———. 1962. The irritable colon syndrome: A study of the clinical features, predisposing causes, and prognosis in 130 cases. Q. J. Med. 31:307–23.

Cheun, L. Y., W. Jùbiz, J. G. Moore, and J. Frailey. 1975. Gastric prostaglandin-E (PGE) output during basal and stimulated acid secretion in normal subjects and patients with peptic ulcer. Gastroenterol. 68:873.

Chey, W. H., C. H. You, K. Y. Lee, and R. Menguy. 1983. Gastric dysrhythmia: Clinical aspects. In Functional disorders of the digestive tract, ed. W. Y. Chey, 175–81. New York: Raven Press.

Chodoff, P. 1975. Psychiatric aspects of the Nazi persecution. In American handbook of psychiatry, vol. 6, 2d ed., ed. S. Arieti, 932–46. New York: Basic Books.

Chopra, I. J., and S. R. Smith. 1975. Circulating thyroid hormones and thyrotropin in adult patients with protein-calorie malnutrition. J. Clin. Endocrinol. Metab. 40:221–27.

Chowdhury, A. R., V. P. Dinoso, and D. H. Lorber. 1976. Characterization of a hyperactive segment at the rectosigmoid function. Gastroenterol. 71:584–88.

Christensen, J. 1971. The control of gastrointestinal movements: Some old and new views. New Engl. J. Med. 285:85–98.

Christian, J. J. 1963. Endocrine adaptive mechanisms and the physiological regulation of population growth. In Physiological mammalogy, vol. 1, ed. W. Mayer and R. van Gelder, 189–253. New York: Academic Press.

Chrysant, S. G. 1979. Effects of high salt intake and meclofenamate on arterial pressure and renal function in the spontaneously hypertensive rat. Clin. Sci. Mol. Med. 57 (Suppl. 5): 251s–53s.

Chung, E. K. 1989. Principles of cardiac arrhythmias. 4th ed. Baltimore: Williams and Wilkins.

Ciaranello, R. D. 1979. Genetic regulation of the catecholamine synthesizing enzymes. In Genetic variation in hormone systems, vol. 2, ed. J. G. M. Shire, 49–61. Boca Raton, FL: CRC Press.

Clarkson, T. B., J. R. Kaplan, M. R. Adams, and S. B. Manuck. 1987. Psychosocial influences on the pathogenesis of atherosclerosis among nonhuman primates. Circulation 76 (Suppl. 1): 1–29–I–40.

Clayton, P. J., M. Herjanic, G. E. Murphy, and R. Woodruff, Jr. 1974. Mourning and depression: Their similarities and differences. Can. J. Psychiat. 19:309–12.

Clouse, R. E., and P. J. Lustman. 1983. Psychiatric illness and contraction abnormalities of the esophagus. New Engl. J. Med. 309:1337–42.

Cobb, S. 1976. Social support as a moderator of life stress. Psychosom. Med. 38:300–314.

Coe, C., L. Rosenberg, and S. Levine. 1988. Immunological consequences of psychological disturbance and maternal loss in infancy. In Advances in infancy research, ed. C. Rovee-Collier and L. Lipsitt, 97–134. Norwood, NJ: Ablex.

Coe, C. L., M. E. Stanton, and S. Levine. 1983. Adrenal response to reinforcement and extinction: Role of expectancy versus instrumental response. Behav. Neurosci. 97:654–57.

Coe, C. L., S. G. Wiener, and S. Levine. 1983. Psychoendocrine responses of mother and infant monkeys to disturbance and separation. In Symbiosis in parent-young interactions, ed. H. Moltz and L. A. Rosenblum, 189–214. New York: Plenum Press.

Cohen, B. R. 1973. Emotional considerations in esophageal disease. In Emotional factors in gastrointestinal disease, ed. A. E. Lindner, 37–44. Amsterdam: Excerpta Medica.

Cohen, D. H. 1981. Cardiovascular neurobiology: The substrate for biobehavioral approaches to hypertension. In 1981 joint USA-USSR symposium, Hypertension: Biobehavioral and epidemiological aspects, 93. Bethesda, MD: U.S. Department of Health and Human Services.

Cohen, F., M. J. Horowitz, R. S. Lazarus, R. H. Moos, L. N. Robins, R. M. Rose, and M. J. Rutter. 1982. Panel report on psychosocial assets and modifiers of stress. In Stress and human health, ed. G. R. Elliott and C. Eisdorfer, 147–88. New York: Springer.

Cohen, M. B., G. Baker, R. A. Cohen, F. Fromm-Reichman, and E. V. Weigert. 1954. An intensive study of twelve cases of manic depressive psychosis. Psychiatry 17:103–7.

Cohen, S. 1979. Motor disorders of the esophagus. New Engl. J. Med. 301:184–92.

Colpaert, F. C., J. Donnerer, and F. Lembeck. 1983. Effects of capsaicin on inflammation and on the substance P content of nervous tissues in rats with adjuvant arthritis. Life Sci. 32:1827–34.

Condon, J. T. 1986. Psychological disability in women who relinquish a baby for adoption. Med. J. Aust. 144:117–19.

Conger, J. J., W. L. Sawrey, and E. S. Turrell. 1958. The role of social experience in the production of gastric ulcers in hooded rats placed in a conflict situation. J. Abn. Soc. Psychol. 57:214–20.

Connell, A. M. 1962. Motility of the pelvic colon, 2: Paradoxical motility in diarrhea and constipation. Gut 3:342–48.

Connell, A. M., M. Gaafer, M. A. Hassanein, and F. A. Jones. 1964. Motility of the pelvic colon, 3: Motility response in patients with symptoms following amoebic dysentery. Gut 5:443–47.

Connell, A. M., F. A. Jones, and E. N. Rowlands. 1965. Motility of the pelvic colon, 4: Abdominal pain associated with colonic hypermotility after meals. Gut 6:105–12.

Cook, D. G., R. O. Cummings, M. J. Bartley, and A. S. Shaper. 1982. The health of unemployed middle-aged men in Great Britain. Lancet 1:1290–91.

Cooke, D. J., and D. J. Hole. 1983. The aetiological importance of stressful life events. Br. J. Psychiat. 143:397–400.

Cools, A. R. 1987. Transformation of emotion into motion: Role of mesolimbic noradrenaline and neostriatal dopamine. In Neuronal control of bodily function: Neurobiological approaches to human disease, ed. D. Hellhammer, I. Florin, and H. Weiner, 15–28. Toronto: Hans Huber.

Copeland, D. D. 1977. Concepts of disease and diagnosis. Perspect. Biol. Med. 20:528–38.

Coryell, W., R. Noyes, and J. Clarcy. 1982. Excess mortality in panic disorder: A comparison with primary unipolar depression. Arch. Gen. Psychiat. 39:701–3.

Coryell, W., R. Noyes, and J. D. House. 1986. Mortality among outpatients with anxiety disorders. Am. J. Psychiat. 143:508–10.

Costello, C. G. 1982. Social factors associated with depression: A retrospective community study. Psychol. Med. 12:329–39.

Courtright, L. G., and W. C. Kuzell. 1965. Sparing effect of neurological deficit and trauma on the course of adjuvant arthritis in the rat. Ann. Rheum. Dis. 24:360–68.

Coyle, J. T., and C. B. Pert. 1976. Ontogenetic development of (H)-Naloxone binding in the rat brain. Neuropharmacol. 15:550–55.

Crabtree, G. R., K. A. Smith, and A. Munck. 1981. Glucocorticoid receptors. In The leukemic cell, ed. D. Catovsky, 252–69. New York: Churchill Livingstone.

Crean, G. P., W. I. Card, A. D. Beattie, R. J. Holden, W. B. James, R. P. Knill-Jones, R. W. Lucas, and D. Spiegelhalter. 1982. Ulcer-like dyspepsia. Scand. J. Gastroenterol. (Suppl.) 79:9–15.

Crews, D. 1975. Psychobiology of reptilian reproduction. Science 189:1059–65.

Crews, D., and M. D. Moore. 1986. Evolution of mechanisms controlling mating behavior. Science 231:121–25.

Crook, J., E. Rideout, and G. Browne. 1984. The prevalence of pain complaints in a general population. Pain 18:299–314.

Crown, S., J. M. Crown, and A. Fleming. 1975. Aspects of the psychology and epidemiology of rheumatoid disease. Psychol. Med. 5:291–99.

Cryer, P. E., and J. E. Gerich. 1985. Glucose counterregulation, hypoglycemia, and intensive insulin therapy in diabetes mellitus. New Engl. J. Med. 313:232–41.

Cullen, J., J. Siegrist, and H. M. Wegman. 1984. Breakdown in human adaptation to stress: Towards a multidisciplinary approach, vol. 1. Boston: Martinus Nijhoff.

Curtis, G. C., M. Buxton, D. Lippman, R. Nesse, and J. Wright. 1976. Flooding in vivo during the circadian phase of minimal cortisol secretion: Anxiety and therapeutic success without adrenal cortical activation. Biol. Psychiat. 11:101–7.

Curtis, G. C., R. Nesse, M. Buxton, and D. Lippman. 1978. Anxiety and plasma cortisol at the crest of the circadian cycle: Reappraisal of a classical hypothesis. Psychosom. Med. 40:368–78.

———. 1979. Plasma growth hormone: Effect of anxiety during flooding in vivo. Am. J. Psychiat. 136:410–14.

DaCosta, J. M. 1871a. On irritable heart: A clinical study of a form of functional cardiac disorder and its consequences. Am. J. Med. Sci. 61:17–52.

———. 1871b. Membranous enteritis. Am. J. Med. Sci. 124:321–28.

Dahl, L. K., M. Heine, and L. Tassinari. 1962. Effects of chronic excess salt ingestion: Evidence that genetic factors play an important role in susceptibility to experimental hypertension. J. Exp. Med. 115:1173–90.

Dallman, M. F., and F. E. Yates. 1969. Dynamic asymmetrics in the corticosteroid feedback path and distribution-metabolism-binding elements of the adrenocortical system. Ann. N.Y. Acad. Sci. 156:696–721.

Daniel, E. E. 1975. Electrophysiology of the colon. Gut 16:298–329.

Darwin, C. R. 1859. On the origin of species by means of natural selection, or, the preservation of favoured races in the struggle for life. London: Murray.

———. 1872. The expression of the emotions in man and animals. Reprint, Chicago: University of Chicago Press, 1965.

Davies, H. A., Jones, D. B., and Rhodes, J. 1982. "Esophageal angina" as the cause of chest pain. JAMA 249:2274–78.

Day, G. 1951. The psychosomatic approach to pulmonary tuberculosis. Lancet 1:1025–28.

Deanfield, J. E., A. Maseri, A. P. Selwyn, P. Ribeiro, S. Chierchia, S. Krikler, and M. Morgan. 1983. Myocardial ischemia during daily life in patients with stable angina: Its relation to symptoms and heart rate changes. Lancet 2:574–78.

Deanfield, J. E., M. Shea, M. Kensett, P. Horlock, R. A. Wilson, C. M. DeLandsheere, and A. P. Selwyn. 1984. Silent myocardial ischaemia due to mental stress. Lancet 2:1001–5.

de Arauyo, G., P. P. Van Arsdel, T. H. Holmes, and D. L. Dudley. 1973. Life change, coping ability, and chronic intrinsic asthma. J. Psychosom. Res. 17:359–63.

DeCherney, G. S., C. R. Debold, R. V. Jackson, W. R. Sheldon, J., D. P. Island, and D. N. Orth. 1985. Diurnal variation in the response of plasma adrenocorticotropin and cortisol to intravenous ovine corticotropin-releasing hormone. J. Clin. Endocrinol. Metab. 61:273–79.

DeLongis, A., J. C. Coyne, G. Dakof, S. Folkman, and R. S. Lazarus. 1982. Relationship of daily hassles, uplifts, and major life events to health status. Hlth. Psychol. 1:119–36.

Denning, P. J. 1990. The science of computing: Modeling reality. Am. Scientist 78:495–98.

Dent, J., W. J. Dodds, R. H. Friedman, T. Sekiguchi, W. J. Hogan, R. C. Arndorfer, and D. J. Petrie. 1980. Mechanism of gastroesophageal reflux in recumbent asymptomatic human subjects. J. Clin. Invest. 65:226–67.

DeQuattro, V., and Y. Miura. 1973. Neurogenic factors in human hypertension: Mechanism or myth? Am. J. Med. 55:362–78.

Dess, N. K., D. Linwick, J. Patterson, J. B. Overmier, and S. Levine. 1983. Immediate and proactive effects on controllability and predictability of plasma cortisol responses to shocks in dogs. Behav. Neurosci. 97:1005–16.

De Waard, F. 1975. Breast cancer incidence and nutritional status with particular reference to body weight. Cancer Res. 35:3351–56.

Dewey, W. L., L. S. Harris, J. F. Howes, and J. A. Nuite. 1970. The effect of various neurohumoral modulators on the activity of morphine and the narcotic antagonist in the tailflick and phenylquinone test. J. Pharmacol. Exp. Ther. 175:435–42.

DeYoe, E. A., and D. C. Van Essen. 1988. Concurrent processing streams in monkey visual cortex. Trends Neurosci. 11:219–28.

Dick, A. P., L. P. Holt, and E. R. Dalton, 1966. Persistence of mucosal abnormality in ulcerative colitis. Gut 7:355–60.

DiMarino, Jr., A. J., and S. Cohen. 1974. Characteristics of lower esophageal sphincter function in symptomatic diffuse esophageal spasm. Gastroenterol. 66:1–6.

Dimsdale, J., and A. Herd. 1982. Variability of plasma lipids in response to emotional arousal. Psychosom. Med. 44:413–30.

Dimsdale, J., and J. Moss. 1980. Plasma catecholamines in stress and exercise. JAMA 243:340–42.

Dinarello, C. A. 1984. Interleukin-I and the pathogenesis of the acute-phase response. New Engl. J. Med. 311:1413–18.

Dinarello, C. A., and J. W. Mier. 1987. Lymphokines. New Engl. J. Med. 317:940–45.

Dinoso, V. P., H. Meshkinpour, S. H. Lorber, J. G. Gutierrez, and W. Y. Chey. 1973. Motor responses of the sigmoid colon and rectum to exogenous cholecystokinin and secretin. Gastroenterol. 65:438–444.

Dixon, F. J. 1982. Murine SLE models and autoimmune disease. Hosp. Pract. 17:63–73.

Doba, N., and D. J. Reis. 1974. Role of the cerebellum and the vestibular apparatus in regulation of orthostatic reflexes in the cat. Circ. Res. 34:9–14.

Dodge, J. A., I. A. Handi, G. M. Burns, and Y. Yamashiro. 1981. Toddler diarrhea and prostaglandins. Arch. Dis. Child. 56:705–7.

Dohrenwend, B. S., and B. P. Dohrenwend. 1974. Stressful life events. New York: Wiley.

Dolly, J. O. 1988. Potassium channels—what can the protein chemistry contribute? Trends Neurosci. 11:186–88.

Dotevall, G. 1985. Stress and common gastrointestinal disorders: A comprehensive approach. New York: Praeger.

———. 1989. The irritable gastrointestinal tract. In Neuronal control of bodily function: Frontiers of stress research, ed. H. Weiner, I. Florin, R. Murison, and D. Hellhammer, 344–54. Toronto: Hans Huber.

Dotevall, G. J., J. Svedlund,and I. Sjödin. 1982. Symptoms in irritable bowel disease. Scand. J. Gastroenterol. (Suppl.) 79:16–19.

Drossman, D. A. 1982. Patients with psychogenic abdominal pain: Six years observation in the medical setting. Am. J. Psychiat. 139:1549–57.

Drossman, D. A., D. W. Powell, and J. T. Sessions, Jr. 1977. The irritable bowel syndrome. Gastroenterol. 73:811–22.

Drugan, R, S. I. Deutsch, A. Weizman, R. Weizman, F. J. Vocci, J. N. Crawley, P. Skolnick, and S. M. Paul. 1989. Molecular mechanisms of stress and anxiety: Alterations in the benzodiazepine/GABA receptor complex. In Neuronal control of bodily function: Frontiers of stress research, ed. H. Weiner, D. Hellhammer, I. Florin, and R. Murison, 148–59. Toronto: Hans Huber.

Dunn, M. J. 1978. Renal prostaglandin production in the Japanese (Kyoto) spontaneously hypertensive rat. Clin. Sci. Mol. Med. 55 (Suppl. 4): 191s–93s.

Eberwine, J. H., and J. R. Roberts. 1984. Glucocorticoid regulation of pro-opiomelanocortin gene transcription in rat pituitary. J. Biol. Chem. 259:2166–70.

Edwards, F. C., and N. F. Coghill. 1968. Clinical manifestations of patients with chronic atrophic gastritis, gastric ulcer, and duodenal ulcer. Q. J. Med. 37:337–60.

Ehlers, C., E. Frank, and D. J. Kupfer. 1988. Social *Zeitgebers* and biological rhythms: A unified approach to understanding the etiology of depression. Arch. Gen. Psychiat. 45:948–52.

Ehrstrom, M. D. 1945. Psychogene blutdrucksteigerung in Kriegshypertonien. Acta Med. Scand. 122:546–61.

Eigen, M. 1971. Self-organization of matter and the evolution of biological macromolecules. Naturwissenschaften 58:465–523.

Eitinger, L. 1965. Concentration camp survivors in Norway and Israel. New York: Humanities Press.

———. 1971. Acute and chronic psychiatric and psychosomatic reactions in concentration camp survivors. In Society, stress and disease. Vol. 1, The psychosocial environment and psychosomatic disease, ed. L. Levi, 219–30. London and New York: Oxford University Press.

Elliott, G. R., and C. Eisdorfer, eds. 1982. Stress and human health: Analysis and implications of research. New York: Springer.

Endicott, N. A. 1989. Psychosocial and behavioral factors in myocardial infarction and sudden cardiac death. In Psychosomatic medicine: Theory, physiology and practice, ed. S. Cheren, 611–59. Madison, CT: International Universities Press.

Engel, G. L. 1955. Studies of ulcerative colitis, 3: The nature of the psychologic processes. Am. J. Med. 19:231–43.

———. 1956. Studies of ulcerative colitis, 4: The significance of headaches. Psychosom. Med. 18:334–46.

———. 1962. Psychological development in health and disease. Philadelphia: Saunders.

————. 1968. A life setting conducive to illness: The giving-up, given-up complex. Arch. Int. Med. 69:293–300.

————. 1973. Ulcerative colitis. In Emotional factors in gastrointestinal illness, ed. A. E. Lindner, 99–112. Amsterdam: Excerpta Medica.

————. 1977. The need for a new medical model: A challenge for biomedicine. Science 196:129–36.

Enos, W. F., R. H. Holmes, and J. Beyer. 1953. Coronary heart disease among United States soldiers killed in action in Korea. JAMA 152:1090–93.

Epstein, S. E., A. A. Quyyumi, and R. O. Bonow. 1989. Sudden cardiac death without warning: Possible mechanisms and implications for screening asymptomatic populations. New Engl. J. Med. 321:320–23.

Erikson, E. 1950. Childhood and society. New York: W. W. Norton.

Erikson, K. T. 1976. Loss of communality at Buffalo Creek. Am. J. Psychiat. 133:302–5.

Erikssen, J. 1987. Prognostic importance of silent ischemia during long-term follow-up of patients with coronary artery disease. Herz 12:359–68.

Esler, M. D., and K. J. Goulston. 1973. Levels of anxiety in colonic disorders. New Engl. J. Med. 288:16–20.

Esler, M., G. Jennings, P. Korner, P. Blombery, N. Sacharias, and P. Leonard. 1984. Measurement of total and organ-specific norepinephrine kinetics in humans. Am. J. Physiol. 247:E21–28.

Esler, M. D., S. Julius, O. S. Randall, C. N. Ellis, and T. Kashima. 1975. Relation of renin status to neurogenic vascular resistance in borderline hyptertension. Am. J. Cardiol. 36:708–15.

Esler, M. D., S. Julius, A. Zweifler, O. Randall, E. Harburg, H. Gardiner, and V. DeQuattro. 1977. Mild high-renin hypertension. New Engl. J. Med. 296:405–11.

Evoniuk, G. E., G. M. Kuhn, and S. M. Schanberg. 1979. The effect of tactile stimulation on serum growth hormone and tissue orinthine decarboxylase activity during maternal deprivation in rat pups. Comp. Psychopharmacol. 3:363–70.

Fabrega, Jr., H. 1987. Psychiatric diagnosis: A cultural perspective. J. Nerv. Ment. Dis. 175:383–94.

Faisal, M., F. Chiappelli, I. I. Ahmed, E. L. Cooper, and H. Weiner. 1989a. Social confrontation "stress" in aggressive fish is associated with an opioid-mediated suppression of proliferative response to mitogens and non-specific cytotoxicity. Brain Behav. Immunol. 3:223–33.

————. 1989b. Evidence for the role of the endogenous opioids in modulatng some immune parameters in *Tilapia*. Aquat. Anim. Hlth. 1:301–6.

Fändriks, L., C. Jönson, and B. Lisander. 1989. Hypothalamic inhibition of duodenal alkaline secretion via a sympatho-adrenergic mechanism in the rat. Acta Physiol. Scand. 137:357–63.

Farber, E. 1984. The multistep nature of cancer development. Cancer Res. 44:4217–23.

Farrow, S. C. 1984. Unemployment and health: A review of methodology. In Breakdown in human adaptation to stress, ed. J. Cullen and J. Siegrist, 149–58. Boston: Martinus Nijhoff.

Fehm, H. L., K. H. Voigt, and J. Bron. 1987. Extrapituitary mechanisms in the regulation of cortisol secretion in man. In Neuronal control of bodily function: Neurobiological approaches to human disease, ed. D. Hellhammer, I. Florin, and H. Weiner, 344–57. Toronto: Hans Huber.

Fehm, H. L., K. H. Voigt, G. W. Kummer, and E. F. Pfeiffer. 1979. Positive rate-sensitive corticosteroid feedback mechanisms of ACTH secretion in Cushing's disease. J. Clin. Invest. 64:102–8.

Feige, J. J., C. Cochet, and E. M. Chambaz. 1986. Type β transforming growth factor is a potent modulator of differential adrenocortical function. Biochem. Biophys. Res. Commun. 139:693–700.

Feldman, E., G. Van Deventer, K. Sabovich, and J. Elashoff. 1985. Psychological factors and duodenal ulcer disease. Relationship to serum pepsinogin-I levels. Gastroenterol. 88:1380.

Feldman, S. 1985. Neural pathways mediating adrenocortical responses. Fed. Proc. FASEB 44:169–75.

———. 1989. Afferent neural pathways and hypothalamic neurotransmitters regulating adrenal cortical secretion. In Neuronal control of bodily function: Frontiers of stress research, ed. H. Weiner, D. Hellhammer, I. Florin, and R. Murison, 201–8. Toronto: Hans Huber.

Felten, D. L., S. Y. Felten, S. L. Carlson, J. A. Olschowka, and S. Livnat. 1985. Noradrenergic and peptidergic innervation of lymphoid tissue. J. Immunol. 135:755–65.

Felten, S. Y., and D. L. Felten. 1989. Are lymphocytes targets of noradrenergic innervation? In Neuronal control of bodily function: Frontiers of stress research, ed. H. Weiner, D. Hellhammer, I. Florin, and R. Murison, 56–71. Toronto: Hans Huber.

Fenz, M. D., and S. Epstein. 1967. Gradients of physiological arousal of experienced and novice parachutists as a function of an approaching jump. Psychosom. Med. 29:33–51.

Fenz, M. D., and G. B. Jones. 1972. Individual differences in a physiological arousal and performance in sport parachutists. Psychosom. Med. 34:1–18.

Fernstrom, J. D., and R. J. Wurtman. 1972. Brain serotonin content: Physiological regulation by plasma neutral amino acids. Science 178:414–16.

Ferrario, C. M., C. J. Dickinson, P. L. Gildenberg, and J. W. McCubbin, 1969. Central vasomotor stimulation by angiotensin. Fed. Proc. FASEB 28:394A.

Fielding, J. S. 1984. Clinical recognition of stress-related gastrointestinal disorders in adults. In Breakdown in human adaptation to stress, ed. R. E. Ballieux, J. S. Fielding, and A. L'Abbate, 799–806. Boston: Martinus Nijhoff.

Fischer, C. 1982. To dwell among friends: Personal networks in town and city. Chicago: University of Chicago Press.

Flemström, G., and L. A. Turnberg. 1984. Gastroduodenal defense mechanisms. Clin. Gastroenterol. 13:327–54.

Folkow, B. 1987. Physiology of behavior and blood pressure regulation in animals. In Handbook of hypertension, vol. 9, ed. S. Julius and D. R. Bassett, 1–18. Amsterdam: Elsevier.

Folkow, B. U. G., and M. I. L. Hallbäck. 1977. Physiopathology of spontaneous hypertension in rats. In Hypertension, ed. J. Genest, E. Koiw, and O. Kuchel, 507–29. New York: McGraw-Hill.

Foote, S. L., F. E. Bloom, and G. Aston-Jones. 1983. Nucleus locus coeruleus: New evidence of anatomical and physiological specificity. Physiol. Rev. 63:844–914.

Forsyth, R. P. 1969. Blood pressure responses to long-term avoidance schedules in the restrained rhesus monkey. Psychosom. Med. 31:300–309.

———. 1971. Regional blood-flow changes during 72-hour avoidance schedules in the monkey. Science 173:546–48.

Fox, A. J., and P. O. Goldblatt. 1982. Longitudinal study, 1971–1975. OPCS London: Her Majesty's Stationery Office.

Frankenhaeuser, M. 1983. The sympathetic-adrenal and pituitary-adrenal response to challenge. In Biobehavioral basis of coronary heart disease, ed. T. M. Dembroski, T. H. Schmidt, and G. Blümchen, 91–105. Basel: Karger.

Frankenhaeuser, M., and B. Gandell. 1976. Underload and overload in working life: Outline of a multidisciplinary approach. J. Hum. Stress 2:35–46.

Frankenhaeuser, M., B. Nordheden, A. L. Myrsent, and V. Post. 1971. Psycho-physiological reactions to under-stimulation and over-stimulation. Acta Psychol. Scand. 35:298–308.

Frankenhaeuser, M., and A. Rissler. 1970. Effects of punishment on catecholamine release and efficiency of performance. Psychopharmacologica 17:378–90.

Frederick, C. J. 1980. Effects of natural versus human induced violence upon victims. Eval. Changes (Special Issue): 71–75.

———. 1981. Violence and disaster: Immediate and long-term consequences. Paper presented at working group conference on the psychosocial consequences of violence. Geneva: World Health Organization.

———. 1987. Psychic trauma in victims of crime and terrorism. In Cataclysms, crises, and catastrophes: Psychology in action, ed. G. R. Van den Bos and B. K. Bryant, 59–107. Washington, DC: American Psychological Association.

Frederickson, D. S., J. L. Goldstein, and M. D. Brown. 1978. The familial hyper-lipoproteinemias. In The metabolic basis of inherited disease, ed. J. B. Stanbury, J. B. Wyngaarden, and D. S. Frederickson, 604–55. New York: McGraw-Hill.

Freeman, L. J. 1987. Hyperventilation and ischaemic heart disease. In Cardiorespiratory and cardiosomatic psychophysiology, ed. P. Grossman, K. H. L. Janssen, and D. Vaitl, 319–26. New York: Plenum Press.

Freeman, L. J., P. G. F. Nixon, C. Legg, and B. H. Timmons. 1987. Hyperventilation and angina pectoris. J. R. Coll. Phys. (London) 21:46–50.

Friedman, M., S. O. Byers, J. Diamant, and R. H. Rosenman. 1979. Plasma catecholamine response of coronary-prone subjects (Type A) to a specific challenge. Metabol. 4:205–10.

Friedman, M., and R. H. Rosenman. 1959. Association of a specific overt behavior pattern with blood and cardiovascular findings. JAMA 169:1286–95.

Friedman, R., and J. Iwai. 1977. Dietary sodium, psychic stress, and genetic predisposition to experimental hypertension. Proc. Soc. Exp. Biol. Med. 155:449–52.

Fries, H., and S. J. Nillius. 1973. Dieting, anorexia nervosa, and amenorrhoea after oral contraceptive treatment. Acta Psychiat. Scand. 49:669–79.

Frohlich, E. D., R. C. Tarazi, and H. P. Dustan. 1971. Clinical-physiological correlation in the development of hypertensive heart disease. Circulation 44:446–55.

Fuster, J. 1980. The prefrontal cortex. New York: Raven Press.

Gann, D. C. 1969. Parameters of the stimulus initiating the adreno-cortical response to hemorrhage. Ann. N.Y. Acad. Sci. 156:740–55.

Ganten, D., A. Marquez-Julio, P. Granger, K. Hayduk, K. P. Karsunsky, R. Boucher, and J. Genest. 1971. Renin in dog brain. Am. J. Physiol. 221:1733–37.

Ganten, D., P. Schelling, and U. Ganten. 1977. Tissue isorenins. In Hypertension, ed. J. Genest, E. Koiw, and O. Kuchel, 240–56. New York: McGraw-Hill.

Gardiner, B. M. 1980. Psychological aspects of rheumatoid arthritis. Psychol. Med. 10:159–63.

Garfinkel, A. 1983. A mathematics for physiology. Am. J. Physiol. 245 (Regul. Integ. Comp. Physiol.) 14:R455–66.

Garfinkel, P. E., and D. M. Garner. 1982. Anorexia nervosa: A multidimensional perspective. New York: Brunner/Mazel.

Garrick, T., S. Buack, and P. Bass. 1986. Gastric motility is a major factor in cold restraint–induced lesion formation in rats. Am. J. Physiol. 250:G191–99.

Garrick, T., S. Buack, A. Veiseh, and Y. Taché. 1987. Thyrotropin-releasing hormone (TRH) acts centrally to stimulate gastric contractility in rats. Life Sci. 40:649–57.

Garrick, T., A. Veiseh, H. Weiner, and Y. Taché. 1988. CRF acts centrally to suppress stimulated gastric contractility in the rat. Reg. Pept. 21:173–81.

Garrity, T. F., G. W. Somes, and M. B. Marx. 1978. Factors influencing self-assessment of health. Soc. Sci. Med. 12:77–81.

Gelshteyn, E. M. 1943. Clinical characteristics of hypertensive disease under wartime conditions. Klin. Med. (Moscow) 21:10–15.

Genest, J., E. Koiw, and O. Kuchel, eds. 1977. Hypertension. New York: McGraw-Hill.

Gennari, F. J., M. B. Goldstein, and W. B. Schwartz. 1972. The nature of the renal adaption to chronic hypocapnia. J. Clin. Invest. 51:1722–30.

Gerster, J. C., and A. Hadj-Djilani. 1984. Hearing and vestibular abnormalities in primary fibrositis syndrome. J. Rheumatol. 11:678–88.

Gibbs, D. M. 1986. Vasopressin and oxytocin: Hypothalamic modulators of the stress response. Psychoneuroendocrinol. 11:131–40.

Giguere, V., H. Meunier, R. Veilleux, and F. Labrie. 1982. Direct effects of sex steroids on prolactin release at the anterior pituitary level: Interactions with dopamine, thyrotropin releasing hormone, and isobutylmethylxanthine. Endocrinol. 111:857–62.

Gildenberg, P. L. 1971. Site of angiotensin vasopressor activity in the brain stem. Fed. Proc. FASEB 30:432A.

Gillies, M., R. Nicks, and A. Skyring. 1967. Clinical manometric and pathological studies in diffuse esophageal spasm. Br. Med. J. 2:527–30.

Gilman, A. G. 1987. G proteins: Transducers of receptor-generated signals. Ann. Rev. Biochem. 56:615–49.

Gindoff, P. R., and M. Ferin. 1987. Endogenous opioid peptides modulate the effect of corticotropin-releasing factor on gonadotropin release in the primate. Endocrinol. 121:837–42.

Glaser, R., J. K. Kiecolt-Glaser, C. E. Speicher, and J. E. Holliday. 1985a. Stress, loneliness, and changes in herpes virus latency. J. Behav. Med. 8:249–60.

Glaser, R., J. K. Kiecolt-Glaser, J. C. Stout, K. L. Tarr, C. E. Speicher, and J. E. Holliday. 1985b. Stress-related impairments of cellular immunity. Psychiat. Res. 16:233–39.

Glaser, R., J. Rice, C. E. Speicher, J. C. Stout, and J. K. Kiecolt-Glaser. 1986. Stress depresses interferon production. Behav. Neurosci. 100:675–78.

Glass, D. C., L. R. Krakoff, R. Contrada, W. F. Hilton, K. Kehoe, E. G. Mannucci, C. Collins, B. Snow, and E. Elting. 1980. Effect of harassment and competition upon cardiovascular and plasma catecholamine responses in Type A and Type B individuals. Psychophysiol. 17:453–63.

Glass, L., and M. C. Mackey. 1979. Pathological conditions resulting from instabilities in physiological control systems. Ann. N.Y. Acad. Sci. 316:214–35.

———. 1988. From clocks to chaos: The rhythms of life. Princeton, NJ: Princeton University Press.

Glavin, G. B. 1985. Effects of morphine and naloxone on restraint-stress ulcers in rats. Pharmacol. 31:57–60.

Glazer, H. I., J. M. Weiss, L. A. Pohorecky, and N. E. Miller. 1975. Monoamines as mediators of avoidance escape behavior. Psychosom. Med. 37:535–43.

Gliner, J. A. 1972. Predictable vs. unpredictable shock: Preference behavior and stomach ulceration. Physiol. Behav. 9:693–98.

Gloor, P. 1978. Inputs and outputs of the amygdala: What the amygdala is trying to tell the rest of the brain. In Limbic mechanisms, ed. K. E. Livingston and O. Hornykiewicz, 189–209. New York: Plenum Press.

Glossi, F. B., B. Messini, T. Del Duca, M. Ricci, and M. Messini. 1966. Peristaltic activity of the colonic mass in sequence after the administration of "cecekin." Clin. Therap. 37:117–21.

Glowinski, J. 1975. Regulation of synthesis and release processes in central catecholaminergic neurons. In Metabolic compartmentation and neurotransmission, ed. S. Berl, D. D. Clarke, and D. Schneider, 187–203. New York: Plenum Press.

Goldberg, E. L., and G. W. Comstock. 1980. Epidemiology of life events: Frequency in general populations. Am. J. Epidemiol. 111:736–52.

Goldberger, L., and S. Breznitz, eds. 1982. Handbook of stress: Theoretical and clinical aspects. New York: Free Press.

Goldblatt, P. B., M. E. Moore, and A. J. Stunkard. 1965. Social factors in obesity. JAMA 192:1039–44.

Goldman, L., G. D. Coover, and S. Levine. 1973. Bidirectional effects of reinforcement shifts on pituitary-adrenal activity. Physiol. Behav. 10:209–14.

Goldstein, A., R. W. Barrett, I. F. James, L. I. Lowney, C. J. Weitz, L. L. Knipmeyer, and H. Rapaport. 1985. Morphine and other opiates from beef brain and adrenal. Proc. Natl. Acad. Sci. (USA) 82:5203–7.

Goldstein, D. S. 1987. Stress-induced activation of the sympathetic nervous system. Ballière's Clin. Endocrinol. Metabol. 1:253–78.

Goldstein, D. S., G. Eisenhofer, F. L. Sax, H. R. Keiser, and I. J. Kopin. 1987. Plasma norepinephrine pharmacokinetics during mental challenge. Psychosom. Med. 49:591–605.

Goldstein, K. 1939. The organism (pp. 35–65). New York: American Book Co.

Gomez, J., and P. Dally. 1977. Psychologically mediated abdominal pain in surgical and medical outpatient clinics. Br. Med. J. 1:1451–53.

Gormley, G. J., M. T. Lowy, A. T. Reder, V. D. Hospelhorn, J. A. Antel, and H. Y. Meltzer. 1985. Glucocorticoid receptors in depression: Relationship to the dexamethasone suppression test and mitogen-induced lymphocyte proliferation. Am. J. Psychiat. 142:1278–84.

Goto, Y., and Y. Taché. 1985. Gastric erosions induced by intracisternal thyrotropin-releasing hormone (TRH) in rats. Peptides 6:153–56.

Gottlieb, D. 1988. GABAergic neurons. Scient. Am. 258:82–89.

Gould, S. J. 1985. The flamingo's smile (pp. 160–65). New York: W. W. Norton.

Graham, D. T. 1978. Hypertensive lower esophageal sphincter: A reappraisal. South. Med. J. 71:31–37.

Graham, J. D. P. 1945. High blood pressure after battle. Lancet 1:239–40.

Grant, I., J. Yager, H. L. Sweetwood, and R. Olshen. 1982. Life events and symptoms: Fourier analyses of time series from a three-year prospective inquiry. Arch. Gen. Psychiat. 39:598–605.

Gray, G. D., A. M. Bergfors, R. Levin, and S. Levine. 1978. Comparison of the effects of restricted morning or evening water intake on adrenocortical activity in female rats. Neuroendocrinol. 25:236–46.

Gray, J. 1971. The psychology of fear and stress. London: Weidenfeld & Nicholson.

Gray, T. S., and J. E. Morley. 1986. Neuropeptide Y: Anatomical distributions and possible function in mammalian nervous system. Life Sci. 38:389–401.

Green, D. J., and R. Gillette. 1982. Circadian rhythm of firing rate recorded from single cells in the rat suprachiasmatic brain slice. Brain Res. 245:198–200.

Greenberg, R., and C. Pearlman. 1968. Sleep patterns in temporal lobe epilepsy. Comp. Psychiat. 9:194–99.

Greene, W. A. 1954. Psychological factors and reticulo-endothelial disease, 1: Preliminary observations on a group of males with lymphomas and leukemias. Psychosom. Med. 16:220–30.

Greene, W. A., S. Conron, D. S. Schalch, and B. F. Schreiner. 1970. Psychological correlates of growth hormone and adrenal secretory responses of patients undergoing cardiac catheterization. Psychosom. Med. 32:599–614.

Griffin, D. R. 1984. Animal thinking. Am. Scient. 72:456–64.

Grijalva, C., and B. Roland. 1989. The involvement of the hypothalamus in the production of stomach ulceration. In Neuronal control of bodily function: Frontier of stress research, ed. H. Weiner, D. Hellhammer, I. Florin, and R. Murison, 72–82. Toronto: Hans Huber.

Grinker, R. R., and J. Spiegel. 1945. Men under stress. Philadelphia: Blakiston.

Groen, J. J. 1976. Psychosomatic aspects of ischaemic (coronary) heart disease. In Modern trends in psychosomatic medicine 3, ed. O. W. Hill, 288–329. London: Butterworths.

Groen, J. J., J. H. Medalie, H. Neufeld, and E. Ris. 1968. An epidemiological investigation of hypertension and ischemic heart disease in Israel. Israel J. Med. Sci. 4:177–94.

Grossarth-Maticek, R., H. J. Eysenck, H. Vetter, and P. Schmidt. 1988. Psychosocial types and chronic diseases: Results of the Heidelberg prospective intervention study. In Topics in health psychology, ed. S. Maes, C. D. Spielberger, P. B. Defares, and I. G. Sarason, 57–75. New York: John Wiley.

Grossberg, J. M., and H. K. Wilson. 1968. Physiological changes accompanying the visualization of fear and neutral situations. J. Person. Soc. Psychol. 10:124–33.

Grossman, C. J. 1984. Regulation of the immune system by sex steroids. Endocr. Rev. 5:435–55.

———. 1989. Stress and the immune system: Interaction of peptides, gonadal steroids, and immune system. In Neuronal control of bodily function: Frontiers of stress research, ed. H. Weiner, D. Hellhammer, I. Florin, and R. Murison, 181–90. Toronto: Hans Huber.

Grossman, M. I. 1978. Abnormalities of acid secretion in patients with duodenal ulcer. Gastroenterol. 75:524–26.

———. 1979. Elevated serum pepsinogen, 1: A genetic marker for duodenal disease. Editorial. New Engl. J. Med. 300:89.

Gu, J., J. M. Polak, T. E. Adrian, J. M. Allen, K. Tatemoto, and S. R. Bloom. 1983. Neuropeptide tyrosine NPY—a major cardiac neuropeptide. Lancet 1:1008–10.

Guillemin, R. 1978. Biochemical and physiological correlates of hypothalamic peptides: The new endocrinology of the neuron. Res. Publ. Assoc. Nerv. Ment. Dis. 56:155–94.

Guillemin, R., and J. E. Gerich. 1976. Somatostatin: Physiological and clinical significance. Ann. Rev. Med. 27:379–88.

Gunderson, E. E., and R. H. Rahe. 1974. Life stress and illness. Springfield, IL: Charles C. Thomas.

Gupta, M., and H. Moldofsky. 1986. Dysthymic disorder and rheumatic pain modulation disorder (fibrositis syndrome): A comparison of symptoms and sleep physiology. Can. J. Psychiat. 31:608–16.

Gutierrez, J. G., W. Y. Chey, and V. P. Dinoso. 1974. Actions of cholecystokinin and secretin on the motor activity of the small intestine in man. Gastroenterol. 67:35–41.

Guyenet, P. G., and G. K. Aghajanian. 1979. ACh, substance P, and met-enkephalin in the locus coeruleus: Pharmacological evidence for different sites of action. Eur. J. Pharmacol. 53:319–28.

Guyre, P. M., M. T. Girard, P. M. Morganelli, and P. D. Manganiello. 1988. Glucocorticoid effects on the production and actions of immune cytokines. J. Steroid Biochem. 30:89–93.

Hackett, D., G. Davies, S. Chierchia, and A. Maseri. 1987. Intermittent coronary occlusion in acute myocardial infarction: Value of combined thrombolytic and vasodilator therapy. New Engl. J. Med. 317:1055–59.

Hackett, T. P., E. H. Cassem, and H. A. Wishnie. 1968. The coronary-care unit: An appraisal of its psychologic hazards. New Engl. J. Med. 279:1365–70.

Haeusler, G., L. Finch, and H. Thoenen. 1972. Central adrenergic neurons and the initiation and development of experimental hypertension. Experientia 28:1200–1203.

Haeusler, G., J. Gerold, and H. Thoenen. 1972. Cardiovascular effects of 6-hydroxydopamine injected into a lateral brain ventricle of the rat. Naunyn Schmiedebergs Arch. Pharmacol. 274:211–28.

Haines, A. P., J. D. Imeson, and T. W. Meade. 1987. Phobic anxiety and ischaemic heart disease. Br. Med. J. 295:297–99.

Halberg, F. 1960. Temporal coordination of physiological function. Cold Spring Harbor Symp. Quant. Biol. 25:289–308.

Hallbäck, M. 1975. Consequence of social isolation on blood pressure, cardiovascular reactivity, and design in spontaneous hypertensive rats. Acta Physiol. Scand. 93:455–65.

Hamburg, D. A., and J. E. Adams. 1967. A perspective on coping behavior. Arch. Gen. Psychiat. 17:277–84.

Hanley, W. B. 1964. Hereditary aspects of duodenal ulceration: Serum pepsinogen level in relation to ABO blood group and salivary ABH secretor status. Br. Med. J. 1:936–40.

Hannum, C. H., C. J. Wilcox, W. P. Arend, F. G. Joslin, O. J. Dripps, P. L. Heimdal, L. G. Armes, A. Sommer, S. P. Eisenberg, and R. C. Thompson. 1990. Inter-leukin-I receptor antagonist activity of a human interleukin-I inhibitor. Nature (London) 343:336–40.

Harburg, E., J. C. Erfurt, L. S. Hauenstein, C. Chape, W. J. Schull, and M. A. Schork. 1973. Socio-ecological stress, suppressed hostility, skin color, and black-white male blood pressure: Detroit. Psychosom. Med. 35:276–96.

Hartmann, H. 1958. Ego psychology and the problem of adaptation. New York: International Universities Press.

Harvey, R. F. 1979. Effects of hormones in normal subjects and patients with the irritable bowel syndrome. Pract. Gastroenterol. 3:10–15.

Harvey, R. F., and A. E. Read. 1973. Effect of cholecystokinin on colonic motility and symptoms in patients with the irritable bowel syndrome. Lancet 1:1–3.

Hayes, R. L., G. J. Bennett, P. G. Newlon, and D. J. Mayer. 1976. Analgesic effects of certain noxious and stressful manipulations in the rat. Soc. Neurosci. Abstr. 2:939.

Haynes, S. G., M. Feinleib, and W. B. Kannel. 1980. The relationship of psycho-social factors in the Framingham study, 3: Eight-year incidence of coronary heart disease. Am. J. Epidemiol. 111:37–58.

Haynes, S. G., S. Levine, N. Scotch, M. Feinlieb, and W. B. Kannel. 1978. The relationship of psychosocial factors to coronary heart disease in the Framingham study, 1: Methods and risk factors. Am. J. Epidemiol. 107:362–83.

Hearst, N., T. Newman, and S. B. Hulley. 1986. Delayed effects of the military draft on mortality: A randomized natural experiment. New Engl. J. Med. 314:620–24.

Heijnen, C. J., N. deFouw, and R. E. Ballieux. 1986. Influence of α-endorphin on the antigen induced PFC response of human blood B lymphocytes in vitro. In Neuroregulation of autonomic, endocrine, and immune systems, ed. R. C. A. Frederickson, H. C. Hendrie, J. N. Hingtgen, and M. H. Aprison, 533–37. Boston: Martinus Nijhoff.

Heistad, D. D., R. C. Wheeler, A. L. Mark, R. G. Schmid, and F. M. Abboud. 1972. Effects of adrenergic stimulation on ventilation in man. J. Clin. Invest. 51: 1469–75.

Helsing, K. J., M. Szklo, and G. W. Comstock. 1981. Factors associated with mortality after widowhood. Am. J. Publ. Hlth. 71:802–9.

Hench, P. S., E. C. Kendall, C. N. Slocumb, and H. F. Polley. 1949. The effect of a hormone of the adrenal cortex (17-hydroxy-11-dehydrocorticosterone: Compound E) and of pituitary adrenocorticotropic hormone on rheumatoid arthritis. Proc. Staff Mtgs. Mayo Clin. 24:181–97.

Henn, F. A., E. Edwards, and J. Johnson. 1988. Research directions in behavioral medicine. In Neurobiological approaches to human disease, ed. D. Hellhammer, I. Florin, and H. Weiner, 215–24. Toronto: Hans Huber.

Henriksen, O., and K. Skagen. 1986. Local and central sympathetic vasoconstrictor reflexes in human limbs during orthostatic stress. In The sympathoadrenal system: Physiology and pathophysiology, ed. N. J. Christensen, O. Henriken, and N. A. Lassen, 83–91. New York: Raven Press.

Henry, J. P., and J. C. Cassel. 1969. Psychosocial factors in essential hypertension. Recent epidemiologic and animal experimental evidence. Am. J. Epidemiol. 90:171–93.

Henry, J. P., J. P. Meehan, and P. M. Stephens. 1967. The use of psychosocial stimuli to induce prolonged systolic hypertension in mice. Psychosom. Med. 29:408–32.

Henry, J. P., and P. M. Stephens. 1977. Stress, health, and the social environment: A sociobiologic approach to medicine. New York: Springer-Verlag.

Henry, J. P., P. M. Stephens, J. Axelrod, and R. A. Mueller. 1971. Effect of psychosocial stimulation on the enzymes involved in the biosynthesis and metabolism of noradrenaline and adrenaline. Psychosom. Med. 33:227–37.

Henry, J. P., P. M. Stephens, and D. Ely. 1986. Psychosocial hypertension and the defense and defeat reactions. J. Hyperten. 4:687–97.

Henry, J. P., and P. Stephens-Larson. 1985. Specific effects of stress on disease processes. In Animal stress, ed. G. Moberg, 161–75. Baltimore, MD: American Psychological Society, Williams & Wilkins.

Herman, S. P., G. B. Stickler, and A. R. Lucas. 1981. Hyperventilation syndrome in children and adolescents: Long-term follow-up. Pediatrics 67:183–87.

Hess, W. R. 1957. The functional organization of the diencephalon, ed. J. R. Hughes. New York: Grune & Stratton.

Hill, O. W., and L. Blendis. 1967. Physical and psychological evaluation of "non-organic" abdominal pain. Gut 8:221–29.

Hilton, S. W. 1975. Ways of viewing the central nervous control of the circulation— old and new. Brain Res. 87:213–19.

Hinkle, Jr., L. E. 1973. The concept of stress in the biological and social sciences. Sci. Med. Man 1:31–48.

———. 1974. The effect of exposure to culture change, social change, and changes in interpersonal relationships on health. In Stressful life events: Their nature and effects, ed. B. S. Dohrenwend and B. P. Dohrenwend, 9–44. New York: Wiley.

———. 1977. Measurement of the effects of the environment on the health and behavior of people. In The effect of the man-made environment on health and behavior, ed. L. E. Hinkle, Jr., and W. C. Loring, 197–239. Washington, DC: U.S. Government Printing Office. DHEW publ. no. (CDC) 77-8318.

———. 1987. Stress and disease: The concept after fifty years. Soc. Sci. Med. 25:561–66.

Hinkle, Jr., L. E., F. D. Kane, W. N. Christenson, and H. G. Wolff. 1959. Hungarian refugees: Life experiences and features influencing participation in the revolution and subsequent flight. Am. J. Psychiat. 116:16–19.

Hinkle, Jr., L. E., and S. Wolf. 1952. A summary of experimental evidence relating life stress to diabetes mellitus. J. Mt. Sinai Hosp. 19:537–70.

Hirata, F., E. Schiffman, K. Venkatasubramanian, D. Solomon, and J. Axelrod. 1980.

A phospholipase A_2 inhibitory protein in rabbit neutrophils induced by glucocorticoids. Proc. Natl. Acad. Sci. (USA) 77:2533–35.

Hislop, I. G. 1971. Psychological significance of the irritable colon syndrome. Gut 12:452–57.

Hodgkin, A. L., and A. F. Huxley. 1952. A quantitative description of membrane current and its application to conduction and excitation in nerve. J. Physiol. (London) 117:500–544.

Hodgson, R., and S. Rachman. 1974. Desynchrony in measures of fear. Behav. Res. Ther. 12:319–26.

Hofer, M. A. 1970. Cardiac and respiratory function during sudden prolonged immobility in young rodents. Psychosom. Med. 340:633–47.

———. 1976. The organization of sleep and wakefulness after maternal separation in young rats. Develop. Psychobiol. 9:189–206.

———. 1981. Toward a developmental basis for disease predisposition: The effects of early maternal separation on brain, behavior, and cardiovascular system. In Brain, behavior, and bodily disease, ed. H. Weiner, M. A. Hofer, and A. J. Stunkard, 209–28. New York: Raven Press.

———. 1983. On the relationship between attachment and separation processes in infancy. In Emotion, theory, research, and experience: Emotions in early development 2, ed. R. Plutchick and H. Kellerman, 199–219. New York: Academic Press.

———. 1984. Relationships as regulators. Psychosom. Med. 46:183–87.

Hofer, M. A., and H. Weiner. 1972. Mechanisms for nutritional regulation of autonomic cardiac control in early development. Psychosom. Med. 34:472–73.

———. 1975. Physiological mechanisms for cardiac control by nutritional intake after early maternal separation in the young rat. Psychosom. Med. 37:8–24.

Hofer, M. A., C. T. Wolff, S. B. Friedman, and J. W. Mason. 1972a. A psychoendocrine study of bereavement, part 1: 17-hydroxycorticosteroid excretion rates of parents following death of their children from leukemia. Psychosom. Med. 34:481–91.

———. 1972b. A psychoendrocine study of bereavement, part 2: Observations on the process of mourning in relation to adrenocortical function. Psychosom. Med. 34:492–504.

Hökfelt, T., J. Fahrenkrug, K. Tatemoto, V. Mutt, S. Werner, A.-L. Hulting, L. Terenius, and K. J. Change. 1983. The PHI (PHI-27)/corticotropin-releasing factor/enkephalin immunoreactive neuron: Possible morphological basis for integrated control of prolactin, corticotrophin, and growth hormone secretion. Proc. Natl. Acad. Sci. (USA) 80:895–98.

Hökfelt, T., O. Johansson, M. Goldstein. 1984. Chemical anatomy of the brain. Science 225:1326–34.

Holaday, J. W. 1985. Endogenous opioids and their receptors: Current concepts. Kalamazoo, MI: Upjohn Company.

———. 1989. Opioid peptides: Physiological and behavioral effects. In Neuronal control of bodily function: Frontiers of stress research, ed. H. Weiner, D. Hellhammer, I. Florin, and R. Murison, 309–20. Toronto: Hans Huber.

Holaday, J. W., and A. I. Faden. 1983. TRH: Autonomic effects upon cardiorespiratory function in endotoxic shock. Reg. Pept. 7:111–25.

Holden, A. V. 1988. What makes them tick? Book review of From clocks to chaos: The rhythms of life by Leon Glass and Michael Mackey. Nature (London) 336:119.

Holdstock, D. J., J. J. Misiewicz, and S. L. Waller. 1969. Observations on the mechanism of abdominal pain. Gut 10:19–31.

Holmes, T. H., and R. H. Rahe. 1967. The social readjustment scale. J. Psychosom. Res. 11:213–18.

Hollenberg, N. K., and D. F. Adams. 1976. The renal circulation in hypertensive disease. Am. J. Med. 60:773–84.

Holzwarth, M. A. 1984. The distribution of vasoactive intestinal peptide in the rat adrenal cortex and medulla. J. Autonom. Nerv. Syst. 11:269–83.

Horowitz, L., and J. T. Farrar. 1962. Intraluminal small intestinal pressure in normal patients and in patients with functional gastrointestinal disorders. Gastroenterol. 42:455–64.

Horowitz, M. J. 1975. Intrusive and repetitive thoughts after experimental stress. Arch. Gen. Psychiat. 32:1457–63.

———. 1976. Stress response syndromes. New York: Aronson.

Horowitz, M. J., C. Schaeffer, D. Hiroto, N. Wilner, and B. Levin. 1977. Life event questionnaires for measuring presumptive stress. Psychosom. Med. 39:413–31.

Horowitz, M. J., and N. Wilner. 1980. Life events, stress, and coping. In Aging in the 1980s: Psychological issues, ed. L. Poon, 363–70. Washington, DC: American Psychological Association.

Horowitz, M. J., N. Wilner, and W. Alvarez. 1979. Impact of event scale: A measure of subjective stress. Psychosom. Med. 41:209–18.

Horrocks, J. C., and F. T. DeDombal. 1978. Clinical presentation of patients with dyspepsia: Detailed symptomatic study of 360 patients. Gut 19:19–26.

Hotchin, J., and R. Buckley. 1977. Latent form of scrapie virus: A new factor in slow-virus disease. Science 196:668–71.

House, J. S., K. R. Landis, and D. Umberson. 1988. Social relationships in health. Science 241:540–45.

Hubel, D. H., and T. N. Wiesel. 1965. Binocular interaction of striate cortex of kittens reared with artificial squint. J. Neurophysiol. 28:1041–59.

Hughes, J., T. W. Smith, H. W. Kosterlitz, L. A. Fothergill, B. A. Morgan, and H. R. Morris. 1975. Identification of two related pentapeptides from the brain with potent opiate agonist activity. Nature (London) 258:577–79.

Hunt, P. S., A. M. Connell, and T. B. Smiley. 1970. The crico-pharyngeal sphincter in gastric reflux. Gut 11:303–6.

Hunt, R. H., J. B. Delawari, and J. J. Misiewicz. 1975. The effect of intravenous prostaglandin F_2a and E_2 on the motility of the sigmoid colon. Gut 16:47–49.

Huxley, J. 1942. Evolution, the modern synthesis. London: Allen & Unwin.

Iberal, A. 1975. A proposal for a force essential to biological organization. Perspect. Biol. Med. 18:399–408.

Ingelfinger, F. J. 1958. Esophageal motility. Physiol. Rev. 38:533–83.

Irwin, M. R., M. Daniels, E. T. Bloom, T. L. Smith, and H. Weiner. 1987. Life events, depressive symptoms, and immune function. Am. J. Psychiat. 144:437–41.

Irwin, M. R., M. Daniels, E. T. Bloom, and H. Weiner. 1986. Life events, depression, and natural killer cell activity. Psychopharmacol. Bull. 22:1093–96.

Irwin, M. R., W. Vale, and K. Britton. 1987. Central corticotropin releasing factor suppresses natural killer cell activity. Brain Beh. Immun. 1:81–87.

Irwin, M. R., and H. Weiner. 1987. Depressive symptoms and immune functions during bereavement. In Biopsychosocial aspects of bereavement, ed. S. Zisook, 157–74. Washington, DC: American Psychiatric Press.

Isenberg, J. I., J. A. Selling, D. L. Hogan, and M. A. Koss. 1987. Impaired proximal duodenal mucosal bicarbonate secretion in patients with duodenal ulcer. New Engl. J. Med. 316:374–79.

Iversen, K. 1948. Temporary rise in the frequency of thyrotoxicosis in Denmark, 1945. Copenhagen: Rosenkilde & Bagger.

Jacob, F., and J. Monod. 1961. Genetic regularity mechanisms in the synthesis of proteins. J. Mol. Biol. 3:318–56.

Jacobs, A., and G. S. Kirkpatrick. 1964. The Paterson-Kelly syndrome. Br. Med. J. 2:79–82.

Jacobs, S. C. 1987. Psychoendocrine aspects of bereavement. In Biopsychosocial aspects of bereavement, ed. S. Zisook, 141–55. Washington, DC: American Psychiatric Press.

Jacobs, S., and A. Ostfeld. 1977. An epidemiological review of the mortality of bereavement. Psychosom. Med. 39:344–57.

Jacobson, E. 1927. Spastic esophagus and mucous colitis. Arch. Int. Med. 30:433–45.

———. 1971. Depression. New York: International Universities Press.

Jahoda, M., and H. Rush. 1980. Work employment and unemployment. Sussex, Eng.: University of Sussex Science Policy Research Unit Report 12.

Jänig, W. 1987. The function of the autonomic nervous system at the interface between body and environment: W. B. Cannon and W. R. Hess revisited. In Neuronal control of bodily function: Neurobiological approaches to human disease, ed. D. Hellhammer, I. Florin, and H. Weiner, 143–73. Toronto: Hans Huber.

Jarrott, B., A. McQueen, L. Graf, and W. J. Louis. 1975. Serotonin levels in vascular tissue and the effects of a serotonin synthesis inhibitor on blood pressure in rats. Clin. Exp. Pharmacol. Physiol. 2 (Suppl.): 201–5.

Jemmott, J. B., M. Borysenko, R. Chapman, J. Z. Borysenko, D. C. McClelland, D. Meyer, and H. Benson. 1983. Academic stress, power motivation, and decrease in secretion rate of salivary secretory immunoglobulin A. Lancet 1:1400–1402.

Jenkins, C. D. 1976. Recent evidence supporting psychologic and social risk factors for coronary heart disease. New Engl. J. Med. 294:987–94, 1033–38.

Joasoo, A., and J. M. McKenzie. 1976. Stress and the immune response in rats. Int. Arch. Allerg. Appl. Immunol. 50:659–63.

Johnson, C. H., and J. W. Hastings. 1986. The elusive mechanism of the circadian clock. Am. Scientist 74:29–36.

Johnson, J., A. D. Sherman, F. Petty, D. Taylor, and F. A. Henn. 1982. Receptor changes in learned helplessness. Soc. Neurosci. Abstr. 8:392.

Johnson, L. F., and T. R. DeMeester. 1974. Twenty-hour four pH monitoring of the distal esophagus: A quantitative measure of gastroesophageal reflux. Am. J. Gastroenterol. 62:325–32.

Johnson, L. F., T. R. DeMeester, and E. C. Haggitt. 1978. Esophageal epithelial response to gastroesophageal reflux: A quantitative study. Am. J. Dig. Dis. 23: 498–509.

Johnson, T. S., J. B. Young, and L. Landsberg. 1983. Sympatho-adrenal responses to acute and chronic hypoxia in the rat. J. Clin. Invest. 71:1263–72.

Jones, V. A., P. McLaughlan, M. Shorthouse, E. Workman, and J. O. Hunter. 1982. Food intolerance: A major factor in the pathogenesis of irritable bowel syndrome. Lancet 2:1115–17.

Jönson, C., and L. Fändriks. 1988. Afferent electrical stimulation of mesenteric nerves inhibits duodenal HCO_3^- secretion via a spinal reflex activation of the splanchnic nerves in the rat. Acta Physiol. Scand. 133:545–50.

———. 1989. Splanchnic nerve stimulation inhibits duodenal HCO_3^- secretion in the rat. Am. J. Physiol. 255 (Gastrointest. Liver Physiol.): G709–12.

Jönson, C., P. Tunbäck-Hansson, and L. Fändriks. 1989. Splanchnic nerve activation inhibits HCO_3^- secretion from the duodenal mucosa induced by luminal acid in the rat. Gastroenterol. 96:45–49.

Jorgensen, L. S., L. Bonlokke, and N. J. Christensen. 1985. Plasma adrenaline and noradrenaline during mental stress and isometric exercise in man: The role of arterial sampling. Scand. J. Clin. Lab. Invest. 45:447–52.

Joy, M. D., and R. D. Lowe. 1970. The site of cardiovascular action of angiotensin II in the brain. Clin. Sci. 39:327–36.

Juli, D., and M. Engelbrecht-Greve. 1978. Stressverhalten ändern lernen: Programm zum abbau psychosomatischen krankheits krisen. Reinbeck: Rowohlt.

Julius, S., and M. D. Esler. 1975. Autonomic nervous cardiovascular regulation in borderline hypertension. Am. J. Cardiol. 36:672–85.

Julius, S., O. S. Randall, M. D. Esler, T. Kashima, C. Ellis, and J. Bennett. 1975. Altered cardiac responsiveness and regulation in the normal cardiac output type of borderline hypertension. Circ. Res. (6 Suppl. 1) 36:199–207.

Kafka, M. S., A. Wirz-Justice, and D. Naber. 1981. Circadian and seasonal rhythms in α- and β-adrenergic receptors in the rat brain. Brain Res. 207:409–19.

Kagan, A. 1971. Epidemiology and society, stress, and disease. In Society, stress, and disease. Vol. 1, The psychosocial environment and psychsomatic disease, ed. L. Levi, 36–48. London and New York: Oxford University Press.

Kaneko, M., K. Kaneko, J. Shinsako, and M. F. Dallman. 1981. Adrenal sensitivity to adrenocorticotropin varies diurnally. Endocrinol. 109:70–75.

Kanki, J. P., and D. B. Adams. 1978. Ventrobasal thalamus necessary for visually released defensive boxing of the rat. Physiol. Behav. 21:7–12.

Kannel, W. B., J. T. Doyle, P. M. McNamara, P. Quickerton, and T. Gordon. 1975. Precursors of sudden coronary deaths. Circulation 51:606–13.

Kanner, A. D., J. C. Coyne, C. Schaeffer, and R. S. Lazarus. 1981. Comparison of two modes of stress measurement: Daily hassles and uplifts versus major life events. J. Behav. Med. 4:1–39.

Kant, G. J., B. N. Bunnell, E. H. Mougey, L. L. Pennington, and J. L. Meyerhoff. 1983. Effects of repeated stress on pituitary cyclic AMP, and plasma prolactin, corticosterone, and growth hormone in male rats. Pharmacol. Biochem. Behav. 18:967–72.

Kant, G. J., T. Eggleston, L. Landman-Roberts, C. C. Kenion, G. C. Driver, and J. L.

Meyerhoff. 1985. Habituation to repeated stress is stressor specific. Pharmacol. Biochem. Behav. 22:631–34.

Kaplan, G. A., and T. Camacho. 1983. Perceived health and mortality: A nine-year follow-up of the human population laboratory cohort. Am. J. Epidemiol. 117: 292–304.

Karasu, T. B., and R. I. Steinmuller. 1978. Psychotherapeutics in medicine. New York: Grune & Stratton.

Karczmar, A. G., and C. L. Scudder. 1967. Behavioral responses to drugs and brain catecholamine levels in mice of different strains and genera. Fed. Proc. FASEB 26:1186–91.

Karli, P., M. Vergnes, and F. Didiergeorges. 1969. Rat-mouse interspecific aggressive behavior and its manipulation by brain ablation and by brain stimulation. In Aggressive behaviour, ed. S. Garattini and E. B. Sigg, 47–55. Amsterdam: Excerpta Medica.

Kasl, S. V. 1977. The effects of the residential environment on health and behavior: A review. In The effects of the man-made environment on health and behavior, ed. L. E. Hinkle, Jr., and W. C. Loring. Washington, DC: U.S. Government Printing Office. DHEW publ. no. (CDC) 77-8318.

———. 1979. Mortality and the business cycle: Some questions about research strategies when utilizing macrosocial and ecological data. Am. J. Publ. Hlth. 64: 784–88.

Kasl, S. V., R. F. Chisholm, and B. Eskenazi. 1981. The impact of the accident at Three Mile Island on the behavior and well-being of nuclear workers. Am. J. Publ. Hlth. 71:472–95.

Kasl, S. V., and S. Cobb. 1970. Blood pressure changes in men undergoing job loss: A preliminary report. Psychosom. Med. 32:19–38.

Kasl, S. V., S. Cobb, and G. W. Brooks. 1968. Changes in serum uric acid and cholesterol levels in men undergoing job loss. JAMA 206:1500–1503.

Katz, J. L. 1982. Three studies in psychosomatic medicine revisited. Psychosom. Med. 44:29–42.

Kay, D. C., W. B. Pickworth, G. L. Neidert, D. Falcone, P. M. Fishman, and E. Othmer. 1979. Opioid effects on computer-derived sleep and EEG parameters in nondependent human addicts. Sleep 2:175–91.

Kehoe, P., and E. M. Blass. 1986. Opioid-mediation of separation distress in 10-day rats: Reversal of stress with maternal stimulation. Develop. Psychobiol. 19: 385–98.

Keller, S. E., J. M. Weiss, S. J. Schleifer, N. E. Miller, and M. Stein. 1983. Stress-induced suppression of immunity in adrenalectomized rats. Science 221:1301–4.

Keller-Wood, M. E., and M. F. Dallman. 1984. Corticosteroid inhibition of ACTH secretion. Endocr. Rev. 5:1–24.

Kellett, J. 1989. Health and housing. J. Psychosom. Res. 33:255–68.

Kellner, R. 1986. Somatization and hypochondriasis. New York: Praeger.

Kelly, D. D., and A.-J. Silverman. 1988. Plasticity of peptidergic neurons in response to stress. Abstract. In Neuronal Control of Bodily Function: Frontiers of Stress Research (program). September 1987.

Kelly, K. A. 1983. Physiology of gastric motility and emptying. In Functional disorders of the digestive tract, ed. W. Y. Chey, 143–49. New York: Raven Press.

Kemeny, M. E., H. Weiner, S. E. Taylor, S. Schneider, B. Visscher, and J. L. Fahey. 1991. Repeated bereavement, depressed mood, and immune response in HIV seropositive and seronegative homosexual men. Psychosom. Med. (submitted).

Kerr, J. W., J. A. Dalton, and P. A. Gliebe. 1937. Some physical phenomena associated with anxiety states and their relation to hyperventilation. Ann. Int. Med. 11:961–62.

Kety, S. S. 1950. Cerebral circulation and metabolism in health and disease. Am. J. Med. 8:205–17.

Khachaturian, H., N. E. Alessi, N. Munfakh, and S. J. Watson. 1983. Ontogeny of opioid and related peptides in the rat CNS and pituitary: An immunocytochemical study. Life Sci. 33:137–40.

Khachaturian, H., M. E. Lewis, M. Shafer, and S. J. Watson. 1985. Anatomy of CNS opioid systems. Trends Neurosci. 8:111–19.

Kidd, K. K., and L. A. Morton. 1989. The genetics of psychosomatic disorders. In Psychosomatic medicine: Theory, physiology, and practice, ed. S. Cheren, 385–424. Madison, CT: International Universities Press.

Kiecolt-Glaser, J. K., W. Garner, C. E. Speicher, G. M. Penn, J. E. Holliday, and R. Glaser. 1984. Psychosocial modifiers of immunocompetence in medical students. Psychosom. Med. 46:7–14.

Kiecolt-Glaser, J. K., R. Glaser, E. Strain, J. Stout, K. Tarr, J. Holliday, and C. Speicher. 1986. Modulation of cellular immunity in medical students. J. Behav. Med. 9:5–21.

Kiss, J. Z., E. Mezey, and L. Skuboll. 1984. Corticotropin-releasing factor-immunoreactive neurons become vasopressin positive after adrenalectomy. Proc. Natl. Acad. Sci. (USA) 81:1854–58.

Kiss, R. 1951. Experimentell-morphologische Analyse der Nebennieren innervation. Acta Anat. (Basel) 13:81–89.

Kissen, D. M. 1967. Psychological factors, personality, and lung cancer in men aged 55–64. Br. J. Med. Psychol. 40:29–43.

Klerman, G. L., and J. E. Izen. 1977. The effects of bereavement and grief on physical health and well-being. Adv. Psychosom. Med. 9:66–104.

Klosterhalfen, W., and S. Klosterhalfen. 1987. Effects of restraint on adjuvant arthritis in two strains of rats. In Neurobiological approaches to human disease, ed. D. Hellhammer, I. Florin, and H. Weiner, 392–96. Toronto: Hans Huber.

Knutsson, A., T. Akerstedt, B. G. Jonsson, and K. Orth-Omer. 1986. Increased risk of ischaemic heart disease in shift workers. Lancet 1:89–92.

Kobasa, S. C. 1979. Stressful life events, personality, and health: An inquiry into hardiness. J. Person. Soc. Psychol. 37:1–11.

Kontos, H. A., D. W. Richardson, A. J. Raper, Zubair-Ul-Hassen, and J. L. Patterson Jr. 1972. Mechanisms of action of hypocapnic alkalosis on limb blood vessels in man and dog. Am. J. Physiol. 223:1296–1307.

Konturek, S. H. 1978. Prostaglandins and gastrointestinal secretion and motility. Adv. Exp. Med. Biol. 106:297–307.

Kopin, I. 1989. Adrenergic responses following recognition of stress. In Molecular biology of stress, UCLA symposia on molecular and cellular biology, new series, vol. 97, ed. S. Breznitz and O. Zinder, 123–32. New York: Alan R. Liss.

Korner, P. I., M. J. West, J. Shaw, and J. B. Uther. 1974. "Steady state" properties of baroreceptor–heart rate reflex in essential hypertension in man. Clin. Exp. Pharmacol. Physiol. 1:65–76.

Kosten, T. R., J. W. Mason, E. L. Geller, R. O. Ostroff, and L. Harkness. 1987. Sustained norepinephrine and epinephrine elevation in post-traumatic stress disorder. Psychoneuroendocrinol. 12:13–20.

Kosterlitz, H. W., L. E. Robson, and S. J. Peterson. 1989. Opioid peptides and their receptors. In Neuronal control of bodily function: Frontiers of stress research, ed. H. Weiner, D. Hellhammer, I. Florin, and R. Murison, 302–8. Toronto: Hans Huber.

Kracht, J. 1954. Fright-thyrotoxicosis in the wild rabbit: A model of thyrotrophic alarm-reaction. Acta Endocrinolog. (Kbh) 15:355–62.

Kraus, A. S., and A. M. Lilienfeld. 1959. Some epidemiological aspects of the high mortality in a young widowed group. J. Chron. Dis. 10:207–17.

Krehl, L. von 1932. Entstehung, Erkennung, und Behandlung innerer Krankheiten. Berlin: F. C. W. Vogel.

Kreisberg, R. A. 1977. Phosphorus deficiency in hypophosphatemia. Hosp. Pract. 12:121–28.

Kreuning, J., F. T. Bosman, G. Kuiper, A. M. v. d. Wal, and J. Lindman. 1978. Gastric and duodenal mucosa in healthy subjects. J. Clin. Pathol. 31:69–77.

Krieger, D. T., and A. S. Liotta. 1979. Pituitary hormones in the brain. Science 205:366–72.

Krieger, D. T., W. Allen, F. Rizzo, and H. P. Krieger. 1971. Characterization of the normal temporal pattern of plasma corticosteroid levels. J. Clin. Endocrinol. 32:266–84.

Kron, L., J. L. Katz, G. Gorzynski, and H. Weiner. 1977. Anorexia nervosa and gonadal dysgenesis: Further evidence of a relationship. Arch. Gen. Psychiat. 34:332–35.

Kruyswijk, H. H., B. ten Hove Jansen, and E. J. Miller. 1986. Hyperventilation-induced coronary artery spasm. Am. Heart J. 112:613–15.

Kubek, M., M. A. Rea, Z. I. Hodes, and M. H. Aprison. 1983. Quantitation and characterization of thyrotropin-releasing hormone in vagal nuclei and other regions of the medulla oblongata of the rat. J. Neurochem. 40:1307–13.

Kuch, K., R. P. Swinson, and M. Kirby. 1985. Post-traumatic stress disorder after car accidents. Can. J. Psychiat. 30:426–27.

Kuchel, O. 1977. Autonomic nervous system in hypertension: Clinical aspects. In Hypertension, ed. J. Genest, E. Koiw, and O. Kuchel, 93–114. New York: McGraw Hill.

Kuhn, C. M., S. R. Butler, and S. M. Schanberg. 1978. Selective depression of serum growth hormone during maternal deprivation in rat pups. Science 201:1034–36.

Kuhn, C. M., and S. M. Schanberg. 1979. Loss of growth hormone sensitivity in brain and liver during maternal deprivation in rats. Soc. Neurosci. Abstr. 5:168.

Kvetnansky, R., and L. Mikulaj. 1970. Adrenal and urinary catecholamines in rats during adaptation to repeated immobilization stress. Endocrinol. 87:738–43.

Kvetnansky, R., V. K. Weise, and I. J. Kopin. 1970. Elevation of adrenal tyrosine hydroxylase and phenylethanolamine-N-methyl transferase by repeated immobilization of rats. Endocrinol. 87:744–49.

L'Abbate, A. 1991. Coronary flow and mental stress in man. Circulation (in press).

Lacey, J. I. 1967. Somatic response patterning and stress: Some revisions of activation theory. In Psychological stress, ed. M. Appley and R. Trumbull, 14–42. New York: Appleton-Century-Crofts.

Lader, M. 1970. Psychosomatic and psychophysiological aspects of anxiety. In Modern trends in psychosomatic medicine 2, ed. O. W. Hill, 35–52. New York: Appleton-Century-Crofts.

———. 1982. Biological differentiation of anxiety, arousal, and stress. In The biology of anxiety, ed. R. J. Matthew, 11–22. New York: Brunner/Mazel.

Lagerspetz, K. Y. H., R. Tirri, and K. M. Lagerspetz. 1968. Neurochemical and endocrinological studies of mice selectively bred for aggressiveness. Scand. J. Psychol. 9:157–60.

Lang, P. J. 1971. The application of psychophysiological methods to the study of psychotherapy and behavior modification. In Handbook of psychotherapy and behavior change, ed. A. E. Bergin and S. L. Garfield, 75–125. New York: Wiley.

Langman, M. J. S. 1973. Blood groups and alimentary disorders. Clin. Gastroenterol. 2:497–506.

Langner, T. S., and S. T. Michael. 1963. Life stress and mental health. Vol. 2, The midtown Manhattan study. New York: Free Press.

Laragh, J. H. 1985. Atrial natriuretic hormone, the renin-aldosterone axis, and blood pressure–electrolyte homeostasis. New Engl. J. Med. 313:1330–40.

Laragh, J. H., L. H. Baer, H. R. Brunner, F. R. Buhler, J. E. Sealy, and E. D. Vaughan, Jr. 1972. Aldosterone in pathogenesis and management of hypertensive vascular disease. Am. J. Med. 52:633–52.

Lasser, R. B., J. H. Bond, and M. D. Levitt. 1975. The role of intestinal gas in functional abdominal pain. New Engl. J. Med. 293:524–26.

Latimer, P. R. 1983. Colonic psychophysiology: Implications for functional bowel disorders. In Psychophysiology of the gastrointestinal tract, ed. R. Hölzl and W. E. Whitehead, 263–88. New York: Plenum Press.

Latimer, P. R., D. Campbell, M. Latimer, S. K. Sarna, E. E. Daniel, and W. E. Waterfall. 1979. Irritable bowel syndrome: A test of the colonic hyperalgesia hypothesis. J. Behav. Med. 2:285–95.

Latimer, P. R., S. K. Sarna, D. Campbell, M. R. Latimer, W. E. Waterfall, and E. E. Daniel. 1981. Colonic motor and myoelectrical activity: A comparative study of normal subjects, psychoneurotic patients, and patients with irritable bowel syndrome (IBS). Gastroenterol. 80:893–901.

Lavie, P., A. Hefez, G. Halperin, and D. Enoch. 1979. Long-term effects of traumatic war-related events on sleep. Am. J. Psychiat. 136:174–78.

Lawton, M. P., and L. Nahemow. 1973. Ecology and the aging process. In The psychology of adult development and aging, ed. C. Eisdorder and P. Lawton, 619–74. Washington, DC: American Psychological Association.

Lazarus, R. S. 1966. Psychological stress and the coping process. New York: McGraw-Hill.

———. 1971. The concepts of stress and disease. In Society, stress, and disease: The psychosocial environment and psychosomatic disease, vol. I, ed. L. Levi, 53–58. London: Oxford University Press.

Lazarus, R. S., and J. B. Cohen. 1977. Environmental stress. In Human behavior and environment: Advances in theory and research, ed. I. Altman and J. F. Wohlwill, 89–127. New York: Plenum Press.

Lazarus, R. S., and A. DeLongis. 1983. Psychological stress and coping in aging. Am. Psychologist 38:245–54.

Lazarus, R. S., and S. Folkman. 1984. Stress, appraisal, and coping. New York: Springer.

Leaf, R. C., L. Lerner, and Z. P. Horovitz. 1969. The role of the amygdala in the pharmacological and endocrinological manipulation of aggression. In Aggressive behaviour, ed. S. Garattini and E. B. Sigg, 120–31. Amsterdam: Excerpta Medica.

LeDoux, J. E. 1989. Central pathways of emotional plasticity. In Neuronal control of bodily function: Frontiers of stress research, ed. H. Weiner, D. Hellhammer, I. Florin, and R. Murison, 122–36. Toronto: Hans Huber.

LeFeuvre, R. A., N. J. Rothwell, and M. J. Stock. 1987. Activation of brown fat thermogenesis in response to central injection of corticotropin releasing hormone in the rat. Neuropharmacol. 26:1217–21.

Lehman, M. N., and D. B. Adams. 1977. A statistical and motivational analysis of the social behaviors of the male laboratory rat. Behavior 61:238–75.

Lehtinen, V., and H. Puhakka. 1976. A psychosomatic approach to the globus hystericus syndrome. Acta Psychiat. Scand. 53:21–28.

Leitenberg, H., S. Agras, R. Butz, and J. Wincze. 1971. Relationship between heart rate and behavioral change during the treatment of phobias. J. Abn. Psychol. 78:59–68.

Lennard-Jones, J. E. 1983. Functional gastrointestinal disorders. New Engl. J. Med. 308:431–35.

Levi, L. 1972. Stress and distress in response to psychosocial stimuli. Acta Med. Scand. 191 (Suppl. 528): 1–166.

Levi-Montalcini, R. 1987. The nerve growth factor 35 years later. Science 237: 1154–62.

Levine, J. D., S. J. Dardick, M. S. Roizen, C. Helms, and A. I. Basbaum. 1986. Contribution of sensory afferents and sympathetic efferents to joint injury in experimental arthritis. J. Neurosci. 6:3423–29.

Levine, J. D., M. A. Moskowitz, and A. I. Basbaum. 1988. Neuroimmunologic mechanisms in arthritis. Prog. Neuroendocrinimmunol. 1:15–18.

Levine, S. 1987. Psychobiologic consequences of disruption in mother-infant relationships. In Perinatal development: A psychobiological perspective, ed. N. A. Krasnegor, E. M. Blass, M. A. Hofer, and W. P. Smotherman, 359–76. Orlando, FL: Academic Press.

Levine, S., and C. L. Coe. 1989. Endocrine regulation. In Psychosomatic medicine: Theory, physiology and practice, vol. 1, ed. S. Cheren, 331–83. Madison, CT: International Universities Press.

Levine, S., J. Madden IV, R. L. Conner, J. R. Moskal, and D. C. Anderson. 1973. Physiological and behavioral effects of prior aversive stimulation (pre-shock) in the rat. Physiol. Behav. 10:467–71.

Levine, S., and D. M. Treiman. 1964. Differential plasma corticosterone response to stress in four inbred strains of mice. Endocrinol. 75:142–44.

Levins, R., and R. Lewontin. 1985. The dialectical biologist. Cambridge, MA: Harvard University Press.

Levitt, M. D., and J. H. Bond. 1983. The role of intestinal gas in functional abdominal pain. In Functional disorders of the digestive tract, ed. W. Y. Chey, 245–49. New York: Raven Press.

Lewis, J. W., G. Baldrighi, S. J. Watson, and H. Akil. 1975. Electrical stimulation of the nucleus tractus solitarius (NTS) causes opioid mediated analgesia in the rat. Soc. Neurosci. Abstr. 11:637.

Lewis, J. W., J. T. Cannon, and J. C. Liebeskind. 1980. Opioid and non-opioid mechanisms of stress-analgesia. Science 208:623–25.

———. 1983. Involvement of central muscarinic cholinergic mechanisms in opioid stress analgesia. Brain Res. 270:289–93.

Lewis, J. W., E. H. Chudler, J. T. Cannon, and J. C. Liebeskind. 1981. Hypophysectomy differentially affects morphine and stress analgesia. Proc. West. Pharmacol. Soc. 24:323–26.

Lewis, J. W., M. E. Lewis, D. J. Loomus, and H. Akil. 1984. Acute systemic adminstration of morphine selectively increases mu opioid receptor binding in the rat brain. Neuropept. 5:117–20.

Lewis, J. W., J. E. Sherman, and J. C. Liebeskind. 1981. Opioid and nonopioid stress analgesia: Assessment of tolerance and cross-tolerance with morphine. J. Neurosci. 1:358–63.

Lewis, J. W., G. W. Terman, L. R. Watkins, D. J. Mayer, and J. C. Liebeskind. 1983. Opioid and nonopioid mechanisms of footshock-induced analgesia: Role of the spinal dorsolateral funiculus. Brain Res. 267:139–44.

Lewis, J. W., M. G. Tordoff, J. C. Liebeskind, and O. H. Viveros. 1982a. Evidence for adrenal medullary opioid involvement in stress analgesia. Soc. Neurosci. Abstr. 8:778.

Lewis, J. W., M. G. Tordoff, J. E. Sherman, and J. C. Liebeskind. 1982b. Adrenal medullary enkephalin-like peptides may mediate opioid stress analgesia. Science 217:557–59.

Lidz, T. 1949. Emotional factors in the etiology of hyperthyroidism. Psychosom. Med. 11:2–10.

Light, K. C. 1981. Cardiovascular responses to effortful coping: Implications for the role of stress in hypertension development. Psychophysiol. 18:216–28.

Light, K., and P. Obrist. 1980. Cardiovascular reactivity to behavioral stress in young males with and without marginally elevated casual systolic pressures: Comparison of clinic, home, and laboratory measure. Hypertension 2:802–8.

Lind, R. W., L. W. Swanson, and P. E. Sawchenko. 1985. Anatomical evidence that neural circuits related to the subfornical organ contain angiotension II. Brain Res. Bull. 15:79–82.

Lindemann, E. 1944. Symptomatology and management of acute grief. Am. J. Psychiat. 101:141–48.

Lipowski, Z. J. 1970. Physical illness, the individual, and the coping process. Psychiat. Med. 1:91–102.

———.1986. Somatization: A borderline between medicine and psychiatry. Can. Med. Assoc. J. 135:609–14.

Livett, B. G., X.-F. Zhou, Z. Khalil, D. C.-C. Wan, S. J. Bunn, and P. D. Marley. 1989. Endogenous neuropeptides maintain adrenal catecholamine output during stress. In Molecular biology of stress, ed. S. Breznitz and O. Zinder, 179–90. New York: Alan R. Liss.

Llinás, R. R. 1988. The intrinsic electrophysiological properties of mammalian neurons: Insights into central nervous system function. Science 242:1654–64.

Lloyd, G. 1983. Medicine without signs. Br. Med. J. 287:539–42.

Loewy, A. D., and H. Burton. 1978. Nuclei of the solitary tract: Efferent connections to the lower brain stem and spinal cord of the cat. J. Comp. Neurol. 181:421–50.

Lolait, S. J., J. A. Clements, A. J. Markwick, C. Cheng, C. McNally, A. I. Smith, and J. Funder. 1986. Pro-opiomelanocortin messenger ribonucleic acid and post-translational processing of β endorphin in spleen macrophages. J. Clin. Invest. 77:1776–79.

London, R. L., A. Ouyang, W. J. Snape, Jr., S. Goldberg, J. W. Hirschfeld, and S. Cohen. 1981. Provocation of esophageal pain by ergonovine or edrophonium. Gastroenterol. 81:10–14.

Lorimer, A. R., P. W. McFarlane, G. Provan, T. Duffy, and T. D. V. Lawrie. 1971. Blood pressure and catecholamine responses to stress in normotensive and hypertensive subjects. Cardiovas. Res. 5:169–75.

Lotz, M., D. A. Carson, and J. H. Vaughan. 1987. Substance P activation of rheumatoid synoviocytes: Neural pathway in pathogenesis of arthritis. Science 235:893–95.

Louis, W. J., A. E. Doyle, S. N. Anavekar, and K. G. Chua. 1973. Sympathetic activity and essential hypertension. Clin. Sci. Mol. Med. 45 (Suppl. 1): 119.

Low, M. G., and A. R. Saltiel. 1987. Structural and functional roles of glycosyl phosphatidylinositol in membranes. Science 239:268–75.

Lown, B. 1977. Role of higher nervous activity in sudden death. In First USA-USSR symposium on sudden death. Washington, DC: U.S. Department of Health, Education, and Welfare Public Health Service, NIH no. 718-1470.

———. 1982. Psychophysiologic and biobehavioral factors and sudden death. Washington, DC: Special Lecture Program, American Pychiatric Association.

Lown, B., R. Verrier, and R. Corbalan. 1973. Psychologic stress and threshold for repetitive ventricular response. Science 182:834–36.

Lowy, M. T., G. J. Gormley, A. T. Reder, and H. Y. Meltzer. 1988. Immune function, glucocorticoid receptor regulation, and depression. In Depressive disorders and immunity, ed. A. H. Miller, 107–33. Washington, DC: APA Press.

Lum, L. C. 1976. The syndrome of chronic habitual hyperventilation. In Modern trends in psychosomatic medicine, ed. O. W. Hill, 196–230. London: Butterworths.

Maas, J. W. 1962. Neurochemical differences between two strains of mice. Science 137:621–22.

McCain, G. A. 1986. The role of physical fitness training in the fibrositis/fibromyalgia syndrome. Am. J. Med. 81 (Suppl. 3A): 73–77.

McCarley, R. W., and J. A. Hobson. 1975. Neuronal excitability modulation over the sleep cycle: A structural and mathematical model. Science 189:58–60.

McClintock, M. K. 1971. Menstrual synchrony and suppression. Nature (London) 229:244–45.

McConnell, R. B. 1963. Associations and linkage in human genetics. Am. J. Med. 34:692–701.

McCubbin, J. W. 1967. Interrelationship between the sympathetic nervous system and the renin-angiotensin system. In Baroreceptors and hypertension, ed. P. Kezdi, 327–30. New York: Pergamon.

McDonald, E. M., A. H. Mann, and H. C. Thomas. 1987. Interferons as mediators of psychiatric morbidity: An investigation in a trial of recombinant A-interferon in hepatitis B carriers. Lancet 2:1175–78.

McDougall, J. 1974. The psychosoma and the psychoanalytic process. Int. Rev. Psychoanal. 1:437–50.

McFarlane, R. C., R. S. Kalucy, and P. M. Brooks. 1987. Psychobiological predictors of disease course in rheumatoid arthritis. J. Psychsom. Res. 31:757–64.

McGuire, M., and M. Raleigh. 1985. Serotonin-behavior interactions in vervet monkeys. Psychopharmacol. Bull. 21:458–63.

McKeown, T. J. 1976. The role of medicine: Dream, mirage, or nemesis. London: Nuffield Provincial Trusts.

Mackey, M. C., and J. G. Milton. 1987. Dynamical diseases. Ann. N.Y. Acad. Sci. 504:16–32.

McLennan, A. D., and S. Grillner. 1984. Activation of "fictive" swimming by microstimulation of brain stem locomotor regions in an *in vivo* preparation of lamprey central nervous system. Brain Res. 300:357–61.

MacLennan, A. J., R. C. Drugan, R. L. Hyson, S. F. Maier, J. Madden, and J. D. Barchas. 1982. Corticosterone: A critical factor in an opioid form of stress-induced analgesia. Science 215:1530–32.

McMichael, H. B., J. Webb, and A. M. Dawson. 1965. Lactase deficiency in adults: Cause of functional diarrhea. Lancet 1:717–20.

McRae, S., K. Younger, D. C. Thomson, and D. L. Wingate. 1982. Sustained mental stress alters human jejunal motor activity. Gut 23:404–9.

Madden, J., H. Akil, R. L. Patrick, and J. D. Barchas. 1977. Stress-induced parallel changes in central opioid levels and pain responsiveness in the rat. Nature (London) 265:358–60.

Maddison, D., and A. Viola. 1968. The health of widows in the year following bereavement. J. Psychosom. Res. 12:297–306.

Magarian, G. J. 1982. Hyperventilation syndromes: Infrequently recognized common expressions of anxiety and stress. Medicine 61:219–36.

———. 1989. Chronic hyperventilation syndrome. In Neuronal control of bodily function: Frontiers of stress research, ed. H. Weiner, D. Hellhammer, I. Florin, and R. Murison, 336–43. Toronto: Hans Huber.

Mahowald, M. W., M. L. Mahowald, S. R. Bundlie, and S. Ytterberg. 1987. Sleep fragmentation and daytime sleepiness in rheumatoid arthritis. Sleep Res. 16:487.

Maier, S. F., and M. E. P. Seligman. 1976. Learned helplessness: Theory and evidence. J. Exp. Psychol. 105:3–46.

Maixner, W., and A. Randich. 1984. Role of the right vagal nerve trunk in antinociception. Brain Res. 298:374–77.

Major, C. T., and B. J. Pleuvry. 1971. Effects of α-methyl-p-tyrosine, p-chlorophenylalanine, L-β (3,4-dihydroxyphenyl) alanine, 5-hydroxytryptophan, and diethyldithiocarbamate on the analgesic activity of morphine and methylamphetamine in the mouse. Br. J. Pharmacol. 42:512–21.

Malliani, A., M. Pagani, and M. Berganaschi. 1979. Positive feedback sympathetic reflexes and hypertension. Am. J. Cardiol. 44:860–65.

Mandler, R. N., W. E. Biddison, R. Mandler, and S. A. Serrate. 1986. Beta-endorphin augments the cytolytic activity and interferon production of natural killer cells. J. Immunol. 136:934–39.

Manning, A. P., W. G. Thompson, K. W. Heaton, and A. F. Morris. 1978. Towards positive diagnosis of the irritable bowel disease. Br. Med. J. 2:653–54.

Mantyh, C. R., T. Gates, R. P. Zimmerman, L. Kruger, J. E. Maggio, S. R. Vigna, A. I. Basbaum, J. Levine, and P. W. Mantyh. 1988. Alterations in density of receptor binding sites for sensory neuropeptides in the spinal cord of arthritic rats. In The arthritic rat as a model of clinical pain, ed. J. M. Besson and G. R. Guilbaud, 139–52. Amsterdam: Elsevier.

Manuck, S. B., J. R. Kaplan, and T. B. Clarkson. 1983a. Social stability and coronary artery atherosclerosis in Cynomolgus monkeys. Neurosci. Biobehav. Rev. 7:485–91.

———. 1983b. Behaviorally induced heart rate reactivity and atherosclerosis in Cynomolgus monkeys. Psychosom. Med. 45:95–108.

Marcus, D. M. 1969. The ABO and Lewis blood-group system. New Engl. J. Med. 280:994–1006.

Marek, P., and J. Szacki. 1991 (submitted). Environmentally induced analgesia in wild mice: Comparison with laboratory mice.

Marmot, M. G. 1982. Socio-economic and cultural factors in ischaemic heart disease. Adv. Cardiol. 29:68–76.

Marmot, M. G., G. Rose, M. Shipley, and P. J. S. Hamilton. 1978. Employment grade and coronary heart disease in British civil servants. J. Epidemiol. Comm. Hlth. 32:244–49.

Marmot, M. G., and S. L. Syme. 1976. Acculturation and coronary heart disease in Japanese-Americans. Am. J. Epidemiol. 104:225–47.

Marmot, M. G., S. L. Syme, and G. Rhoads. 1975. Epidemiologic studies of coronary heart disease and stroke in Japanese men living in Japan, Hawaii, and California: Prevalence of coronary and hypertensive heart disease and associated risk factors. Am. J. Epidemiol. 102:514–25.

Marr, D. 1982. Vision. San Francisco: Freeman & Co.

Martin, J. B., P. Brazeau, G. S. Tannenbaum, J. O. Willoughby, J. Epelbaum, L. C. Terry, and D. Durand. 1978. Neuroendocrine organization of growth hormone regulation. Res. Publ. Assoc. Nerv. Ment. Dis. 56:329–57.

Marty, P., and M. de M'Uzan. 1963. Le pensée opératoire. Rev. Franc. Psychoanal. 27 (Suppl.): 1345.

Maseri, A., S. Severi, M. DeNes, A. L'Abbate, S. Chierchia, M. Marzilli, A. M. Ballestra, O. Parodi, A. Biagini, and A. Distante. 1978. Variant angina: One aspect of a continuous spectrum of vasospastic myocardial ischemia. Am. J. Cardiol. 42:1019–35.

Mason, J. W. 1968. Organization of psychoendocrine mechanisms. Psychosom. Med. 30:565–808.

———. 1971. A re-evaluation of the concept of nonspecificity in stress theory. J. Psychiatr. Res. 8:323–33.

———. 1975. An historical view of the stress field. J. Human Stress 1:6–12, 22–35.

Mason, J. W., E. L. Giller, T. R. Kosten, and L. Harkness. 1988. Elevation of urinary norepinephrine/cortisol ratio in post traumatic stress disorder. J. Nerv. Ment. Dis. 176:498–502.

Mason, J. W., E. L. Giller, T. R. Kosten, R. O. Ostroff, and L. Podd. 1986. Urinary free-cortisol levels in post-traumatic stress disorder patients. J. Nerv. Ment. Dis. 174:145–49.

Mason, M. A., and Berkson, G. 1974. Effects of maternal mobility on the development of rocking and other behaviors in rhesus monkeys. Develop. Psychobiol. 8:197–211.

Mathew, R. J., M. L. Weinman, and J. L. Claghorn. 1982. Anxiety and cerebral blood flow. In The biology of anxiety, ed. R. J. Mathew, 23–33. New York: Brunner/Mazel.

Matsumoto, Y. S. 1970. Social stress and coronary heart disease in Japan: A hypothesis. Milbank Mem. Fund Q. 48:9–36.

Matthews, P. M., C. J. Froehlich, W. L. Sibbit, and A. D. Bankhurst. 1983. Enhancement of natural cytotoxicity by beta-endorphin. J. Immunol. 130:1658–62.

Mayer, D. J., T. L. Wolfle, H. Akil, B. Carder, and J. C. Liebeskind. 1971. Analgesia from electrical stimulation in the brainstem of the rat. Science 174:1351–54.

Mayr, E. 1982. The growth of biological thought: Diversity, evolution, and inheritance. Cambridge, MA: Belknap Press of Harvard University.

Mazur, A., and T. A. Lamb. 1980. Testosterone, status, and mood in human males. Horm. Behav. 14:236–46.

Mechanic, D. 1980. The experience and reporting of common physical complaints. J. Hlth. Soc. Behav. 21:146–55.

Medalie, J., M. Snijder, J. J. Groen, H. Neufeld, E. Ris, and U. Goldboult. 1973. Angina pectoris among 10,000 men, 5 years incidence and univariate analyses. Am. J. Med. 55:583–94.

Medawar, P. B., and J. S. Medawar. 1977. The life science. New York: Harper and Row.

Meister, B., and T. Hökfelt,. 1989. Interaction of peptides and classical neurotransmitters: Focus on neuroendocrine multimessenger systems. In Neuronal control of bodily function: Frontiers of stress research, ed. H. Weiner, D. Hellhammer, I. Florin, and R. Murison, 160–80. Toronto: Hans Huber.

Mellman, T. A., and G. C. Davis. 1985. Combat-related flashbacks in post-traumatic stress disorder: Phenomenology and similarity to panic attacks. J. Clin. Psychiat. 46:379–82.

Mellow, M. 1977. Diffuse esophageal spasm: Manometric follow-up and response to cholinergic stimulation and cholinesterase inhibition. Gastroenterol. 77:472–77.

Melnechuk, T. 1978. Cell receptor disorders. La Jolla, CA: Western Behavioral Sciences Institute.

Mendeloff, A. I. 1983. Epidemiology of functional gastrointestinal disorders. In Functional disorders of the digestive tract, ed. W. Y. Chey, 13–19. New York: Raven Press.

Mendeloff, A. I., M. Monk, C. I. Siegel, and A. Lilienfeld. 1970. Illness experience and life stresses in patients with irritable colon and with ulcerative colitis. New Engl. J. Med. 282:14–17.

Mendlewicz, J., P. Linkowski, M. Kerkhofs, D. Desmedt, J. Golstein, G. Copinschi, and E. Van Ceuter. 1985. Diurnal hypersecretion of growth hormone in depression. J. Clin. Endocrinol. Metab. 60:505–12.

Mendoza, S. P., C. L. Coe, E. L. Lowe, and S. Levine. 1979. The physiological response to group formation in adult male squirrel monkeys. Psychoneuroendocrinol. 3:221–29.

Miczek, K. A., M. L. Thompson, and L. Shuster. 1982. Opioid-like analgesia in defeated mice. Science 215:1520–22.

Millan, M. J., R. Przewlocki, and A. Herz. 1980. A non-β-endorphinergic adenohypophyseal mechanism is essential for an analgetic response to stress. Pain 8:343–53.

Miller, B. V., and D. A. Bernstein. 1972. Instructional demand in a behavioral avoidance test for claustrophobic fears. J. Abn. Psychol. 80:206–10.

Miller, R. G., R. T. Rubin, B. R. Clark, R. E. Poland, and R. J. Arthur. 1970. The stress of aircraft carrier landings, 1: Corticosteroid responses in naval aviators. Psychosom. Med. 32:581–88.

Miller, T. W., ed. 1989. Stressful life events. Madison, CT: International Universities Press.

Mirra, A. P., P. Cole, and B. MacMahon. 1971. Breast cancer in an area of high parity: São Paulo, Brazil. Cancer Res. 31:77–83.

Mirsky, I. A. 1958. Physiologic, psychologic, and social determinants in the etiology of duodenal ulcer. Am. J. Dig. Dis. 3:285–314.

Misiewicz, J. J. 1975. Colonic motility. Gut 16:311–15.

Misiewicz, J. J., A. M. Connell, and F. A. Pontes. 1966. Comparison of the effect of meals and prostigmine on the proximal and distal colon in patients with and without diarrhea. Gut 7:468–73.

Möhring, J., J. Kinz, and J. Schoun. 1978. Role of vasopressin in blood pressure control of spontaneously hypertensive rats. Clin. Sci. Mol. Med. 55 (Suppl. 4): 246s–50s.

Moldofsky, H. 1989. Stress, disordered sleep, and fibrositis syndrome. In Neuronal control of bodily function: Frontiers of stress research, ed. H. Weiner, D. Hellhammer, I. Florin, and R. Murison, 355–65. Toronto: Hans Huber.

Moldofsky, H., and F. A. Lue. 1980. The relationship of alpha delta EEG frequencies to pain and mood in "fibrositis" patients with chlorpromazine and L-tryptophan. Electroencephalogr. Clin. Neurophysiol. 50:71–80.

Moldofsky, H., F. A. Lue, and P. Saskin. 1987. Sleep and morning pain in primary osteoarthritis. J. Rheumatol. 14:124–28.

Moldofsky, H., F. A. Lue, and H. A. Smythe. 1983. Alpha EEG sleep and morning symptoms in rheumatoid arthritis. J. Rheumatol. 10:373–79.

Moldofsky, H., P. Saskin, L. Salem, and F. A. Lue, and H. A. Smythe. 1983. Alpha EEG sleep and morning symptoms in rheumatoid arthritis. J. Rheumatol. 10:373–79.

Moldofsky, H. P. Saskin, L. Salem, and F. A. Lue. 1987. Sleep and symptoms in postinfectious neuromyasthenia and fibrositis syndrome. Sleep Res. 16:492.

Moldofsky, H., and P. Scarisbrick. 1976. Induction of neurasthenic musculoskeletal pain syndrome by selective sleep stage deprivation. Psychosom. Med. 38:35–44.

Moldofsky, H., P. Scarisbrick, R. England, and H. A. Smythe. 1975. Musculoskeletal symptoms and non-REM sleep disturbance in patients with "fibrositis" syndrome and healthy subjects. Psychosom. Med. 37:341–51.

Moldofsky, H., C. Tullis, F. A. Lue, G. Quance, and J. Davidson. 1984. Sleep-related myoclonus in rheumatic pain modulation disorder (fibrositis syndrome) and in excessive daytime somnolence. Psychosom. Med. 46:145–51.

Moldofsky, H., and J. J. Warsh. 1978. Plasma tryptophan and musculoskeletal pain in non-articular rheumatism (fibrositis syndrome). Pain 5:65–71.

Möllman, K.-M., O. Bonnevie, E. Gudmand-Hoyer, and H. R. Wulff. 1976. Nosography of X-ray negative dyspepsia. Scand. J. Gastroenterol. 11:193–97.

Molnar, G. D., W. F. Taylor, and A. L. Langworthy. 1972. Plasma immunoreactive insulin patterns in insulin-treated diabetes. Mayo Clin. Proc. 47:709–29.

Molony, R. R., D. M. MacPeek, P. L. Schiffman, M. Frank, J. A. Neubauer, M. Schwartzberg, and J. R. Seibold. 1986. Sleep, sleep apnea, and the fibromyalgia syndrome. J. Rheumatol. 13:797–98.

Monod, J., J. P. Changeux, and F. Jacob. 1963. Allosteric proteins and cellular control systems. J. Mol. Biol. 6:306–28.

Moore, R. Y., A. Heller, R. J. Wurtman, and J. Axelrod. 1967. Visual pathway mediating pineal response to environmental light. Science 155:220–23.

Moore, R. Y., and N. J. Lenn. 1972. A retinohypothalamic projection in the rat. J. Comp. Neurol. 146:1–14.

Moore-Ede, M. C. 1973. Circadian effects of drug effectiveness and toxicity. Clin. Pharmacol. Ther. 14:925–35.

———. 1986. Physiology of the circadian timing system: Predictive versus reactive homeostasis. Am. J. Physiol. 250:R735–52.

Moore-Ede, M. C., F. M. Sulzman, and C. A. Fuller. 1982. The clocks that time us. Cambridge, MA: Harvard University Press.

Moos, R. H. 1976. The human context: Environmental determinants of behavior. New York: Wiley.

———. 1979. Evaluating educational environments: Procedures, measures, findings, and policy implications. San Francisco: Jossey-Bass.

Moos, R. H., and G. F. Solomon. 1964. Personality correlates of the rapidity of progression of rheumatoid arthritis. Ann. Rheum. Dis. 23:145–51.

———. 1965. Psychologic comparisons between women with rheumatoid arthritis and their nonarthritic sisters, 2: Content analysis of interviews. Psychosom. Med. 27:150–64.

Morera, A. M., A. M. Cathiard, M. Laburthe, and J. M. Saez. 1979. Interaction of vasoactive intestinal peptide (VIP) with a mouse adrenal cell line (Y-1): Specific binding and biological effects. Biochem. Biophys. Res. Commun. 90:78–85.

Morgan, M. M., J. H. Sohn, and J. C. Liebeskind. 1987. Microinjection of glutamate into the nucleus tractus solitarius produces analgesia in the rat. Soc. Neurosci. Abstr. 13:988.

Morita, H., and S. F. Vatner. 1985. Effects of hemorrhage on renal nerve activity in conscious dogs. Circ. Res. 57:788–93.

Morley, J. E. 1983. Neuroendocrine effects of endogenous opioid peptides in human subjects: A review. Psychoneuroendocrinol. 8:361–79.

———. 1989. Neuropeptide-Y: A new stress hormone? In Neuronal control of bodily function: Frontiers of stress research, ed. H. Weiner, D. Hellhammer, I. Florin, and R. Murison, 286–301. Toronto: Hans Huber.

Morley, J. E., N. Kay, and G. F. Solomon. 1989. Opioid peptides, stress, and immune function. In Neuropeptides and stress, ed. Y. Taché, J. E. Morley, and M. R. Brown, 222–34. New York: Springer-Verlag.

Morley, J. E., and A. S. Levine. 1982. Corticotropin-releasing factor, grooming, and ingestive behavior. Life Sci. 31:1459–64.

Morrell, D. C. 1978. The epidemiological imperative for primary care. In Primary health care in industrialized nations 310:2–10. New York: New York Academy of Sciences.

Morrow, B. R., and A. H. Labrum. 1978. The relationship between psychological and physiological measures of anxiety. Psychol. Med. 8:95–101.

Mortensen, S. A., R. Vilhelmson, and E. Sande. 1981. Prinzmetal's variant angina (PVA): Circadian variation in response to hyperventilation. Acta. Med. Scand. Suppl. 644:38–41.

Mortola, J. F., J. H. Liu, J. C. Gillin, D. D. Rasmussen, and S. S. C. Yen. 1987. Pulsatile rhythms of adrenocorticotropin (ACTH) and cortisol in women with endogenous depression: Evidence for increased ACTH pulse frequency. J. Clin. Endocrinol. Metab. 65:962–68.

Moskowitz, A. S., G. W. Terman, and J. C. Liebeskind. 1985. Stress-induced analgesia in the mouse: Strain comparisons. Pain 2:67–72.

Mueller, D. P. 1980. Social networks: A promising direction for research on the relationship of the social environment to psychiatric disorder. Soc. Sci. Med. 14A:147–61.

Mueller, R. A., H. Thoenen, and J. Axelrod. 1969a. Increase in tyrosine hydroxylase activity after reserpine administration. J. Pharmacol. Exp. Ther. 169:74–79.

———. 1969b. Inhibition of transsynaptically increased tyrosine hydroxylase activity by cycloheximide and actinomycin D. Molec. Pharmacol. 5:463–69.

Mugford, R. A., and N. W. Navell. 1970a. Pheromones and their effect on aggression in mice. Nature (London) 226:967–68.

———. 1970b. The aggression of male mice against androgenized females. Psychonom. Sci. 20:191–92.

Munck, A., P. M. Guyre, and N. Holbrook. 1984. Physiological functions of glucocorticoids in stress and their relation to pharmacological actions. Endocr. Rev. 5:25–44.

Murison, R., and E. Isaksen. 1982. Gastric ulceration and adrenocortical activity after inescapable and escapable preshock in rats. Scand. J. Psychol. Suppl. 1:133–37.

Murphy, H. M., C. H. Wideman, and T. S. Brown. 1979. Plasma corticosterone levels and ulcer formation in rats with hippocampal lesions. Neuroendocrinol. 28:123–30.

Murray, H. W., and M. W. Kirschner. 1989. Dominoes and clocks: The union of two views of the cell cycle. Science 246:614–21.

Murray, H. W., B. Y. Rubin, H. Masur, and R. B. Roberts. 1984. Impaired production of lymphokines and immune (gamma) interferon in the acquired immunodeficiency syndrome. New Engl. J. Med. 310:883–89.

Murrell, T. G. C., and D. J. Deller. 1967. Intestinal motility in man: The effects of bradykinin on the motility of the distal colon. Am. J. Dig. Dis. 12:568–76.

Nagler, R., and H. M. Spiro. 1961. Heartburn in late pregnancy: Manometric studies of esophageal motor function. J. Clin. Invest. 40:954–70.

Najman, J. M. 1980. Theories of disease causation and the concept of general susceptibility: A review. Soc. Sci. Med. 14:231–37.

National Center for Health Statistics. 1970. Mortality from selected causes by marital status. Vital and Health Statistics, series 20, nos. 8A and B. Washington, DC: U.S. Dept. of Health, Education, and Welfare.

Neill, W. A., and M. Hattenhauer. 1975. Impairment of myocardial supply due to hyperventilation. Circulation 52:854–58.

Nemiah, J. C., and P. E. Sifneos. 1970. Affect and fantasy in patients with psychosomatic disorders. In Modern trends in psychosomatic medicine 2, ed. O. W. Hill, 26–34. London: Butterworths.

Nepom, G. T., J. A. Hansen, and B. S. Nepom. 1987. The molecular basis for HLA class II associations with rheumatoid arthritis. J. Clin. Immunol. 7:1–7.

Nesse, R. M., G. C. Curtis, G. M. Brown, and R. T. Rubin. 1980. Anxiety induced by flooding therapy for phobias does not elicit a prolactin secretory response. Psychosom. Med. 42:25–31.

Neuhäuser, G., R. F. Daly, N. C. Magnelli, R. F. Barreras, R. M. Donaldson Jr., and J. M. Optiz. 1976. Essential tremor, nystagmus, and duodenal ulceration. Clin. Genetics 9:81–91.

Newsom-Davis, J. 1988. Autoimmunity in neuromuscular disease. Ann. N.Y. Acad. Sci. 540:25–38.

Nicholl, R. A., and J. L. Barker. 1971. Excitation of supraoptic neurosecretory cells by angiotensin II. Nature New Biol. (London) 233:172–74.

Nieschlag, E. 1979. The endocrine function of the human testis in regard to sexuality. In Sex hormones and behavior, Ciba Foundation symposium 62, 183–97. Amsterdam: Excerpta Medica.

Nikolicz, K., A. J. Mason, E. Szonyi, J. Ramachandran, and P. Seeburg. 1985. A prolactin-inhibiting factor within the precursor for human gonadotropin-releasing hormone. Nature (London) 316:511–17.

Nishizuka, Y. 1986. Studies and perspectives of protein kinase C. Science 233:305–12.

Noel, G. L., R. C. Dimond, J. M. Earll, and A. G. Frantz. 1976. Prolactin, thyrotropin, and growth hormone release during stress associated with parachute jumping. Aviat. Space Environ. 47:543–47.

Norman, G. R., A. H. McFarlane, and D. L. Streiner. 1985. Patterns of illness among individuals reporting high and low stress. Can. J. Psychiat. 30:400–405.

Nossal, G. J. V. 1987. The basic components of the immune system. New Engl. J. Med. 316:1320–25.

Notkins, A. L. 1979. The causes of diabetes. Sci. Am. 241:62–73.

Notman, M., and C. C. Nadelson. 1976. The rape victim: Psychodynamic considerations. Am. J. Psychiat. 133:408–12.

Nuckolls, K. B., J. Cassel, and B. H. Kaplan. 1972. Psychosocial assets, life crisis, and the prognosis of pregnancy. Am. J. Epidemiol. 95:431–41.

Odio, M. R., and R. P. Maickel. 1985. Comparative biochemical responses of rats to different stimuli. Physiol. Behav. 34:595–99.

O'Hara, M. W., L. P. Rehm, and S. B. Campbell. 1983. Postpartum depression: A role for social network and life stress variables. J. Nerv. Ment. Dis. 171:336–41.

Okamoto, K. 1972. Spontaneous hypertension. Tokyo: Igaku Shoin.

Okamoto, K., and K. Aoki. 1963. Development of a strain of spontaneously hypertensive rats. Jap. Circ. J. 27:282–93.

Okamoto, K., S. Nosaka, Y. Yamori, and M. Matsumoto. 1967. Participation of neural factor in the pathogenesis of hypertension in the spontaneously hypertensive rat. Jap. Heart J. 8:168–80.

Okel, B. B., and J. W. Hurst. 1961. Prolonged hyperventilation in man: Associated electrolyte changes and subjective symptoms. Arch. Int. Med. 108:757–62.

Okuma, Y., Y. Osumi, T. Ishigawa, and T. Mitsuma. 1987. Enhancement of gastric acid output and mucosal blood flow by tripeptide thyrotropin releasing hormone microinjected into the dorsal motor nucleus of the vagus in rats. Jap. J. Pharmacol. 43:173–78.

Okuma, M., Y. Yamori, K. Ohta, and H. Uchino. 1979. Enhanced generation of prostacyclin (PGI_2) in spontaneously hypertensive rats (SHR). Jap. Heart J. 20 (Suppl. 1): 177–79.

Oley, N., C. C. Cordova, M. Kelly, and J. D. Bronzino. 1982. Morphine administration to the region of the nucleus tractus solitarius produces analgesia in rats. Brain Res. 236:511–15.

Oliver, M. F., V. A. Kurien, and T. W. Greenwood. 1968. Relation between serum free fatty acids and death after acute myocardial infarction. Lancet 1:710–15.

Olivier, B. 1977. The ventromedial hypothalamus and aggressive behavior in rats. Aggr. Behav. 3:47–56.

Oparil, S., C. Vassaux, C. A. Sanders, and E. Haber. 1970. Role of renin in acute postural hypotension. Circulation 41:89–95.

Orr, W. C. 1983. Studies of esophageal function during waking and sleep. In Psychophysiology of the gastrointestinal tract, ed. R. Hölzl and W. E. Whitehead, 5–20. New York: Plenum Press.

Orr, W. C., M. G. Robinson, and L. F. Johnson. 1981. Acid clearance during sleep in the pathogenesis of reflux esophagitis. Dig. Dis. Sci. 26:423–27.

Orth-Gomer, K., and A. Ahlbom. 1980. Impact of psychological stress on idiopathic heart disease when controlling for conventional risk factors. J. Human Stress 6:7–15.

Orth-Gomer, K., C. Hogstedt, L. Bodin, and B. Soderholm. 1986. Frequency of extrasystoles in healthy male employees. Br. Heart J. 55:259–64.

Osborne, F. H., B. A. Mattingly, W. K. Redman, and J. S. Osborne. 1975. Factors affecting the measurement of classically conditioned fear in rats following exposure to escapable versus inescapable signalled shock. J. Exper. Psychol.: Anim. Behav. Proc. 1:364–73.

Ostfeld, A. 1979. The role of stress in hypertension. J. Human Stress 5:20.

Overmier, J. B., and M. E. P. Seligman. 1967. Effects of inescapable shock on subsequent escape and avoidance responding. J. Consult. Clin. Psychol. 63:28–33.

Painter, N. S., and S. C. Truelove. 1964. The intraluminal pressure patterns in diverticulosis, 3: The effect of prostigmine. Gut 5:365–69.

Parati, G., R. Casadei, and G. Mancia. 1989. Cardiovascular effects of emotional behavior in animals and humans. In Neuronal control of bodily function: Frontiers of stress research, ed. H. Weiner, D. Hellhammer, I. Florin, and R. Murison, 100–11. Toronto: Hans Huber.

Pardee, A. B. 1989. G$_1$ events and regulation of cell proliferation. Science 246: 603–8.

Paré, W. P., and G. B. Glavin. 1986. Restraint stress in biomedical research: A review. Neurosci. Biobehav. Rev. 10:339–70.

Parker, L. N., E. R. Levin, and E. T. Lifrat. 1985. Evidence of adrenocortical adaptation to severe illness. J. Clin. Endocrinol. Metab. 60:947–52.

Parkes, C. M. 1964. Recent bereavement as a cause of mental illness. Br. J. Psychiat. 110:198–204.

———. 1970. The first year of bereavement. Psychiatry 33:444–67.

———. 1971. Determination of outcome following bereavement. Proc. Royal Soc. Med. 64:279.

Parkes, C. M., B. Benjamin, and R. G. Fitzgerald. 1969. Broken heart: A statistical study of increased mortality among widowers. Br. Med. J. 1:740–43.

Parkes, C. M., and R. J. Brown. 1972. Health after bereavement. Psychosom. Med. 34:449–61.

Pasnau, R. O., ed. 1975. Consultation-liaison psychiatry. New York: Grune & Stratton.

Paul, O. 1987. DaCosta's syndrome or neurocirculatory asthenia. Br. Heart J. 58: 306–15.

Paulley, J. W. 1983. Pathological mourning: A key factor in the psychopathogenesis of autoimmune disorders. Psychotherap. Psychosom. 40:181–90.

Pavlidis, N., and M. Chirigos. 1980. Stress-induced impairment of macrophage tumoricidal function. Psychosom. Med. 42:47–54.

Pavlov, I. P. 1910. The work of the digestive glands, trans. W. H. Thompson. London: Griffin.

Payan, D. G., J. D. Levine, and E. J. Goetzl. 1984. Modulation of immunity and hypersensitivity by sensory neuropeptides. J. Immunol. 132:1601–4.

Paykel, E. S. 1976. Life stress, depression, and attempted suicide. J. Human Stress 2:3–12.

Pearlin, L. I. 1980. The life cycle and life strains. In Sociological theory and research: A critical appraisal, ed. H. M. Blalock, 349–60. New York: Free Press.

Pearlin, L. I., and M. A. Lieberman. 1979. Social sources of emotional distress. In Research in community and mental health, ed. R. Simmons, 217–48. Greenwich, CT: JAI Press.

Pearlin, L. I., M. A. Lieberman, E. G. Menaghan, and J. T. Mullan. 1981. The stress process. J. Hlth. Soc. Behav. 22:337–56.

Peña, A. S., and S. C. Truelove. 1972. Hypolactasia and the irritable colon syndrome. Scand. J. Gastroenterol. 7:433–38.

Perlman, L. V., S. Ferguson, K. Bergum, E. L. Isenberg, and J. F. Hammarstein. 1971. Precipitation of congestive heart failure: Social and emotional factors. Ann. Int. Med. 75:1–7.

Perry, F., and A. D. Sherman. 1981. GABAergic modulation of learned helplessness. Pharmacol. Biochem. Behav. 15:567–70.

Peters, G., M. Faisal, T. Lang, and I. I. Ahmed. 1988. Stress caused by social interaction and its effect on the susceptibility to *Aeromonas hydrophila* infection in the rainbow trout, *Salmo giardineri* (Rich). Dis. Aquat. Org. 4:369–80.

Peters, G., and L. Q. Hong. 1985. Gill structure and electrolyte level of European eels under stress. In Fish and poultry pathology, ed. A. E. Ellis, 183–96. New York: Academic Press.

Peters, M. N., and C. T. Richardson. 1983. Stressful life events, acid hyper-secretion, and ulcer disease. Gastroenterol. 84:114–19.

Petraglia, F., W. Vale, and C. Rivier. 1986. Opioids act centrally to modulate stress-induced decrease in luteinizing hormone in the rat. Endocrinol. 119:2445–50.

Phillips, M. I., J. F. E. Mann, H. Haebara, R. Dietz, P. Schelling, and D. Ganten. 1977. Lowering of hypertension by central saralasin in the absence of plasma renin. Nature (London) 270:445–47.

Pilowsky, I. 1967. Dimensions of hypochondriasis. Br. J. Psychiat. 113:89–93.

Pilowsky, I., Q. P. Smith, and M. Katsikitis. 1987. Illness, behavior, and general practice utilization: A prospective study. J. Psychosom. Res. 31:177–83.

Piris, J., and R. Whitehead. 1975. Quantitation of G-cells in fibreoptic biopsy specimens and serum gastrin levels in healthy normal subjects. J. Clin. Pathol. 28: 636–38.

Pittendrigh, C. S. 1962. On temporal organization in living systems (Harvey Lectures, ser. 56), pp. 93–125. New York: Academic Press.

Platt, S., and N. Kreitman. 1984. Trends in parasuicide and unemployment among men in Edinburgh, 1968–1982. Br. Med. J. 289:1029–32.

Plotnick, R., D. Mir, and J. M. R. Delgado. 1970. Aggression, noxiousness, and brain stimulation in unrestrained rhesus monkeys. In Physiology of aggression and defeat, ed. B. F. Eleftherion, 143–221. New York: Plenum Press.

Plotsky, P. M., T. O. Bruhn, and W. Vale. 1985. Evidence for multifactor regulation of the adrenocorticotropin secretory response to hemodynamic stimuli. Endocrinol. 116:633–39.

Popovic, M., and D. Petrovic. 1964. After the earthquake. Lancet 2:1169–71.

Porreca, F., R. J. Sheldon, and T. F. Burks. 1989. Central and peripheral visceral actions of bombesin. In Neuronal control of bodily function: Frontiers of stress research, ed. H. Weiner, D. Hellhammer, I. Florin, and R. Murison, 276–85. Toronto: Hans Huber.

Powell, D. W. 1977. Intestinal motility: The irritable bowel syndrome. Gastroenterol. 73:812–14.

Preston, D. M., T. E. Adrian, N. D. Christofides, J. E. Lennard-Jones, and S. R. Bloom. 1983. Gut hormone response in functional bowel disease. Scand. J. Gastroenterol. 18 (Suppl. 82): 199–200.

Prigogine, I. 1980. From being to becoming: Time and complexity in the physical sciences. San Francisco: W. H. Freeman.

Prince, H. E., V. Kermani-Arab, and J. L. Fahey. 1984. Depressed interleukin-2 receptor expression in acquired immune deficiency and lymphadenopathy syndrome. J. Immunol. 133:1313–17.

Quirion, R. 1988. Atrial natriuretic factors and the brain: An update. Trends Neurosci. 11:58–62.

Raab, A., R. Dantzer, B. Michaud, P. Mormede, K. Taghoutzi, H. Simon, and M. LeMoal. 1985. Behavioral, physiological, and immunological consequences of social status and aggression in chronically coexisting resident-intruder dyads of male rats. Physiol. Behav. 36:223–28.

Raab, W. 1970. Preventive myocardiology. Springfield, IL: Thomas.

Rabkin, J. G., and E. L. Struening. 1976. Life events, stress, and illness. Science 194:1013–20.

Rachman, S., and R. I. Hodgson. 1974. Synchrony and desynchrony in fear and avoidance. Behav. Res. Ther. 12:311–18.

Raleigh, M., M. McGuire, G. Brammer, and A. Yuwiler. 1984. Social and environmental influences on blood serotonin concentration in monkeys. Arch. Gen. Psychiat. 41:405–10.

Randich, A., and W. Maixner. 1986. The role of sinoaortic and cardiopulmonary baroreceptor reflex arcs in nociception and stress-induced analgesia. Ann. N.Y. Acad. Sci. 467:385–401.

Raphael, B. 1975. The management of pathological grief. Aust. New Zealand J. Psychiat. 9:173–80.

———. 1977. Preventive intervention with the recently bereaved. Arch. Gen. Psychiat. 34:1450–54.

Rapp, J. P., and L. K. Dahl. 1976. Mutant forms of cytochrome P-450 controlling both 18 and 11 beta-steroid hydroxylation in the rat. Biochemist. 15:1235–42.

Rapp, J. P., and J. Iwai. 1976. Characteristics of rats selectively bred for susceptibility or resistance to the hypertensive effect of high salt diet. Clin. Exp. Pharmacol. Physiol. Suppl. 3:11–14.

Rapp, P. E. 1979. Bifurcation theory, control theory, and metabolic regulation. In Biological systems, modeling and control, ed. D. Linkens, 1–83. New York: Peregrinus.

Rapp, P. E., A. I. Mees, and C. T. Sparrow. 1981. Frequency encoded biochemical regulation is more accurate than amplitude dependent control. J. Theor. Biol. 90:531–44.

Rasmussen, H. 1986. The calcium messenger system. New Engl. J. Med. 314:1094–1101, 1163–70.

Rasmussen, K., J. P. Bagger, J. Bottzauw, and P. Henningsen. 1985. Prevalence of vasospastic ischaemia induced by the cold pressor test or hyperventilation in patients with severe angina. Eur. Heart J. 5:354–61.

Rasmussen, K., S. Juul, J. P. Bagger, and P. Henningsen. 1987. Usefulness of ST deviation induced by prolonged hyperventilation as a predictor of cardiac death in angina pectoris. Am. J. Cardiol. 59:763–68.

Read, N. W. 1980. Disordered transit of a meal through the small and large bowel in the irritable bowel syndrome. Gut 21:A906.

Rees, L. 1964. The importance of psychological, allergic, and infective factors in childhood asthma. J. Psychosom. Res. 7:253–62.

Rees, W., and S. G. Lutkins. 1967. Mortality of bereavement. Br. Med. J. 4:13–16.

Reinberg, A. 1967. The hours of changing responsiveness or susceptibility. Perspect. Biol. Med. 11:111–28.

Reis, D. J. 1981. Brain stem mechanisms in experimental hypertension. In Brain behavior and bodily disease, ed. H. Weiner, M. A. Hofer, and A. J. Stunkard, 229–57. New York: Raven Press.

Reis, O. J., and J. E. LeDoux. 1987. Some central neural mechanisms governing resting and behaviorally coupled control of blood pressure. Circulation 76 (Suppl. 1):2–9.

Reiser, M. F., and E. G. Ferris. 1951. Life situations, emotions, and the course of patients with arterial hypertension. Psychosom. Med. 13:133–42.

Reisine, T. 1989. Molecular mechanisms controlling ACTH release. In Neuronal control of bodily function: Frontiers of stress research, ed. H. Weiner, D. Hellhammer, I. Florin, and R. Murison, 240–49. Toronto: Hans Huber.

Reisine, T., S. Heisler, V. Hook, and J. Axelrod. 1983. Activation of β_2-adrenergic receptors on mouse anterior pituitary cells increases cAMP synthesis and adrenocorticotropin release. J. Neurosci. 3:725–32.

Reite, M., I. C. Kaufman, J. D. Pauley, and A. J. Stynes. 1974. Depression in infant monkeys: Physiological correlates. Psychosom. Med. 36:363–67.

Reite, M., and R. Short. 1978. Nocturnal sleep in separated monkey infants. Arch. Gen. Psychiat. 35:1247–53.

Renaud, L. P. 1978. Neurophysiological organization of the endocrine hypothalamus. Res. Publ. Assoc. Nerv. Ment. Dis. 56:269–201.

Reppert, S. M., M. J. Duncan, and D. R. Weaver. 1987. Maternal influences on the developing circadian system. In Perinatal development: A psychobiological perspective, ed. N. A. Krasnegor, E. M. Blass, M. A. Hofer, and W. P. Smotherman, 343–56. Orlando, FL: Academic Press.

Reynolds, D. V. 1969. Surgery in the rat during electrical analgesia induced by focal brain stimulation. Science 164:444–45.

Rich, B. H., R. L. Rosenfield, A. W. Lucky, J. C. Helke, and P. Otto. 1981. Adrenarche: Changing adrenal response to adrenocorticotropin. J. Clin. Endocrinol. Metab. 52:1129–35.

Richards, D. W. 1952. Homeostasis versus hyperexis, or, Saint George and the dragon. Reprinted in Medical priesthoods and other essays, 46–57. Connecticut Printers, 1970.

———. 1957. Homeostasis: Its dislocations and perturbations. Reprinted in Medical priesthoods and other essays, 58–72. Connecticut Printers, 1970.

Richter, C. P. 1949. Domestication of the Norway rat and its implications for the problem of stress. In Life stress and bodily disease, ed. H. G. Wolff, S. G. Wolf, Jr., and C. C. Hare. Res. Publ. Assoc. Nerv. Ment. Dis. 29:19–47.

Richter, J. E., C. F. Barish, and D. Castell. 1986. Abnormal sensory perception in patients with esophageal chest pain. Gastroenterol. 91:845–51.

Rimón, R. A. 1969. A psychosomatic approach to rheumatoid arthritis: A clinical study of 100 female patients. Acta Rheumat. Scand. 13 (Suppl. 1): 1–154.

———. 1973. Rheumatoid factor and aggression dynamics in female patients with rheumatoid arthritis. Scand. J. Rheumatol. 2:119–22.

Rioch, D. McK. 1971. Transition states as stress. In Society, stress, and disease. Vol. 1, The psychosocial environment and psychosomatic disease, ed. L. Levi, 85–90. London and New York: Oxford University Press.

Ritchie, A. W. S., I. Oswald, H. S. Micklem, J. E. Boyd, R. A. Elton, E. Jazwinska, and K. James. 1983. Circadian variation of lymphocyte subpopulations: A study with monoclonal antibodies. Brit. Med. J. 286:1773–75.

Ritchie, J. 1973. Pain from distension of the pelvic colon by inflating a balloon in the irritable colon syndrome. Gut 14:125–32.

Rivier, C. 1989. Effect of the age of the rat and the duration of the stimulus on stress-induced ACTH secretion. In Neuronal control of bodily function: Frontiers of stress research, ed. H. Weiner, D. Hellhammer, I. Florin, and R. Murison, 223–32. Toronto: Hans Huber.

Rivier, C., R. Rivier, and W. Vale. 1986. Stress-induced inhibition of reproductive functions: Role of endogenous corticotropin-releasing factor. Science 231:607–9.

Rivier, C., and W. Vale. 1984. Influence of corticotropin-releasing factor on reproductive functions in the rat. Endocrinol. 114:914–21.

———. 1985. Involvement of corticotropin-releasing factor and somatostatin in stress-induced inhibition of growth hormone secretion in the rat. Endocrinol. 117: 2478–82.

Robert, A., and J. E. Nezamis. 1964. Histopathology of steroid-induced ulcers: An experimental study in the rat. Arch. Pathol. 77:407–23.

Roberts, W. W. 1962. Fear-like behavior elicited from dorsomedial thalamus of cat. J. Comp. Physiol. Psychol. 55:191–97.

Roess, D. A., C. J. Bellone, M. R. Ruh, E. M. Nadel, and T. S. Ruh. 1982. The effect of glucocorticoids on mitogen stimulated B lymphocytes: Thymidine incorporation and antibody secretion. Endocrinol. 110:169–75.

Rogers, M. P., D. E. Trentham, R. Dynesius-Trentham, K. Daffner, and P. Reich. 1984. Exacerbation of collagen arthritis by noise stress. J. Rheumatol. 10:651–54.

Rogers, M. P., D. E. Trentham, W. J. McCune, B. I. Ginsberg, H. G. Rennke, P. Reich, and J. R. David. 1980a. Abrogation of type II collagen-induced arthritis by psychological stress. Trans. Assoc. Am. Physic. 92:218–28.

———. 1980b. Effect of psychological stress on the induction of arthritis in rats. Arth. Rheumat. 23:1337–42.

Rogers, R. C., and G. E. Hermann. 1985. Dorsal medullary oxytocin, vasopressin, oxytocin antagonist, and TRH effects on gastric acid secretion and heart rate. Peptides 6:1143–48.

Rola-Pleszczynski, M., D. Bolduc, and S. St.-Pierre. 1985. The effects of VIP on human natural killer cells. J. Immunol. 135:2569–73.

Roll, M., and T. Theorell. 1987. Acute chest pain without obvious organic cause before age 40—personality and recent events. J. Psychosom. Res. 31:215–21.

Rook, A. H., H. Masur, H. C. Lane, W. Frederick, T. Kasahara, A. M. Macher, J. Y. Djeu, J. F. Manischewitz, L. Jackson, A. S. Fauci, and G. V. Quinnan, Jr. 1983. Interleukin-2 enhances the depressed natural killer and CMV-specific cytotoxic activation of lymphocytes from patients with the acquired immunodeficiency syndrome. J. Clin. Invest. 72:398–403.

Rose, D. S. 1986. "Worse than death": Psychodynamics of rape victims and the need for psychotherapy. Am. J. Psychiat. 143:817–24.

Rose, R. 1979. The crisis in stress research. J. Human Stress 5:4–48.

Rose, R. M., I. S. Bernstein, and T. P. Gordon. 1975. Consequences of social conflict on plasma testosterone levels in rhesus monkeys. Psychosom. Med. 37:50–61.

Rosenblatt, J. S. 1978. Behavioral regulation of reproductive physiology: A selective review. In Comparative endocrinology, ed. P. J. Galliard and H. H. Boer, 177–88. Amsterdam: Elsevier.

Rosenheck, R. 1985. Malignant post-Vietnam stress syndrome. Am. J. Orthopsychiat. 55:166–76.

Ross, R. 1986. The pathogenesis of atherosclerosis—an update. New Engl. J. Med. 314:488–500.

Rossellini, R. A., and M. E. P. Seligman. 1978. Role of shock intensity in the learned helplessness paradigm. Anim. Learn. Behav. 6:143–46.

Rossier, J., E. D. French, C. Rivier, N. Ling, F. E. Bloom, and R. Guillemin. 1977. Footshock-induced stress increases beta-endorphin levels in blood but not brain. Nature (London) 270:618–20.

Rossier, J., R. Guillemin, and F. E. Bloom. 1978. Footshock-induced stress decreases leu^5-enkephalin immunoreactivity in rat hypothalamus. Eur. J. Pharmacol. 48: 465–66.

Roth, H. P., and B. Fleshler. 1964. Diffuse esophageal spasm. Ann. Int. Med. 61:914–23.

Roth, J. L. A. 1973. Aerophagia. In Emotional factors in gastrointestinal illness, ed. A. E. Lindner, 16–30. Amsterdam: Excerpta Medica.

Rotter, J. B. 1966. Generalized expectancies for internal versus external control of reinforcement. Psychol. Mono. 80:1–28.

Rotter, J. I., and D. L. Rimoin. 1977. Peptic ulcer disease—a heterogeneous group of disorders? Gastroenterol. 73:604–7.

Rotter, J. I., D. L. Rimoin, J. M. Gursky, and I. M. Samloff. 1977a. The genetics of peptic ulcer disease—segregation of serum group I pepsinogen concentrations in families with peptic ulcer disease. Clin. Res. 25:114A.

Rotter, J. I., D. L. Rimoin, J. M. Gursky, P. Terasaki, and R. A. L. Sturdevant. 1977b. HLA-B5 associated with duodenal ulcer. Gastroenterol. 73:438–40.

Rotter, J. I., J. Q. Sones, C. T. Richardson, D. L. Rimoin, and I. M. Samloff. 1977c. The genetics of peptic ulcer disease—segregation of serum group I pepsinogen concentrations in families with peptic ulcer disease. Clin. Res. 25:325A.

Rotter, J. I., J. Q. Sones, I. M. Samloff, C. T. Richardson, J. J. Gursky, J. H. Walsh, and D. L. Rimoin. 1979. Duodenal-ulcer disease associated with elevated serum pepsinogen I: An inherited autosomal dominant disorder. New Engl. J. Med. 300:63–66.

Roy, A. 1987. Five risk factors for depression. Br. J. Psychiat. 150:536–41.

Rozanski, A., C. N. Bairey, D. S. Krantz, J. Friedman, K. J. Resser, M. Morell, S. Hilton-Chalfen, L. Hestrin, J. Bietendorf, and D. S. Berman. 1988. Mental stress and the induction of silent myocardial ischemia in patients with coronary artery disease. New Engl. J. Med. 318:1005–12.

Rubenstein, E. 1980. Diseases caused by impaired communication among cells. Scient. Am. 242:102–21.

Rubin, J., R. Nagler, H. M. Spiro, and M. L. Pilot. 1962. Measuring the effect of emotions on esophageal motility. Psychosom. Med. 24:170–76.

Rubin, R. T., R. G. Miller, B. R. Clark, R. E. Poland, and R. J. Arthur. 1970. The stress of aircraft carrier landings, 2: 3-methoxy-4-hydroxyphenylglycol excretion in naval aviators. Psychosom. Med. 32:589–97.

Rubin, R. T., R. H. Rahe, R. J. Arthur, and B. R. Clark. 1969. Adrenal cortical activity changes during underwater demolition team training. Psychosom. Med. 31:553–64.

Ruesch, J. 1948. The infantile personality: The core problem of psychosomatic medicine. Psychosom. Med. 10:133–44.

Ruesch, J., C. Christiansen, L. C. Patterson, S. Dewees, and A. Jacobson. 1947. Psychological invalidism in thyroidectomized patients. Psychosom. Med. 9:77–91.

Ruskin, A., O. W. Beard, and R. L. Schaffer. 1948. Blast hypertension: Elevated arterial pressure in victims of the Texas City diaster. Am. J. Med. 4:228–35.

Russell, D. C. 1984. Clinical clues to psychological and neurohumoral mechanisms of arrhythmogenesis. In Breakdown in human adaptation to stress, ed. A. L'Abbate, 961–74. Boston: Martinus Nijhoff.

Russell, I. J., C. L. Bowden, J. Michalek, E. Fletcher, and G. A. Hester. 1987. Imipramine receptor density on platelets of patients with fibrositis syndrome: Correlation with disease severity and response to therapy. Arth. Rheumat. 4 (Suppl. 30): S63.

Rutter, M. 1979. Protective factors in children's responses to stress and disadvantage. In Primary prevention of psychopathology, vol. 3, ed. M. Whalen and J. E. Rolfe, 49–74. Hanover, NH: University Press of New England.

Saavedra, J. M., H. Grobecker, and J. Axelrod. 1978. Changes in central catecholaminergic neurons in the spontaneously (genetic) hypertensive rat. Circ. Res. 42:529–34.

Saavedra, J. M., R. Kvetnansky, and I. J. Kopin. 1979. Adrenaline, noradrenaline, and dopamine levels in specific brainstem areas of acutely immobilized rats. Brain Res. 160:271–80.

Sacerdoti, D., B. Escalante, N. G. Abraham, J. C. McGiff, R. D. Levere, and M. L. Schwartz. 1989. Treatment with tin prevents the development of hypertension in spontaneously hypertensive rats. Science 243:388–90.

Safar, M. E., H. A. Kamieniecka, J. A. Levenson, V. M. Dimitriu, and N. F. Pauleau. 1978. Hemodynamic factors and Rorschach testing in borderline and sustained hypertension. Psychosom. Med. 40:620–30.

Sager, R. 1989. Tumor suppressor genes: The puzzle and the promise. Science 246:1406–12.

Saito, M., E. Murakami, and M. Suda. 1976. Circadian rhythms in disaccharidases of rat small intestine and its relation to food intake. Biochem. Biophy. Acta 421:177–79.

Salit, I. E. 1985. Sporadic postinfectious neuromyasthenia. Can. Med. Assoc. J. 133:659–63.

Samloff, I. M. 1971a. Immunologic studies of human group I pepsinogens. J. Immunol. 106:962–68.

———. 1971b. Cellular localization of group I pepsinogens in human gastric mucosa by immunofluorescence. Gastroenterol. 61:185–88.

———. 1977. Radioimmunoassay of group II pepsinogens in serum. Gastroenterol. 72:A–102/1125.

Samloff, I. M., and W. M. Liebman. 1974. Radioimmunoassay of group I pepsinogens in serum. Gastroenterol. 66:494–502.

Samloff, I. M., W. M. Liebman, and M. Panitch. 1975. Serum group I pepsinogens by radioimmunoassay in control subjects and patients with peptic ulcer. Gastroenterol. 69:83–90.

Saper, C. B. 1989. Role of atrial natriuretic peptide (atriopeptin) in cardiovascular response to stress. In Neuronal control of bodily function: Frontiers of stress research, ed. H. Weiner, D. Hellhammer, I. Florin, and R. Murison, 191–98. Toronto: Hans Huber.

Sapolsky, R. M. 1982. The endocrine stress response and social status in the wild baboon. Horm. Behav. 15:279–84.

———. 1985. Stress-induced suppression of testicular function in the wild baboon: Role of glucocorticoids. Endocrinol. 116:2273–78.

———. 1988. Lessons of the Seregenti: Why some of us are more susceptible to stress. The Sciences (May/June): 38–42.

———. 1989. Hypercortisolism among socially subordinate wild baboons originates at the CNS level. Arch. Gen. Psychiat. 46:1047–51.

———. 1990. Stress in the wild. Scient. Am. 252:116–23.

Sapolsky, R. M., L. C. Krey, and B. S. McEwen. 1984. Glucocorticoid-sensitive hippocampal neurons are involved in terminating the adrenocortical stress response. Proc. Natl. Acad. Sci. (USA) 81:6174–77.

———. 1986. The neuroendocrinology of stress and aging: The glucocorticoid cascade hypothesis. Endocrine Rev. 7:284–301.

Sapolsky, R. M., and G. Mott. 1987. Social subordinance in a wild primate is associated with suppressed HDL-cholesterol concentrations. Endocrinol. 121:1605–10.

Sarna, S. K. 1983. The control of colonic motility. In Functional disorders of the gastrointestinal tract, ed. W. Y. Chey, 277–85. New York: Raven Press.

Sarna, S. K., B. L. Bardakjian, W. E. Waterfall, J. F. Lind, and E. E. Daniel. 1980. The organization of human colonic electrical control activity. In Gastrointestinal motility, ed. J. Christensen, 403–10. New York: Raven Press.

Saskin, P., H. Moldofsky, and F. A. Lue. 1986. Sleep and post-traumatic pain modulation disorder (fibrositis syndrome). Psychosom. Med. 48:319–23.

Saskin, P., H. Moldofsky, L. Salem, M. Anch, and F. A. Lue. 1987. Sleep and symptoms in psychophysiologic insomnia and fibrositis. Sleep Res. 16:421.

Sawchenko, P. E. 1989. The functional neuroanatomy of stress related circuitry in the rat brain. In Neuronal control of bodily function: Frontiers of stress research, ed. H. Weiner, D. Hellhammer, I. Florin, and R. Murison, 139–47. Toronto: Hans Huber.

Sawchenko, P. E., L. W. Swanson, and W. Vale. 1984. Co-expression of corticotropin releasing factor and vasopressin immunoreactivity in parvocellular neurosecretory neurons of the adrenalectomized rat. Proc. Natl. Acad. Sci. (USA) 81:1883–87.

Sawrey, W. L., and J. D. Weisz. 1956. An experimental method of producing gastric ulcers. J. Comp. Physiol. Psychol. 49:269–70.

Saxena, K. 1980. Physiological effects of job loss. Paper presented at the annual meeting of the International Society for the Prevention of Stress.

Schanberg, S., G. Evoniuk, and C. Kuhn. 1984. Tactile and nutritional aspects of maternal care: Specific regulators of neuroendocrine function and cellular development. Proc. Soc. Exp. Med. Biol. 175:135–46.

Schanberg, S., and T. Field. 1987. Sensory deprivation stress and supplemental stimulation in the rat pup and preterm human neonate. Child Develop. 58:1431–47.

Scheibel, M. E., U. Tomiyasu, and A. B. Scheibel. 1977. The aging human Betz cell. Exp. Neurol. 56:598–609.

Scheuler, W., D. Stinshoff, and S. Kubicki. 1983. The alpha sleep pattern. Neuropsychobiol. 10:183–89.

Schiffenbauer, J., and B. D. Schwartz. 1987. The HLA complex and its relationship to rheumatic diseases. Rheumat. Dis. Clin. N. Am. 13:463–85.

Schiffer, F., L. H. Hartley, C. L. Schulman, and W. H. Abelman. 1980. Evidence for emotionally induced coronary arterial spasm in patients with angina pectoris. Br. Heart J. 44:62–66.

Schleifer, S. J., S. E. Keller, M. Camarino, J. C. Thornton, and M. Stein. 1983. Suppression of lymphocyte stimulation following bereavement. JAMA 250:374–77.

Schless, A. P., and J. Mendels. 1978. The values of interviewing family and friends in assessing life stressors. Arch. Gen. Psychiat. 35:565–67.

Schmale, Jr., A. H. 1958. Relation of separation and depression to disease, 1: A report on a hospitalized medical population. Psychosom. Med. 20:259–77.

Schneiderman, N. 1983. Behavior, autonomic function, and animal models of cardiovascular pathology. In Biobehavioral basis of coronary heart disease, ed. T. M. Dembroski and T. H. Schmidt, 304–64. Basel: Karger.

Schramm, M., and Z. Selinger. 1984. Message transmission: Receptor controlled adenylate cyclase system. Science 225:1350–56.

Schüle, R., M. Muller, H. Olsuka-Murakami, and R. Renkawitz. 1988. Cooperativity of the glucocorticoid receptor and the CACCC-box binding factor. Nature (London) 332:87–90.

Schumann, S. H. 1972. Patterns of urban heat-wave deaths and implications for prevention: Data from New York and St. Louis during July 1966. Environ. Res. 5:59–75.

Schuster, M. M. 1983. Disorders of the esophagus: Application of psychophysiological methods to treatment. In Psychophysiology of the gastrointestinal tract, ed. R. Hölzl and W. E. Whitehead, 33–42. New York: Plenum Press.

Schuster, M. M., P. Nikoomanesh, and D. Wells. 1973. Biofeedback control of lower esophageal sphincter contraction. Rend. di Gastroenterol. 5:14–18.

Schwartz, G. E., D. A. Weinberger, and B. A. Singer. 1981. Cardiovascular differentiation of happiness, sadness, anger, and fear following imagery and exercise. Psychosom. Med. 43:343–64.

Schwartz, P. J. 1991. Mental stress and sudden cardiac death: The case of the long QT syndrome. Circulation (Suppl.) in press.

Schwartz, W. J., S. M. Reppert, S. M. Eagan, and M. C. Moore-Ede. 1983. In vivo metabolic activity of the suprachiasmatic nuclei: A comparative study. Brain Res. 274:184–87.

Scroop, G. C., and R. D. Lowe. 1968. Central pressor effect of angiotensin mediated by the parasympathetic nervous system. Nature (London) 220:1331–32.

Scudds, R. A., G. B. Rollman, M. Harth, and G. A. McCain. 1987. Pain perception and personality measures as discriminators in the classification of fibrositis. J. Rheumatol. 14:563–69.

Seeger, T. F., G. A. Sforzo, C. B. Pert, and A. Pert. 1984. In vivo autoradiography: Visualization of stress-induced changes in opiate receptor occupancy in the rat brain. Brain Res. 305:303–12.

Segal, M. 1979. Serotonergic innervation of the locus coeruleus from the dorsal raphe and its action on responses to noxious stimuli. J. Physiol. (London) 286:401–5.

Seligman, M. E. P. 1974. Depression and learned helplessness. In The psychology of depression: Contemporary theory and research, ed. R. J. Friedman and M. M. Katz, 83–125. Washington, DC: V. H. Winston.

———. 1975. Learned helplessness: On depression, development and death. San Francisco: W. H. Freeman.

Selye, H. 1936. A syndrome produced by diverse nocuous agents. Nature (London) 148:84–85.

———. 1946. The general adaptation syndrome and the diseases of adaptation. J. Clin. Endocrinol. 6:117–96.

———. 1950. Stress: The physiology and pathology of exposure to stress. Montreal: Acta Medica.

———. 1956. The stress of life. New York: McGraw-Hill.

———. 1971. The evolution of the stress concept—stress and cardiovascular disease. In Society, stress, and disease. Vol. 1, The psychosocial environment and psychosomatic disease, ed. L. Levi, 299–311. London and New York: Oxford University Press.

———. 1973. The evolution of the stress concept. Am. Scientist 61:692–99.

Selye, H., and C. Fortier. 1950. Adaptive reactions to stress. Res. Publ. Assoc. Nerv. Ment. Dis. 29:3–18.

Seward, J., and G. L. Humphrey. 1967. Avoidance learning as a function of pretraining in the cat. J. Comp. Physiol. Psychol. 88:542–47.

Shackell, B. S., and J. A. Horne. 1987. The alpha sleep anomaly and related phenomena. Sleep Res. 16:432.

Shanahan, F., and P. Anton. 1988. Neuroendocrine modulation of the immune system. Dig. Dis. Sci. 33:41s–49s.

Shavit, Y., J. W. Lewis, G. W. Terman, R. P. Gale, and J. C. Liebeskind. 1984. Opioid peptides mediate the suppressive effect of stress on natural killer cell cytotoxicity. Science 223:188–90.

Shavit, Y., G. Terman, F. Martin, J. W. Lewis, J. Liebeskind, and R. P. Gale. 1985. Stress, opioid peptides, the immune system, and cancer. J. Immunol. 135:834s–37s.

Shipley, J. E., and B. Kolb. 1977. Neural correlates of species-typical behavior in the Syrian golden hamster. J. Comp. Physiol. Psychol. 91:1056–73.

Shire, J. G. M. 1974. Endocrine genetics of the adrenal gland. J. Endocrinol. 62:173–207.

———. 1979. Corticosteroids and adrenocortical function in animals. In Genetic variation in hormone systems, vol. 1, ed. J. G. M. Shire, 43–67. Boca Raton, FL: CRC Press.

Shively, C., and J. Kaplan. 1984. Effects of social factors on adrenal weight and related physiology. Physiol. Behav. 33:777–83.

Shore, J. H., E. L. Tatum, and W. M. Vollmer. 1986. Psychiatric reactions to disaster: The Mount St. Helen's experience. Am. J. Psychiat. 143:590–95.

Siegrist, J. 1984. Interaction between short- and long-term stress in cardiovascular disease. In Breakdown in human adaptation to stress, ed. A. L'Abbate, 892–99. Boston: Martinus Nijhoff.

Siegrist, J., D. Klein, and H. Matschinger. 1989. Occupational stress, coronary risk factors, and cardiovascular responsiveness. In Neuronal control of bodily function:

Frontiers of stress research, ed. H. Weiner, D. Hellhammer, I. Florin, and R. Murison, 323–35. Toronto: Hans Huber.

Siegrist, J., H. Matschinger, and K. Siegrist. 1987. Socioemotional inputs to central neuronal regulation of the cardiovascular system. In Neurobiological approaches to human disease, ed. D. Hellhammer, I. Florin, and H. Weiner, 174–90. Toronto: Hans Huber.

Sievers, M. L. 1959. Hereditary aspects of gastric secretory function: Race and ABO blood groups in relationship to acid and pepsin production. Am. J. Med. 27: 246–55.

Simantov, R. 1979. Glucocorticoids inhibit endorphin synthesis by pituitary cells. Nature (London) 280:684–85.

Simson, P. G., J. M. Weiss, M. J. Ambrose, and A. Webster. 1986a. Infusion of a monoamine oxidase inhibitor into the locus coeruleus can protect against stress-induced depression. Biol. Psychiat. 21:724–34.

———. 1986b. Reversal of behavioral depression by infusion of an alpha$_2$ adrenergic agonist into the locus coeruleus. Neuropharmacol. 25:385–89.

Skolnick, N. J., S. H. Ackerman, M. A. Hofer, and H. Weiner. 1980. Vertical transmission of acquired ulcer susceptibility in the rat. Science 208:1161–63.

Smelik, P. G. 1985. Stress and hormones. Organorama 22:16–18.

———. 1987. Differential control of ACTH-related peptides and the importance of the behavioral situation. In Neurobiologic approaches to human disease, ed. D. Hellhammer, I. Florin, and H. Weiner, 286–89. Toronto: Hans Huber.

Smelik, P. G., F. J. H. Tilders, and F. Berkenbosch. 1989. Participation of adrenaline and vasopressin in the stress response. In Neuronal control of bodily function: Frontiers of stress research, ed. H. Weiner, D. Hellhammer, I. Florin, and R. Murison, 94–99. Toronto: Hans Huber.

Smith, E. M., and J. E. Blalock. 1981. Human lymphocyte production of corticotropin and endorphin-like substances: Association with leukocyte interferon. Proc. Natl. Acad. Sci. (USA) 78:7530–34.

Smith, Jr., G. R., R. A. Munson, and D. C. Ray. 1986a. Psychiatric consultation in somatization disorder: A randomized controlled study. New Engl. J. Med. 314: 1407–13.

———. 1986b. Patients with multiple unexplained symptoms: Their characteristics, functional health, and health care utilization. Arch. Int. Med. 146:69–72.

Smith, K. A. 1988. Interleukin-2: Inception, impact, and implications. Science 240:1169–76.

Smith, O. A., C. A. Astley, J. L. DeVito, J. M. Stein, and K. E. Walsh. 1980. Functional analysis of hypothalamic control of the cardiovascular responses accompanying emotional behavior. Fed. Proc. FASEB 39:2487–96.

Smith, P., K. Ohura, H. Masur, H. C. Lane, A. S. Fauci, and S. M. Wahl. 1984. Monocyte function in the acquired immune deficiency syndrome. Defective chemotaxis. J. Clin. Invest. 74:2121–28.

Smith, W. 1980. Hypothalamic regulation of pituitary secretion of luteinizing hormone, 2: Feedback control of gonadotropin secretion. Bull. Math. Biol. 42:57–78.

Snape, W. J., G. M. Carlson, and S. C. Cohen. 1976. Colonic myoelectric activity in the irritable bowel syndrome. Gastroenterol. 70:326–30.

Snape, W. J., G. M. Carlson, S. A. Matarazzo, and S. Cohen. 1977. Evidence that abnormal myoelectrical activity produces colonic motor dysfunction in the irritable bowel syndrome. Gastroenterol. 72:383–87.

Snape, W. J., and S. Cohen. 1979. How colonic motility differs in normal subjects and patients with IBS. Pract. Gastroenterol. 3:21–25.

Snyder, S. H. 1978. Peptide neurotransmitter candidates in the brain: Focus on enkephalin, angiotension II, and neurotensin. Res. Publ. Assoc. Nerv. Ment. Dis. 56:233–43.

Sofia, R. D. 1980. The effect of overcrowding on the development of adjuvant-induced polyarthritis in the rat. J. Pharm. Pharmacol. 32:874–75.

Soll, A. H. 1981. Physiology of isolated canine parietal cells: Receptors and effectors regulating function. In Physiology of the gastrointestinal tract, ed. L. R. Johnson, 673–91. New York: Raven Press.

Souetre, E., E. Salvati, T. A. Wehr, D. A. Sack, B. Krebs, and G. Darcourt. 1988. Twenty-four-hour profiles of body temperature and plasma TSH in bipolar patients during depression and during remission and in normal control subjects. Am. J. Psychiat. 145:1133–37.

Sporn, M. B., and A. B. Roberts. 1988. Peptide growth factors are multifunctional. Nature (London) 332:217–19.

Stacher, G. 1983. The responsiveness of the esophagus to environmental stimuli. In Psychophysiology of the gastrointestinal tract, ed. R. Hölzl and W. E. Whitehead, 21–31. New York: Plenum Press.

Standaert, D. G., C. B. Saper, and P. Needleman. 1985. Atrio-peptin: Potent hormone and potential neuromediator. Trands Neurosci. 8:509–11.

Stastny, P. 1978. Association of the B-cell antigen DRw4 and rheumatoid arthritis. New Engl J. Med. 298:869–71.

Stein, M., S. E. Keller, and S. J. Schleifer. 1985. Stress and immunomodulation: The role of depression and neuroendocrine function. J. Immunol. 135:827s–33s.

Stein, S. P., and E. Charles. 1971. Emotional factors in juvenile diabetes mellitus. A study of early life experience of adolescent diabetics. Am. J. Psychiat. 128:700–704.

Stephens, R. L., T. Garrick, H. Weiner, and Y. Taché. 1989. Serotonin depletion potentiates gastric secretory and motor responses to vagal but not peripheral gastric stimulants. J. Pharmacol. Exp. Ther. 251:524–30.

Stephens, R. L., T. Ishikawa, H. Weiner, D. Novin, and Y. Taché. 1988. TRH analogue, RX 77368, microinjected into dorsal vagal complex stimulates gastric secretion in rats. Am. J. Physiol. 254:G639–43.

Stephenson, R. B., O. A. Smith, A. M. Scher. 1981. Baroreceptor regulation of heart rate in baboons during different behavioral states. Am. J. Physiol. 241:R277.

Steptoe, A. 1987. The assessment of sympathetic nervous function in human stress research. J. Psychosom. Res. 31:141–52.

Sterman, M. D. 1982. EEG biofeedback in the treatment of epilepsy: An overview circa 1980. In Clinical biofeedback: Efficacy and mechanisms, ed. L. White and B. Tursky, 311–30. New York: Guilford Press.

Sternberg, E. M., W. S. Young, R. Bernardini, A. E. Calogero, G. P. Chrousos, P. W. Gold, and R. L. Wilder. 1989. A central nervous system defect in biosynthesis of corticotropin-releasing hormone is associated with susceptibility to streptococcal cell wall–induced arthritis in Lewis rats. Proc. Natl. Acad. Sci. (USA) 86: 4771–75.

Stevenson, N. R., and J. S. Firestein. 1976. Circadian rhythms of intestinal sucrase and glucose transport: Cued by time of feeding. Am. J. Physiol. 230:731–35.

Stewart, D. N., and D. M. R. Winser. 1942. Incidence of perforated peptic ulcer: Effect of heavy air raids. Lancet 1:259–61.

Stobo, J. D. 1982. The influence of immune response genes on the expression of disease. J. Clin. Lab. Med. 100:822–28.

Stone, E. A. 1976. Central noradrenergic activity and the formation of glycol sulfate metabolites of brain norepinephrine. Life Sci. 16:1491–98.

Stone, E., K. Bonnet, and M. A. Hofer. 1975. Survival and development of maternally deprived rats: Role of body temperature. Psychosom. Med. 38:242–49.

Strain, J., and S. Grossman, eds. 1975. Psychological care of the medically ill. New York: Appleton-Century-Crofts.

Streimer, J. H., J. Coststick, and C. Tennant. 1985. The psychosocial adjustment of Australian Vietnam veterans. Am. J. Psychiat. 142:616–18.

Strober, M. 1983. Stressful life events associated with bulimia in anorexia nervosa: Empirical findings and theoretical speculations. Int. J. Eat. Dis. 3:3–16.

Strom, A., ed. 1968. Norwegian concentration camp survivors. Oslo: Oslo University Press.

Stunkard, A. J. 1975. From explanation to action in psychosomatic medicine: The case of obesity. Psychosom. Med. 37:195–236.

Sullivan, M. A., S. Cohen, and W. J. Snape. 1978. Colonic myoelectrical activity in irritable-bowel syndrome: Effect of eating and anticholinergics. New Engl. J. Med. 298:878–83.

Swartz, M., D. Blazer, M. Woodbury, L. George, and R. Landerman. 1986. Somatization disorder in a U.S. southern community: Use of a new procedure for analysis of medical classification. Psychol. Med. 16:595–609.

Swartz, M., D. Hughes, D. Blazer, and L. George. 1987. Somatization disorder in the community: A study of diagnostic concordance among three diagnostic systems. J. Nerv. Ment. Dis. 175:26–33.

Sweet, C. S., and M. J. Brody. 1971. Arterial hypertension elicited by prolonged intravertebral infusion of angiotensin in the conscious dog. Fed. Proc. FASEB 30:432A.

Syme, S. L. 1979. The role of stress in hypertension. J. Human Stress 5:10–11.

Syme, S. L., and L. F. Berkman. 1976. Social class, susceptibility, and sickness. Am. J. Epidemiol. 104:1–8.

Syvalähti, E., R. Lammintausta, and A. Pekkarinen. 1976. Effect of psychic stress of examination on serum growth hormone, serum insulin, and plasma renin activity. Acta Pharmacol. Toxicol. Scand. 38:344–52.

Szafarczyck, A., F. Malaval, A. Laurent, R. Gibaud, and I. Assenmacher. 1987. Further evidence for a central stimulatory action of catecholamines on ACTH release in the rat. Endocrinol. 121:883–92.

Taché, Y. 1985. Role of brain neuropeptides in the regulation of gastric secretion. In specialty conference: Neurobiologic and psychobiologic mechanisms in gastric function and ulceration, moderated by H. Weiner. West. J. Med. 143:215–18.

————. 1987. Central nervous system regulation of gastric acid secretion. In Physiology of the gastrointestinal tract, ed. L. R. Johnson, 911–30. New York: Raven Press.

————. 1988. Central nervous system action of neuropeptides to induce or prevent experimental gastroduodenal ulcerations. In Perspectives in behavioral medicine. Vol. 5, Eating regulation and discontrol, ed. H. Weiner and A. Baum, 101–12. Hillsdale, NJ: Lawrence Erlbaum.

Taché, Y., Y. Goto, D. LeSiege, and D. Novin. 1983. Central nervous system action of thyrotropin-releasing hormone (TRH) to stimulate gastric acid and pepsin secretion in rats. Endocrinol. 112:149.

Taché, Y., and T. Ishikawa. 1989. Role of brain peptides in the ulcerogenic response to stress. In Neuropeptides and stress, ed. Y. Taché, J. E. Morley, and M. R. Brown, 146–57. New York: Springer-Verlag.

Taché, Y., M. Maeda-Hagiwara, Y. Goto, and T. Garrick. 1988. Central nervous system action of TRH to stimulate gastric function and the development of gastric ulceration. Peptides 9 (Suppl. 1): 9–13.

Taché, Y., M. Maeda-Hagiwara, and C. M. Turkelson. 1987. Central nervous action of corticotropin-releasing factor to inhibit gastric emptying in rats. Am. J. Physiol. 253:G241–45.

Taché, Y., J. E. Morley, and M. R. Brown, eds. 1988. Neuropeptides and stress: Hans Selye symposia on neuroendocrinology and stress. New York: Springer-Verlag.

Taché, Y., R. L. Stephens, and T. Ishikawa. 1989. Stress-induced alterations of gastrointestinal function: Involvement of brain CRF and TRH. In Neuronal control of bodily function: Frontiers of stress research, ed. H. Weiner, D. Hellhammer, I. Florin, and R. Murison, 265–75. Toronto: Hans Huber.

Taché, Y., W. Vale, and M. Brown. 1980. Thyrotropin-releasing hormone: Central nervous system action to stimulate gastric acid secretion. Nature (London) 287:149–51.

Tager, H., B. Given, D. Baldwin, M. Mako, J. Markese, A. Rubenstein, J. Olefsky, M. Kobayashi, O. Kolterman, and R. A. Poucher. 1979. A structurally abnormal insulin causing human diabetes. Nature (London) 281:122–25.

Taggart, P., and M. Carruthers. 1971. Endogenous hyperlipedemia induced by emotional stress of racing driving. Lancet 1:363–66.

Taggart, P., M. Carruthers, and W. Somerville. 1973. Electrocardiogram, plasma catecholamines, lipids, and their modification by oxprenolol when speaking before an audience. Lancet 2:341–46.

Taggart, P., D. Gibbons, and W. Somerville. 1969. Some effects of motor car driving on the normal and abnormal heart. Br. Med. J. 4:130–34.

Takeuchi, K., O. Furukawa, and S. Okabe. 1986. Induction of duodenal ulcers in rats under water-immersion stress conditions: Influence of stress on gastric acid and duodenal alkaline secretion. Gastroenterol. 91:554–63.

Tanaka, M., R. Kohno, Y. Ida, S. Takeda, and N. Nagasaki. 1982. Time-related differences in noradrenaline turnover in rat brain regions by stress. Pharmacol. Biochem. Behav. 16:315–19.

Tarazi, R. C., H. P. Dustan, E. D. Frohlich, R. W. Gifford, Jr., and G. C. Hoffman. 1970. Plasma volume and chronic hypertension: Relationship to arterial pressure levels in different hypertensive diseases. Arch. Int. Med. 125:835–42.

Tarnapolsky, A., G. Watkin, and D. J. Hand. 1980. Aircraft noise and mental health, 1: Prevalence of individual symptoms. Psychol. Med. 10:683–98.

Taylor, A. L., and L. M. Fishman. 1988. Corticotropin-releasing hormone. New Engl. J. Med. 319:213–22.

Taylor, G. J. 1987. Psychosomatic medicine and contemporary psychoanalysis. Madison, CT: International Universities Press.

Taylor, I., C. Darby, and P. Hammond. 1978. Comparison of rectosigmoid myoelectrical activity in the irritable colon syndrome during relapses and remissions. Gut 19:923–29.

Taylor, I., C. Darby, P. Hammond, and P. Basu. 1978. Is there a myoelectrical abnormality in the irritable colon syndrome? Gut 19:391–95.

Taylor, I., H. L. Duthie, R. Smallwood, B. H. Brown, and D. A. Linkens. 1974. The effect of stimulation on the myoelectrical activity of the rectosigmoid in man. Gut 15:599–607.

Taylor, I., H. L. Duthie, R. Smallwood, and D. Linkens. 1975. Large bowel myoelectrical activity in man. Gut 16:808–14.

Tazi, A., R. Dantzer, M. LeMoal, J. Rivier, W. Vale, and G. F. Koob. 1987. Corticotropin-releasing factor antagonist blocks stress-induced fighting in rats. Reg. Pept. 18:37–42.

Teicher, M. H., W. B. Stewart, J. S. Kauer, and G. M. Shepherd. 1980. Suckling pheromone stimulation of a modified glomerular region in the developing rat olfactory bulb revealed by the 2-deoxy-glucose method. Brain Res. 194:530–35.

Tennant, C. C., K. J. Goulston, and O. F. Dent. 1986. The psychological effects of being a prisoner of war: Forty years after release. Am. J. Psychiat. 143:618–21.

Terman, G. W. 1985. Intrinsic mechanisms of pain inhibition and their activation by stress. Doctoral dissertation, University of California, Los Angeles.

Terman, G. W., J. W. Lewis, and J. C. Liebeskind. 1983. Opioid and nonopioid mechanisms of stress analgesia: Lack of cross-tolerance between stressors. Brain Res. 260:147–50.

Terman, G., Y. Shavit, J. W. Lewis, J. T. Cannon, and J. Liebeskind. 1984. Intrinsic mechanism of pain inhibition: Activation by stress. Science 226:1270–77.

Terr, L. C. 1979. Children of Chowchilla: A study of psychic trauma. Psychoanal. Study Child. 34:547–623.

Texter, Jr., E. C., and R. C. Butler. 1975. The irritable bowel syndrome. Am. Fam. Phys. 11:169–73.

Thailer, S. A., R. Friedman, G. A. Harshfield, and T. G. Pickering. 1985. Psychologic differences between high-, normal-, low-renin hypertensives. Psychosom. Med. 47:294–97.

Thayson, E. H., and L. Pederson. 1976. Idiopathic bile salt catharsis. Gut 17:965–70.

Theorell, T. 1986. Stress at work and risk of myocardial infarction. Postgrad. Med. J. 62:791–95.

———. 1989. Spontaneously occurring stressors. In Neuronal control of bodily function: Frontiers of stress research, ed. H. Weiner, D. Hellhammer, I. Florin, and R. Murison, 111–21. Toronto: Hans Huber.

Thoenen, H., R. A. Mueller, and J. Axelrod. 1969. Increased tyrosine hydroxylase activity after drug-induced alteration of sympathetic transmission. Nature (London) 221:1264.

Thoits, P. A. 1982. Conceptual methodological and theoretical problems in studying social support as a buffer against life stress. J. Hlth. Soc. Behav. 23:145–59.

Thompson, D. G., J. M. Laidlaw, and D. L. Wingate. 1979. Abnormal small bowel motility demonstrated by radiotelemetry in a patient with irritable colon. Lancet 1:1321–23.

Thompson, W. G., and K. W. Heaton. 1979. Functional bowel disorders in apparently healthy people. Gastroenterol. 79:283–88.

———. 1982. Heartburn and globus in apparently healthy people. Can. Med. Assoc. J. 126:46–48.

Thygesen, P., K. Hermann, and R. Willanger. 1970. Concentration camp survivors in Denmark: Persecution, disease, disability, compensation. Dan. Med. Bull. 17:65–108.

Tinbergen, N. 1951. The study of instinct. Oxford: Clarendon Press.

Todd, J. A., H. Acha-Obrea, J. I. Bell, N. Chao, Z. Fronek, C. O. Jacob, M. McDermott, A. A. Sinha, L. Timmerman, L. Steinman, and H. O. McDevitt. 1988. A molecular basis for MHC class-II-associated autoimmunity. Science 240:1003–9.

Traub, R. D., R. Miles, and R. K. S. Wong. 1989. Model of the origin of rhythmic population oscillations in the hippocampal slice. Science 248:1319–25.

Truelove, S. C. 1966. Movement of the large intestines. Physiol. Rev. 46:457–512.

Truelove, S. C., and P. C. Reynell. 1972. Diseases of the digestive system. 2d ed. Oxford: Blackwell Scientific Publications.

Turiel, J., and D. Wingard. 1985. Estrogens and cancer: A multidisciplinary focus on diethylstilbestrol (DES). Berkeley: University of California Press.

Tyhurst, J. S. 1953. The role of transition states—including disasters—in mental illness. In Symposium on preventive and social psychiatry. Washington, DC: Walter Reed Army Institute of Research.

———. 1957. Psychological and social aspects of civilian disasters. Can. Med. Assoc. J. 76:385–93.

Tzivoni, D., A. Stein, A. Keren, and S. Stern. 1980. Electrocardiographic characteristics of neurocirculatory asthenia during everyday activities. Br. Heart J. 44:426–32.

Udelsman, R., J. P. Harwood, M. A. Millan, G. P. Chrousos, D. S. Goldstein, R. Zinlichman, K. J. Catt, and G. Aguilera. 1986. Functional corticotropin releasing factor receptors in the primate peripheral sympathetic nervous system. Nature (London) 319:147–50.

Uehara, A., P. E. Gottschall, R. R. Dahl, and A. Arimura. 1987a. Stimulaton of ACTH release by human interleukin 1β, but not by interluekin 1α, in conscious, freely moving rats. Biochem. Biophys. Res. Comm. 146:1286–90.

———. 1987b. Interleukin-1 stimulates ACTH release by an indirect action which requires endogenous corticotropin releasing factor. Endocrinol. 121:1580–82.

Unger, R. N., L. Orci, and R. E. Dobbs. 1978. Insulin, glucagon, and somatostatin secretion in the regulation of metabolism. Ann. Rev. Physiol. 40:307–43.

Ungerleider, L. G., and M. Mishkin. 1982. Two cortical visual systems. In Analysis of visual behavior, ed. D. J. Ingle, M. A. Goodale, and R. J. W. Mansfield, 549–86. Cambridge, MA: MIT Press.

Unsicker, K. 1971. On the innervation of the rat and pig adrenal cortex. Z. Zellforsch. 116:151–56.

Ursin, H., E. Baade, and S. Levine. 1978. Psychobiology of stress: A study of coping men. New York: Academic Press.

Vaillant, G. 1977. Adaptation to life. Boston: Little, Brown.

Vale, W., M. Brown, and C. Rivier. 1977. Regulatory peptides of the hypothalamus. Ann. Rev. Physiol. 39:473–527.

Vale, W., and C. Rivier. 1977. Substances modulating the secretion of ACTH by cultured anterior pituitary cells. Fed. Proc. FASEB 36:2094–99.

Valori, R. M., D. Kumar, and D. L. Wingate. 1986. Effects of different types of stress and of "prokinetic" drugs on the control of the fasting motor complex in humans. Gastroenterol. 90:1890–1900.

Vantrappen, G., and J. Hellemans. 1983. Esophageal motility disorders. In Functional disorders of the digestive tract, ed. W. Y. Chey, 117–24. New York: Raven Press.

Verrier, R. L. 1991. Autonomic nervous system and coronary flow changes related to emotional activation and sleep. Circulation. In press.

Vesely, K. T., K. T. Kubickova, and M. Dvorakova. 1968. Clinical data and characteristics differentiating types of peptic ulcer. Gut 9:57–68.

Vizi, E. S. 1980. Modulation of cortical release of acetylcholine by noradrenaline released from nerves arising from the rat locus coeruleus. Neurosci. 5:2139–44.

Vollhardt, B. R., S. H. Ackerman, A. I. Grayzel, and P. Barland. 1982. Psychologically distinguishable groups of rheumatoid arthritis patients: A controlled, single blind study. Psychosom. Med. 44:353–62.

Volpicelli, N. A., J. H. Yardley, and T. R. Hendrix. 1977. The association of heartburn with gastritis. Am. J. Dig. Dis. 22:333–39.

von Holst, D. 1972. Renal failure as the cause of death in Tupaia belangeri tree shrews exposed to persistent social stress. J. Comp. Physiol. 78:236–43.

von Uexküll, T., ed. 1979. Lehrbuch der psychosomatischen medizin. Munich: Urban and Schwarzenberg.

von Uexküll, T., and E. Wick. 1962. Die Situations hypertonie. Arch. für Kreislauf Forschung 39:236–42.

Wadsorth, M. E. J., W. J. H. Butterfield, and R. Blaney. 1971. Health and sickness: The choice of treatment. London: Tavistock.

Wahler, R. 1980. The insular mother: Her problems in parent-child treatment. J. Appl. Behav. Anal. 13:207–19.

Wall, P. D., and M. Gutnick. 1974. Ongoing activity in peripheral nerves: The physiology and pharmacology. Exp. Neurol. 43:580–93.

Wallace, D. J. 1984. Fibromyalgia: Unusual historical aspects and new pathogenic insights. J. Mt. Sinai Hosp. 51:124–31.

Wallach, D., M. Fellous, and M. Revel. 1982. Preferential effect of gamma-interferon on the synthesis of HLA antigens and their mRNAs in human cells. Nature (London) 299:833–36.

Waller, S. L., J. J. Misiewicz, and N. Kiley. 1972. Effect of eating on motility of the pelvic colon in constipation and diarrhea. Gut 13:805–11.

Wallin, B. G. 1987. Recording of postganglionic sympathetic impulse traffic in man: What can it tell us about health and disease? In Neuronal control of bodily function: Neurobiological approaches to human disease, ed. D. Hellhammer, I. Florin, and H. Weiner, 225–30. Toronto: Hans Huber.

Wallin, B. G., and J. Fagins. 1986. The sympathetic nervous system in man—aspects derived from microelectrode recordings. Trends Neurosci. 9:63–67.

Wangel, A. G., and D. J. Deller. 1965. Intestinal motility in man, 3: Mechanisms of constipation and diarrhea with particular reference to the irritable bowel syndrome. Gastroenterol. 48:69–84.

Ward, I. 1984. The pre-natal stress syndrome: Current status. Psychoneuroendocrinol. 9:3–11.

Ward, I., and O. B. Ward. 1989. Reproductive behavior and physiology in prenatally stressed males. In Neuronal control of bodily function: Frontiers of stress research, ed. H. Weiner, D. Hellhammer, I. Floin, and R. Murison, 9–20. Toronto: Hans Huber.

Ware, J. C., J. Russell, and E. Campos. 1986. Alpha intrusions into the sleep of depressed and fibromyalgia syndrome (fibrositis) patients. Sleep Res. 15:210.

Watkins, L. R., Y. Katayama, I. B. Kinschek, D. J. Mayer, and R. L. Hayes. 1984. Muscarinic cholinergic mediation of opiate and non-opiate environmentally induced analgesias. Brain Res. 300:231–42.

Watkins, L. R., and D. J. Mayer. 1982. The organization of endogenous opiate and nonopiate pain control systems. Science 216:1185–92.

Weder, A. B., and S. Julius. 1985. Editorial: Behavior, blood pressure variability, and hypertension. Psychosom. Med. 47:406–14.

Wehr, T. A., and F. K. Goodwin, eds. 1983. Circadian rhythms in psychiatry. Pacific Grove, CA: Boxwood Press.

Weinberg, J., and S. Levine. 1980. Psychobiology of coping in animals: The effects of predictability. In Coping and health, ed. S. Levine and H. Ursin, 39–59. New York: Plenum Press.

Weinberg, S. 1987. Newtonianism, reductionism, and the art of congressional testimony. Nature (London) 330:433–37.

Weiner, H. 1972. Some comments on the transduction of experience by the brain: Implications for our understanding of the relationship of mind to body. Psychosom. Med. 34:355–80.

———. 1975. Are psychosomatic diseases, diseases of regulation? Psychosom. Med. 37:289–91.

———. 1977. Psychobiology and human disease. New York: Elsevier.

———. 1978. The illusion of simplicity: The medical model revisited. Am. J. Psychiat. 135 (Supp.): 27–33.

———. 1979a. Psychobiological markers of disease. In Psychiatric Clinics of North America, ed. C. P. Kimball, 227–42. Philadelphia: W. B. Saunders.

———. 1979b. Psychobiology of essential hypertension. New York: Elsevier.

———. 1982. The prospects for psychosomatic medicine: Selected topics. Psychosom. Med. 44:488–517.

———. 1983. Gesundheit, Krankheitsgefühl, und Krankheit—Ansatze zu einem integrativen Verständnis. Psychother. med. Psychol. 33:15–34.

———. 1984. What the future holds for psychosomatic medicine. Psychotherap. Psychosom. 42:15–25.

———. 1985a. The concept of stress in the light of studies on disasters, unemployment, and loss: A critical analysis. In stress in health and disease, ed. M. R. Zales, 24–94. New York: Brunner/Mazel.

————. 1985b. The psychobiology and pathophysiology of anxiety and fear. In Anxiety and the anxiety disorders, ed. A. H. Tuma and J. D. Maser, 333–54. Hillsdale, NJ: Lawrence Erlbaum.

————. 1986. Die Geschichte der psychosomatischen Medizin und das Leib-Seele-Problem in der Medizin. Psychother. Med. Psychol. 36:361–91.

————. 1987. Human relationships in health, illness, and disease. In Psychopathology: An interactional perspective, ed. D. Magnusson and A. Öhman, 305–23. Orlando, FL: Academic Press.

————. 1988. The functional bowel disorders. In Perspectives in behavioral medicine. Vol. 5, Eating regulation and discontrol, ed. H. Weiner and A. Baum, 137–61. Hillsdale, NJ: Lawrence Erlbaum.

————. 1989a. Overview of the fourth symposium in Trier, Germany. In Neuronal control of bodily function: Frontiers in stress research, ed. H. Weiner, D. Hellhammer, I. Florin, and R. Murison, 405–18. Toronto: Hans Huber.

————. 1989b. The dynamics of the organism. Psychosom. Med. 51:608–35.

————. 1989c. Psychoendocrinology of anorexia nervosa. Psychiatr. Clin. North Am. 12:187–206.

————. 1990a. Social and psychobiological factors in autoimmune disease. In Psychoneuroimmunology 2, ed. R. Ader, D. L. Felten, and N. Cohen, 955–1011. San Diego: Academic Press.

————. 1990b. Application of psychosomatic concepts to psychiatry. In Lehrbuch der psychosomatischen medizin, 4th ed., ed. T. von Uexküll, 916–40. Munich: Urban and Schwarzenberg.

————. 1991a. Stressful experience and cardiorespiratory disorders. Circulation 83 (Suppl. 2): 2-2–2-8.

————. 1991b. The revolution in stress theory and research. In Stress in psychiatry and medicine, ed. R. Liberman and J. Yager. New York: Plenum Press. In press.

Weiner, H., and F. Fawzy. 1989. An integrative model of health, illness and disease. In Psychosomatic medicine: Theory, physiology and practice, vol. 1, ed. S. Cheren, 9–44. Madison, CT: International Universities Press.

Weiner, H., D. Hellhammer, I. Florin, and R. Murison, eds. 1989. Neuronal control of bodily function: Frontiers in stress research. Toronto: Hans Huber.

Weiner, H., M. A. Hofer, and A. J. Stunkard, eds. 1980. Brain, behavior, and bodily disease. New York: Raven Press.

Weiner, H., and E. Mayer. 1990. Der organismus in gesundheit und krankheit. Auf dem weg zu einem integrierten biomedizinischen modell: Folgerungen für die theorie der psychosomatischen medizin. Psychother. Med. Psychol. 40:81–101.

Weiner, H., M. Thaler, M. F. Reiser, and I. A. Mirsky. 1957. Etiology of duodenal ulcer, 1: Relation of specific psychological characteristics to rate of gastric secretion. Psychosom. Med. 19:1–10.

Weiss, J. M. 1968. Effects of coping responses on stress. J. Comp. Physiol. Psychol. 65:251–60.

————. 1970. Somatic effects of predictable and unpredictable shock. Psychosom. Med. 32:397–408.

————. 1971. Effects of coping behavior with and without a feedback signal on stress pathology in rats. J. Comp. Physiol. Psychol. 77:22–30.

————. 1972. Psychological factors in stress and disease. Scient. Am. 226:104–13.

Weiss, J. M., W. H. Bailey, P. A. Goodman, L. J. Hoffman, M. J. Ambrose, S. Salman, and J. M. Charry. 1982. A model for neurochemical study of depression. In Behavioral models and the analysis of drug action, ed. M. Y. Spiegelstein and A. Levy, 195–223. Amsterdam: Elsevier.

Weiss, J. M., W. H. Bailey, L. A. Pohorecky, D. Korzeniowski, and G. Grillione. 1980. Stress-induced depression of motor activity correlates with regional changes in brain norepinephrine but not in dopamine. Neurochem. Res. 5:9–22.

Weiss, J. M., and H. I. Glazer. 1975. Effects of acute exposure to stressors on subsequent avoidance-escape behavior. Psychosom. Med. 37:499–521.

Weiss, J. M., H. I. Glazer, L. A. Pohorecky, J. Brick, and N. E. Miller. 1975. Effects of chronic exposure to stressors on avoidance-escape behavior and on brain norepinephrine. Psychosom. Med. 37:522–33.

Weiss, J. M., H. I. Glazer, L. A. Pohorecky, W. H. Bailey, and D. Schneider. 1979. Coping behavior and stress-induced behavioral depression: Studies of the role of brain catecholamines. In The psychobiology of the depressive disorders: Implications for the effects of stress, ed. E. Depue, 125–160. New York: Academic Press.

Weiss, J. M., P. A. Goodman, B. G. Losito, S. Corrigan, J. M. Charry, and W. H. Bailey. 1981. Behavioral depression produced by an uncontrollable stressor: Relationship to norepinephrine, dopamine, and serotonin levels in various regions of rat brain. Brain Res. Rev. 3:167–205.

Weiss, J. M., L. A. Pohorecky, S. Salman, and M. Gruenthal. 1976. Attenuation of gastric lesions by psychological aspects of aggression in rats. J. Comp. Physiol. Psychol. 90:252–59.

Weiss, J. M., and P. G. Simson. 1985. Neurochemical mechanisms underlying stress-induced depression. In Stress and coping, vol. 1, ed. T. Field, P. McCabe, and N. Schneiderman, 93–116. Hillsdale, NJ: Lawrence Erlbaum.

Weiss, J. M., P. G. Simson, M. J. Ambrose, A. Webster, and L. J. Hoffman. 1985. Neurochemical basis of behavioral depression. In Advances in behavioral medicine, vol. 1, ed. E. Katkin and S. Manuck, 233–75. Greenwich, CT: JAI Press.

Weiss, J. M., P. G. Simson, and P. E. Simson. 1989. Neurochemical basis of stress-induced depression. In Neuronal control of bodily function: Frontiers of stress research, ed. H. Weiner, D. Hellhammer, I. Florin, and R. Murison, 37–50. Toronto: Hans Huber.

Weiss, J. M., E. A. Stone, and N. Harrell. 1970. Coping behavior and brain norepinephrine level in rats. J. Consult. Clin. Psychiat. 72:153–60.

Weissman, M. M., E. S. Paykel, R. French, H. Mark, K. Fox, and R. A. Prusoff. 1973. Suicide attempts in an urban community: 1955–1970. Soc. Psychiat. 8: 82–89.

Welch, A. S., and B. L. Welch. 1968a. Effect of stress and p-chlorophenylalanine upon brain serotonin, 5-hydroxyindoleacetic acid, and catecholamines in grouped and isolated mice. Biochem. Pharmacol. 17:699–708.

———. 1968b. Reduction of norepinephrine in the lower brainstem by psychological stimulus. Proc. Natl. Acad. Sci. (USA) 60:478–81.

———. 1971. Isolation reactivity and aggression: Evidence for an involvement of brain catecholamines and serotinin. In The physiology of aggression and defeat, ed. B. E. Eleftheriou and J. P. Scott, 91–142. New York: Plenum Press.

Welch, B. L., and A. S. Welch. 1965. Effect of grouping on the level of brain nor-epinephrine in white swiss mice. Life Sci. 4:1011–18.

———. 1966. Graded effect of social stimulation upon d-amphetamine toxicity, aggressiveness, and heart and adrenal weight. J. Pharmacol. Exp. Ther. 151:331–38.

———. 1968. Differential activation by restraint stress of a mechanism to conserve brain catecholamines and serotonin in mice differing in excitability. Nature (London) 218:575–77.

———. 1969. Aggression and the biogenic amine neurohumors. In Aggressive behaviour, ed. S. Garattini and E. B. Sigg, 188–22. Amsterdam: Excerpta Medica.

Wesemann, W., N. Weiner, M. Rotsch, and E. Schultz. 1983. Serotonin binding in rat brain: Circadian rhythm and effect of sleep deprivation. J. Neur. Trans. (Suppl.) 18:287–94.

Weser, E., W. Rubin, L. Ross, and M. H. Sleisinger. 1965. Lactase deficiency in patients with "irritable colon syndrome." New Engl. J. Med. 273:1070–75.

Wexler, B. C., and B. P. Greenberg. 1978. Pathophysiological differences between paired and communal breeding of male and female Sprague Dawley rats. Circ. Res. 42:126–35.

Wheeler, E. O., P. D. White, E. W. Reed, and M. E. Cohen. 1950. Neurocirculatory asthenia (anxiety neurosis, effort syndrome, neurasthenia): A twenty-year follow-up study of 173 patients. JAMA 142:878–89.

Whitehead, W. E., B. T. Engel, and M. M. Schuster. 1980. Irritable bowel syndrome: Physiological and psychological differences between diarrhea-predominant and constipation-predominant patients. Dig. Dis. Sci. 25:404–13.

Whitehead, W. E., and M. M. Schuster. 1985. Gastrointestinal disorders: Behavioral and physiological basis for treatment. New York: Academic Press.

Whorwell, P. J., C. Clouter, and C. L. Smith. 1981. Oesophageal motility in the irritable bowel syndrome. Br. Med. J. 282:1101–2.

Wiesel, T. N., and D. H. Hubel. 1965. Comparison of the effects of unilateral and bilateral eye closure on cortical unit responses in kittens. J. Neurophysiol. 28:1029–40.

Wildenthal, K., D. S. Fuller, and W. Shapiro. 1968. Paroxysmal atrial fibrillation induced by hyperventilation. Am. J. Cardiol. 21:436–41.

Williams, A. W., F. Edwards, T. H. C. Lewis, and N. F. Coghill. 1957. Investigation of non-ulcer dyspepsia by gastric biopsy. Br. Med. J. 1:372–77.

Windholz, M. J., C. R. Marmar, and M. J. Horowitz. 1985. A review of the research on conjugal bereavement: Impact on health and efficacy of intervention. Comp. Psychiat. 26:433–47.

Winfree, A. T. 1983. Sudden cardiac death: A problem in topology. Scient. Am. 248:144–60.

———. 1987. When time breaks down. Princeton, NJ: Princeton University Press.

Wingate, D. L., R. M. Valori, and D. Kumar. 1989. The influence of psychological stress on intestinal motility. In Stress and digestive motility, ed. L. Buéno, S. Collins, and J.-L. Junien, 85–92. London: John Libbey.

Wirz-Justice, A., and T. A. Wehr. 1983. Neuropsychopharmacology and biological rhythms. Adv. Biol. Psychiat. 11:20–34.

Wolf, S. 1969. Psychosocial forces in myocardial infarction and sudden death. Circulation 39–40 (Suppl. 4): 74–83.

Wolfe, E., M. A. Cathey, and S. M. Kleinheksel. 1984. Fibrositis (fibromyalgia) in rheumatoid arthritis. J. Rheumatol. 11:814–18.

Wolfe, E., M. A. Cathey, S. M. Kleinheksel, S. P. Amos, R. G. Hoffman, D. Y. Young, and D. J. Hawley. 1984. Psychological status in primary fibrositis and fibrositis associated with rheumatoid arthritis. J. Rheumatol. 11:500–506.

Wolff, C. T., S. B. Friedman, M. A. Hofer, and J. W. Mason. 1964. Relationship between psychological defenses and mean urinary 17-hydroxycorticosteroid excretion rates, 1: A predictive study of parents with fatally ill children. Psychosom. Med. 26:576–91.

Wolff, C. T., M. A. Hofer, and J. W. Mason. 1964. Psychological defenses and mean urinary 17-hydroxycorticosteroid excretion rates, 2: Methodologic and theoretical considerations. Psychosom. Med. 26:592–609.

Wolff, H. G. 1953. Stress and disease. Springfield, IL: Charles C. Thomas.

Wortman, C. B., and R. C. Silver. 1989. The myths of coping with loss. J. Consult. Clin. Psychol. 57:349–57.

Wortsman, J., S. Frank, W. B. Wehrenberg, P. H. Petra, and J. E. Murphy. 1985. Gamma$_3$-melanocyte-stimulating hormone immunoreactivity is a component of the neuroendocrine response to maximal stress (cardiac arrest). J. Clin. Endocrinol. Metab. 61:355–60.

Wurtman, R. J., and J. Axelrod. 1966. Control of enzymatic synthesis of adrenaline in the adrenal medulla by adrenal cortical steroids. J. Biol. Chem. 241:2301–5.

Wynder, E. L., G. C. Escher, and N. A. Mantel. 1966. An epidemiological investigation of cancer of the endometrium. Cancer 19:489–520.

Yamori, Y. 1976. Neural and non-neural mechanisms in spontaneous hypertension. Clin. Sci. Mol. Med. 51 (Suppl.): 431s–34s.

———. 1981. Environmental influences on the development of hypertensive vascular diseases in SHR and related models, and their relation to human disease. In New trends in arterial hypertension (INSERM Symposium no. 17), ed. E. Worcel, J. P. Bonvalet, S. Z. Langer, J. Menard, and J. Sassard, 305–20. Amsterdam: Elsevier/North-Holland Biomedical Press.

———. 1983. Physiopathology of the various strains of spontaneously hypertensive rats. In Hypertension: Physiopathology and treatment, 2d ed., ed. J. Genest, O. Kuchel, P. Hamet, and M. Cantin, 556–81. Montreal: McGraw-Hill.

Yamori, Y. K., Ikeda, M. Kihara, Y. Nara, R. Horie, and A. Ooshima. 1980. Analysis of the heredity of stroke in stroke-prone SHR (SHRSP). Jap. Heart J. 21:558.

Yamori, Y., K. Ikeda, A. Ooshima, and M. Fukase. 1979. Inheritance of hypertension in stroke-prone spontaneously hypertensive rats. In Prophylactic approach to hypertensive diseases, ed. Y. Yamori, W. Lovenberg, and E. D. Freis, 121–25. New York: Raven Press.

Yamori, Y., M. Matsumoto, H. Yamabe, and K. Okamoto. 1969. Augmentation of spontaneous hypertension by chronic stress in rats. Jap. Circ. J. 33:399–409.

Yasue, H., M. Nagao, S. Omote, A. Takizawa, J. K. Miwa, and S. Tanbaka. 1978. Coronary arterial spasm and Prinzmetal's variant form of angina induced by hyperventilation and tris-buffer infusion. Circulation 58:56–62.

Yates, F. E. 1982. Outline of a physical theory of physiological systems. Can. J. Physiol. Pharmacol. 60:217–48.

Yen, T. T., P. Yu, H. Roeder, and P. W. Willard. 1974. A genetic study of hypertension in Okamoto-Akoi spontaneously hypertensive rats. Heredity 33:309–16.

You, C. H., W. H. Chey, K. T. Lee, R. Menguy, and A. Bortoff. 1981. Gastric and small intestinal myoelectric dysrhythmia associated with chronic intractable nausea and vomiting. Ann. Int. Med. 95:449–51.

You, C. H., K. T. Lee, W. H. Chey, and R. Menguy. 1980. Electrogastrographic study of patients with unexplained nausea, bloating, and vomiting. Gastroenterol. 79:311–14.

Young, M., B. Benjamin, and C. Wallis. 1963. The mortality of widowers. Lancet 2:454–56.

Young, S. J., D. H. Alpers, C. C. Norland, and R. A. Woodruff. 1976. Psychiatric illness and the irritable bowel syndrome: Practical implications for the primary physician. Gastroenterol. 70:162–66.

Yuwiler, A. 1976. Stress, anxiety, and endocrine function. In Biological foundations of psychiatry, ed. R. G. Grenell and S. Galay, 889–943. New York: Raven Press.

———. 1982. Biobehavioral consequences of experimental early life stress: Effects of neonatal hormones on monoaminergic systems. In Critical issues in behavioral medicine, ed. L. J. West and M. Stein, 59–78. Philadelphia: J. B. Lippincott.

Zales, M. R., ed. 1985. Stress in health and disease. New York: Brunner/Mazel.

Zanchetti, A., G. Baccelli, and G. Mancia. 1976. Fighting, emotion, and exercise: Cardiovascular effects in the cat. In Regulation of blood pressure by the central nervous system, ed. G. Onesti, M. Fernandez, and K. E. Kim, 87–104. New York: Grune & Stratton.

Zeki, S. 1984. The construction of colours by the cerebral cortex. Proc. Royal Inst. Gr. Britain 56:231–57.

Zigmond, M., and J. Harvey. 1970. Resistance to central norepinephrine depletion and decreased mortality in rats chronically exposed to electric footshock. J. Neuro-Visc. Relations 31:373–81.

Zisook, S. 1987. Unresolved grief. In Biopsychosocial aspects of bereavement, ed. S. Zisook, 23–34. Washington, DC: American Psychiatric Press.

Zuckerman, M. 1984. Sensation seeking: A comparative approach to a human trait. Behav. Brain Sci. 7:413–71.

Zuckerman, M., S. Levine, and V. D. Biase. 1964. Stress response in total and partial perceptual isolation. Psychosom. Med. 26:250–60.

Zumoff, B., R. Freeman, S. Coupey, P. Saenger, M. Markowitz, and J. Kream. 1983. A chronobiological abnormality in luteinizing hormone secretion in teenage girls with the polycystic ovary syndrome. New Engl. J. Med. 309:1206–9.

Index

351